Recent Advances

Cardio
14

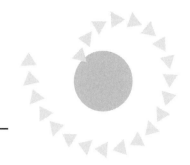

Recent Advances in

Cardiology
14

Edited by

Derek J Rowlands BSc MD FRCP FACC FESC

Honorary Consultant Cardiologist, Manchester Heart Centre,
Manchester Royal Infirmary, Manchester, UK.
Consultant Cardiologist, Alexandra Hospital,
The Beeches Consulting Centre, Cheadle, Cheshire, UK

Bernard Clarke BSc MD FRCP(Lond.) FRCP(Edin.) FESC FACC

Consultant Cardiologist, Manchester Heart Centre, Manchester
Royal Infirmary, Central Manchester and Manchester Children's
University Hospitals NHS Trust, Manchester, UK.
Honorary Lecturer in Medicine, University of
Manchester, UK

The ROYAL
SOCIETY *of*
MEDICINE
PRESS *Limited*

© 2007 Royal Society of Medicine Press Ltd

Published by the Royal Society of Medicine Press Ltd
1 Wimpole Street, London W1G 0AE, UK
Tel: +44 (0)20 7290 2921
Fax: +44 (0)20 7290 2929
Email: publishing@rsm.ac.uk
Website: www.rsmpress.co.uk

British Library Cataloguing in Publication Data
A catalogue record for this book is available from the British Library
ISBN 978–1–85315–715–8

Distribution in Europe and Rest of World:

Marston Book Services Ltd
PO Box 269, Abingdon
Oxon OX14 4YN, UK
Tel: +44 (0)1235 465500
Fax: +44 (0)1235 465555
Email: direct.order@marston.co.uk

Distribution in the USA and Canada:

Royal Society of Medicine Press Ltd
c/o BookMasters Inc
30 Amberwood Parkway
Ashland, OH 44805, USA
Tel: +1 800 247 6553/+1 800 266 5564
Fax: +1 419 281 6883
Email: order@bookmasters.com

Distribution in Australia and New Zealand:

Elsevier Australia
30-52 Smidmore Street
Marrikville NSW 2204, Australia
Tel: +61 2 9517 8999
Fax: +61 2 9517 2249
Email: service@elsevier.com.au

Editorial services and typesetting by GM & BA Haddock, Ford, Midlothian, UK
Printed in Great Britain by Bell & Bain, Glasgow, UK

Contents

Contents

Contributors

Mimi R. Bhattacharyya BSc MBBS MRCP
Clinical Research Fellow, Psychobiology Group, Department of Epidemiology
and Public Health, University College London, London, UK

Elisabetta Cerbai PhD
Professor of Pharmacology, Center of Molecular Medicine CIMMBA, Department
of Pharmacology, University of Florence, Firenze, Italy

Bernard Clarke BSc(Hons) MB ChB MD FRCP(Lond.) FRCP(Edin) FESC FACC
Consultant Cardiologist, Manchester Heart Centre, Manchester Royal Infirmary,
Central Manchester and Manchester Children's University Hospitals NHS Trust,
Manchester, UK. Honorary Lecturer in Medicine, University of Manchester, UK

Ihab Diab MB BS MSc MD
Clinical Electrophysiology Fellow, Manchester Heart Centre, Manchester Royal
Infirmary, Manchester, UK

David A. Eisner MA DPhil DMedSci
British Heart Foundation Professor of Cardiac Physiology, Unit of Cardiac
Physiology, Core Technology Facility, University of Manchester, Manchester, UK

Farzin Fath-Ordoubadi BSc MB BCh MD FRCP
Consultant Cardiologist, Manchester Heart Centre, Manchester Royal Infirmary,
Manchester, UK

Clifford Garratt DM FRCP FESC
Professor of Cardiology, Manchester Heart Centre, Manchester Royal Infirmary,
Manchester, UK

Melanie Greaves MB BS MRCP FRCR
Consultant Radiologist, University Hospitals of South Manchester NHS Foundation
Trust, Manchester, UK

Tony M. Heagerty MD FRCP FMedSci
Professor of Medicine, Division of Cardiovascular and Endocrine Sciences,
University of Manchester, Manchester, UK

Cara Hendry MB ChB MRCP
Clinical Fellow in Interventional Cardiology and Specialist Registrar in Cardiology,
Manchester Heart Centre, Manchester Royal Infirmary, Manchester, UK

J. Andreas Hoschtitzky MSc MRCS(Ed)
Specialist Registrar in Cardiothoracic Surgery, Manchester Heart Centre,
Manchester Royal Infirmary, Manchester, UK

Daniel J.M. Keenan BSc MB BCh FRCS
Consultant Cardiothoracic Surgeon, Manchester Heart Centre, Manchester Royal Infirmary, Manchester, UK

Vaikom S. Mahadevan MD MRCP
Consultant Cardiologist and Interventionist in Adult Congenital Heart Disease, Manchester Heart Centre, Manchester Royal Infirmary, Manchester, UK

Mamas A. Mamas MA DPhil MRCP
Clinical Lecturer in Cardiology, Manchester Heart Centre, Manchester Royal Infirmary, Manchester, UK

William J. McKenna DSc FACC FESC FRCP
Professor of Cardiac Medicine, Centre of Cardiology in the Young, The Heart Hospital, London, UK

Ghada W. Mikhail BSc MD MRCP
Consultant Cardiologist and Honorary Senior Lecturer, Imperial College London, St Mary's Hospital NHS Trust, London, UK

J. Paul Miller BM BCh MSc DPhil FRCP
Consultant Gastroenterologist, University Hospital of South Manchester NHS Foundation Trust, Wythenshawe Hospital, Manchester, UK

Philip R. Moore MRCP PhD
SpR in Cardiology, Harefield Hospital, Royal Brompton & Harefield NHS Trust, Harefield, Middlesex, UK

Alessandro Mugelli MD
Professor of Pharmacology, Center of Molecular Medicine CIMMBA, Department of Pharmacology, University of Florence, Firenze, Italy

Ludwig Neyses MD
Professor of Medicine/Cardiology, Manchester Heart Centre, Manchester Royal Infirmary, Manchester, UK

Derek J. Rowlands BSc MD FRCP FACC FESC
Honorary Consultant Cardiologist, Manchester Heart Centre, Manchester Royal Infirmary, Manchester, UK. Consultant Cardiologist, Alexandra Hospital, The Beeches Consulting Centre, Cheadle, Cheshire, UK

Sanjay Sharma BSc FRCP MD)
Consultant Cardiologist, Department of Cardiology, King's College Hospital, London, UK

Andrew Steptoe MA DPhil DSc
British Heart Foundation Professor of Psychology, Deputy Head, Department of Epidemiology and Public Health, University College London, London, UK

Sarah Vause MD MRCOG
Consultant in Fetal and Maternal Medicine, Department of Obstetrics, St Mary's Hospital, Hathersage Road, Manchester M13 0JH, UK

Luigi A. Venetucci MB ChB MRCP PhD
Lecturer in Cardiovascular Medicine, Unit of Cardiac Physiology, Core Technology Facility, University of Manchester, Manchester, UK

Elisabetta Cerbai Alessandro Mugelli

1

I$_f$ inhibition: the concept and its possible role in the treatment of congestive heart failure

MECHANISMS OF PHYSIOLOGICAL PACEMAKER ACTIVITY IN THE HEART

In the normal heart, impulses are generated in the sinoatrial node (SAN); from there, they propagate to activate the atria and then, travelling in the conducting system, the ventricles.

'Pacemaker' cells in the SAN are endowed with the property of spontaneous activity: as opposed to normal cells of the working myocardium, they generate repetitive action potentials since they spontaneously depolarise during diastole (Fig. 1). In this way, a self-sustained rhythm is produced which determines the cardiac rate. Other cells of the specialised conducting system have the property of automaticity, but in the normal heart their rhythm is generally suppressed by that of the SAN.[1] The rhythm of the 'secondary pacemakers' is only expressed when the rate of the SAN is markedly reduced or arrested or in the presence of a block of the atrioventricular (AV) node.

IONIC CURRENTS IMPLICATED IN THE DIASTOLIC DEPOLARISATION PHASE (PHASE 4)

Several mechanisms contribute to provide the cellular and molecular elements necessary for pacemaking to occur (Fig. 1): the spontaneous depolarisation is initiated by I$_f$, the so-called 'funny current' (see below). This initial depolarisation is due to an 'inward' (*i.e.* depolarising) current due to a flow of Na$^+$ ions, which

Elisabetta Cerbai PhD
Professor of Pharmacology, Center of Molecular Medicine CIMMBA, Department of Pharmacology, University of Florence, Viale G. Pieraccini 6, Firenze, Italy

Alessandro Mugelli MD (for correspondence)
Professor of Pharmacology, Center of Molecular Medicine CIMMBA, Department of Pharmacology, University of Florence, Viale G. Pieraccini 6, Firenze, Italy
E-mail: alessandro.mugelli@unifi.it

1

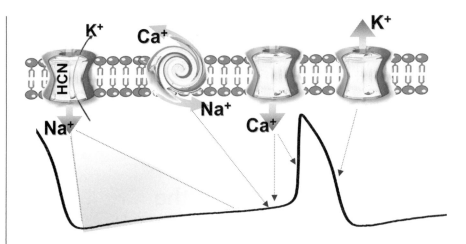

Fig. 1 Pacemaker mechanisms in the sinoatrial node (SAN). The scheme shows a typical action potential (lower trace) and a representation of major ionic conductances contributing to SAN automaticity. From the left, I_f current (HCN), the sodium–calcium exchanger, calcium currents and repolarising potassium currents.

brings the membrane potential to more positive potentials.[2] Inward Ca^{2+} currents contribute to the latter portion of the diastolic depolarisation phase and to the upstroke of the action potential (Fig. 1). Finally, an inward current generated by the Na/Ca exchanger contributes to the depolarisation phase.[3] These inward currents are counteracted by outward (repolarising) currents carried by K ions that play a major role in the repolarisation phase of the action potential and that tend to maintain the membrane potential at negative values.

The multiplicity of currents contributing to pacemaking may be seen as a safety factor: even if one of the currents is completely blocked, the others will continue to be activated thus ensuring that pacemaker activity will continue, albeit at a lower rate.

PROPERTIES OF THE 'FUNNY CURRENT' I_f

As previously stated, multiple currents are involved in phase 4 depolarisation, but it is now generally recognised that I_f is critical for its initiation. We will describe the main properties of I_f.

I_f has been named 'funny' because it has peculiar properties: (i) it is a mixed (Na^+ and K^+ ions) inward current activated upon hyperpolarisation (all the other currents are activated on depolarisation); and (ii) it is directly modulated by cyclic nucleotides. These properties are summarised in Figure 2.

The channels that carry the 'funny current' are designated as hyperpolarisation-activated, cyclic nucleotide gated (HCN) channels,[4] reflecting the fact that the I_f is activated on hyperpolarisation and that cyclic adenosine monophosphate (cAMP), i.e. the second messenger of the β-adrenergic receptors, binds to special sites of the channel shifting the activation curve of I_f toward more positive voltages. The direct regulation of the channel (and consequently of the current) by cAMP highlights another property of I_f, that is its exquisite responsiveness to the autonomic nervous system: this is obviously

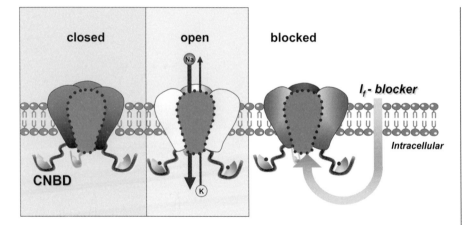

Fig. 2 The structure and functional states of the pacemaker channel. The channel is formed by four subunits, coded by HCN gene(s); each subunit contains a cAMP binding domain (CNBD) in the intracellular site. Upon hyperpolarisation, the channel passes from the closed to the open state, thus allowing Na$^+$ and K$^+$ ions to cross the channel in the inward and outward direction, respectively. Heart-rate lowering drugs (I$_f$ blocker) are lipophilic compounds able to cross the sarcolemma and enter f-channel from the inner site of the pore when in the open state.

essential for rapidly adapting the heart rate in response to exercise, emotion, and stress. There are four isoforms of the HCN channels (HCN1–4), the HCN4 being the most represented in the sinus node.

It is important to have some elementary knowledge of the structure, functioning and modulation by neurotransmitters of the HCN channels. Drugs may interact differently with the different isoforms and it is important to know how a drug, such as ivabradine, interacts with the channel since this will allow understanding its pharmacological profile.

HCN CHANNELS: STRUCTURE, FUNCTIONING AND REGULATION

The f-channels are constituted by tetrameric association of four α-subunits, *i.e.* the transcript of HCN genes (Fig. 2).[4,5] The subunits combine in diverse ways to form homomeric or heteromeric channels; the exact stoichiometry of native channels is unknown, but the predominant isoform in the SAN is HCN4, followed by HCN1 and HCN2.[6] Each α-subunit displays the typical topology of voltage-gated K$^+$ channels, with six transmembrane domains (S1–6), a selectivity filter between S5 and S6,[4] and a voltage-sensor motif in S4. The movement of the sensor (outward upon depolarisation and inward upon hyperpolarisation) corresponds, respectively, to channel closing and opening, at variance with voltage-gated K$^+$ channels where the outward movement is coupled to channel opening.[7] The basic properties (activation upon hyperpolarisation and modulation by intracellular cAMP) are common to the four HCN transcripts; however, when heterologously re-expressed, these properties are quite different between channels encoded by the four genes. Of the three isoforms expressed in the heart, HCN1 (almost limited to the sinus node) shows rapid activation kinetics (tens of milliseconds) and weakly sensitivity to cAMP; HCN2 and HCN4 (present throughout the heart,

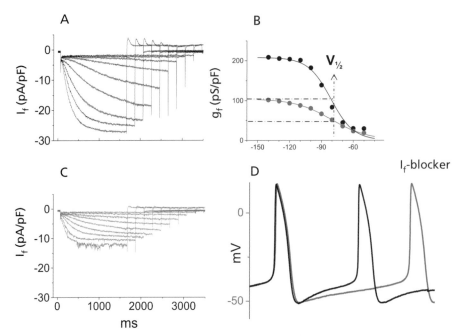

Fig. 3 Bradycardic agents inhibit I_f. Family of I_f currents elicited by hyperpolarising steps in the absence (A) and presence (C) of a heart-rate lowering drug. (B) Current-voltage relationships measured in the absence (black line and symbols) and presence (grey line and symbols) of drug. (D) As a result, the spontaneous rate is reduced in SAN cells.

including non-pacemaker cells where they are not expressed in physiological conditions) give currents activating in hundreds of milliseconds and are highly sensitive to cAMP. Thus, the properties of native I_f in different cell types probably arise from the different proportion of HCN isoforms.

The cytosolic C-terminal of each monomer contains a cyclic nucleotide binding domain (CNBD; Fig. 2). The maximal effect on the voltage-dependence is achieved when all four CNBD bind to cAMP. However, the allosteric gating model resulting from the dual voltage and ligand regulation is a complex one, which is described in detail elsewhere.[8] In addition to these utmost regulatory mechanisms, HCN isoforms are sensitive to intracellular pH and can be phosphorylated by serine/threonine as well as tyrosine kinase activity. A recently appreciated difference among HCN isoforms consists in the sensitivity to HCN blockers. This topic will be addressed below, after a description of the chemical and pharmacological properties of these drugs.

As shown in Figure 3, f-channels open during hyperpolarisation thus allowing Na^+ ions to enter SAN cells and generate a depolarising current, which contributes to diastolic depolarisation. A family of currents evoked in SAN cells is reported in Figure 3A: inward currents activate with a typical mono-exponential kinetics, whose time constant becomes progressively faster from less to more negative voltages. Plotting steady-state current amplitude as a function of voltage gives a sigmoidal current–voltage relationship (Fig. 3B), with current increasing at more negative potentials as expected for a hyperpolarisation-activated channel.

MECHANISM OF ACTION OF IVABRADINE

DEVELOPMENT OF SELECTIVE HEART-RATE LOWERING DRUGS: A BRIEF HISTORY

Heart-rate lowering drugs derive from alinidine, an analogue of the antihypertensive agent clonidine with peculiar bradycardic and analgesic properties (see Baruscotti et al.[9] for a review). In vitro studies demonstrated that alinidine slowed the spontaneous rate of SAN preparations and decreased the steepness of diastolic depolarisation phase of sheep Purkinje fibres. Both effects were accompanied by a reduction of I_f conductance and a shift of its activation curve to more negative voltages.

Notwithstanding its bradycardic effects, alinidine proved to have limited selectivity (it also prolonged repolarisation due to blockade of K+-currents) and multiple side-effects; therefore, alinidine and its derivatives did not succeed as heart-rate lowering agents but paved the way to structure–action relationship studies.

These studies led to verapamil derivatives, such as falipamil (AQ-A39), zatebradine (UL-FS-49), and cilobradine (DK-AH26), able to block f-channels and thus to reduce heart rate (Fig. 4).[9] UL-FS-49 (zatebradine) was the first compound undergoing extensive in vitro and in vivo characterisation, and differs from falipamil in the lattamic 7-atom ring (Fig. 4), which confers bradycardic properties. The basic –NH residue (Fig. 4, arrow) is required for activity, since the protonated form of the drug enters the channel pore and binds to the receptor.[10] The selectivity of zatebradine as f-channel blocker was higher than that of alinidine, although the compound exerted inhibitory effects on Ca2+ and K+ currents.[11] Ivabradine (S 16257-2), derives from zatebradine and possesses a chiral centre (Fig. 4, asterisk), the S-enantiomer being the active one.

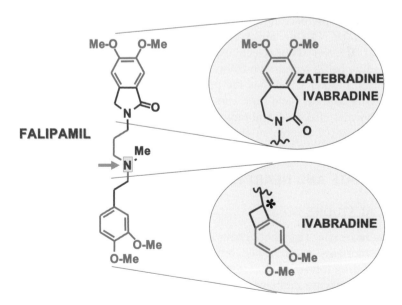

Fig. 4 Structure of falipamil and its derivatives, ivabradine and zatebradine. The asterisk indicates the presence of a chiral centre in the ivabradine structure.

PHARMACOLOGY OF HEART-RATE LOWERING DRUGS

The common feature of heart-rate lowering drugs is the capability to block I_f. Zatebradine and newer derivatives (ivabradine, cilobradine) share common mechanisms of action: their effect on I_f mainly consists in a reduction of current conductance, with no effect on voltage-dependence. Owing to their lipophilicity, heart-rate lowering drugs freely cross the membrane and enter the pore from the cytoplasmic site when the channel is in the open state (Fig. 2, right panel).[10]

Figure 3C shows what happens to f-currents when a SAN cell is challenged with a heart-rate lowering drug. This drug reduces I_f at any voltage (Fig. 3C); thus the I–V curve is similar to the control but of smaller amplitude (Fig. 3B). Notably, the midpoint ($V_{1/2}$) of I_f activation lies around similar voltages in the absence and in the presence of the drug. All these features are displayed by ivabradine and analogues, which reduce current conductance without modifying its voltage-dependence.[12] The result is a slowing of the spontaneous discharge of SAN cells, thus leading to bradycardia (Fig. 3D).

Another essential property of heart-rate lowering drugs is the use-dependence of their effect: the rate and amount of blockade is related to the frequency of SAN discharge, and it is a direct consequence of the dependence of blockade upon channel state.[13] From a physiological and pharmacological point of view, the result is that the higher the heart rate (such as in pathological conditions), the greater is the drug effect.

The most striking difference between ivabradine and the first-generation derivatives, namely zatebradine, is selectivity: the latter also affects potassium currents controlling action potential repolarisation, such as Kv1.5.[12,14] Moreover, a high incidence of adverse side effects of zatebradine on vision was reported,[15] due to the block of neuronal type of f-channels (I_h) in photo-receptors and retinal cells.[16] Conversely, the effect of ivabradine on retinal HCN channels seems to be less pronounced and promptly reversible.[17] Possibly, this difference resides in a differential molecular interaction of the drug with HCN4 (the major SAN isoform) or HCN1 (the predominant neuronal isoform).[2] Poor selectivity and high incidence of side effects led to zatebradine being withdrawn from clinical studies. Ivabradine is, at present, the only I_f blocker which has the properties for therapeutic use. Large, on-going, clinical trials have been carried out to evaluate the anti-anginal and anti-ischaemic effects of ivabradine with respect to placebo or other anti-anginal drugs (*i.e.* atenolol or amlodipine).[18,19]

HEART RATE AND HEART FAILURE

CLINICAL STUDIES

Resting heart rate is thought to have an independent prognostic value in heart failure: mortality trials carried out in heart failure patients with different classes of drug (phosphodiesterase inhibitors, hydralazine-nitrate, angiotensin converting enzyme inhibitors, β-blockers) have documented a relationship between the reduction in resting heart rate and the reduction in mortality.[20] Base-line heart rate has been reported to be an important determinant of the response to enalapril[21] and amiodarone[22] in patients with severe heart failure.

In fact, the benefit in terms of reduction in mortality was only obtained in patients with high heart rate at base-line and with a significant decrease in heart rate during treatment. The concept that heart rate reduction *per se* is associated with survival improvement in patients with heart failure has been more recently confirmed with β-blocker treatment.[23] Thus, heart rate reduction appears to be a central mechanism in the beneficial effects of β-blockers in heart failure.[24]

EXPERIMENTAL STUDIES

The effect of long-term 'pure' heart rate reduction on left ventricular (LV) function and remodelling was recently studied in a rat model of congestive heart failure (CHF), the post-myocardial infarction (post-MI) in rats.[25] The rats with CHF were treated with the selective I_f current inhibitor ivabradine (as food administration for 90 days starting 7 days after coronary artery ligation). Ivabradine decreased heart rate over the 90-day treatment period (−18% versus untreated at 10 mg/kg/day), without modifying blood pressure, LV end-diastolic pressure, or $dP/dt_{max}/min$. Ivabradine significantly reduced LV end-systolic but not end-diastolic diameter, which resulted in preserved cardiac output due to increased stroke volume. In the Langendorff preparation, ivabradine shifted LV systolic but not end-diastolic pressure–volume relationships to the left. Ivabradine decreased LV collagen density and increased LV capillary density without modifying LV weight. Three days after interruption of treatment, the effects of ivabradine on LV geometry, shortening, and stroke volume persisted despite normalisation of heart rate.

Thus experimental and clinical data are consistent with the view that the heart rate reduction *per se* may be beneficial in heart failure. The effect of 'pure' heart rate reduction with ivabradine on morbidity/mortality in patient with coronary artery disease and LV systolic dysfunction is being evaluated in a large, on-going clinical trial.[26,27] The effects of ivabradine on morbidity/mortality in patients with moderate-to-severe heart failure will be assessed in a large-scale, randomised, clinical trial called SHIFT.

To get an insight into the possible mechanism of the probable beneficial effect of heart rate reduction, an experimental study in a rat model of congestive heart failure (CHF) similar to the one previously described is on-going. The study will also investigate the effect of long-term ivabradine administration on ventricular electrophysiological remodelling. The reason for this kind of investigation will be clarified in the next session.

'FUNNY CURRENT' IN NON-PACEMAKER CELLS

We have recently reviewed the possible role of I_f in non-pacemaker cells.[28] Here, we shall focus on the expression of the 'funny current' in ventricular myocytes, since this aspect is more relevant to this article.

In practice, I_f is abundantly expressed in ventricular myocytes during fetal and neonatal life.[29] I_f is also detected in human embryonic stem cells and in beating myocytes derived from these cells.[30] Obviously, during the process of electrophysiological maturation toward the adult ventricular phenotype, these cells at some point lose their capacity to generate spontaneous activity. This

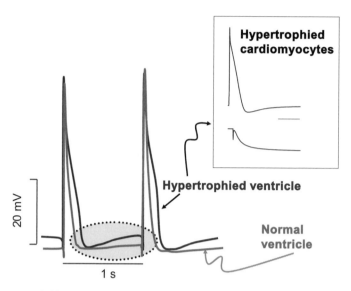

Fig. 5 Myocardial hypertrophy is accompanied by I_f overexpression. The traces represent typical action potentials recorded from ventricular muscles of normal (grey lines) and hypertrophied rat hearts; note the presence of a diastolic depolarisation phase in the action potential of hypertrophied hearts. Cells dissociated from these hearts (inset) also show a diastolic depolarisation phase, which is due to I_f activation (bottom trace).

phenomenon is associated with a progressive reduction of I_f current expression both in mouse and rat ventricles.[29] In our experience, the I_f current occurs in all ventricular myocytes early after birth, but is present in half after 2 weeks and in 30% at 4 weeks of age; at this age, the amplitude of I_f is much smaller than in newborn rats.[29] In the adult heart, I_f occurrence has long been considered a feature of a few specialised sites, such as SAN cells. The first demonstration of its occurrence in ventricular cardiomyocytes was obtained in the 1990s.[31] Electrophysiological studies designed to elucidate the molecular mechanisms for enhanced arrhythmogenesis in a rat model of cardiac hypertrophy showed the presence of an unusual diastolic depolarisation in ventricular muscles (Fig. 5).[32] Subsequent measurements demonstrated that the diastolic depolarisation was indeed attributable to the occurrence of I_f in hypertrophied ventricular cardiomyocytes (Fig. 5, inset),[33] whose functional expression (I_f density) was linearly related to the severity of myocardial hypertrophy.[33] In the following 10 years, evidence from our own and others' laboratories demonstrated the overexpression of I_f in animal models of cardiac disease[34] as well as in human cardiomyopathies.[35-37] Some of these results are schematically reported in Figure 6 from which it is apparent that a relationship exists between the amplitude of I_f and the severity of hypertrophy. Interestingly, functional expression of I_f in human ventricular cardiomyocytes seems to be related to the aetiology of the disease, current density being higher in ischaemic than in dilated cardiomyopathy (Fig. 6B),[35-37] as confirmed also by measurements of mRNA transcripts and protein expression for HCN isoforms (unpublished data).

In the complex, all these alterations lead to an enhanced susceptibility of the diseased heart to fatal arrhythmias.[38] This propensity may be due also to the anomalous presence of I_f in ventricular cells. The possibility that this current –

A. Rat

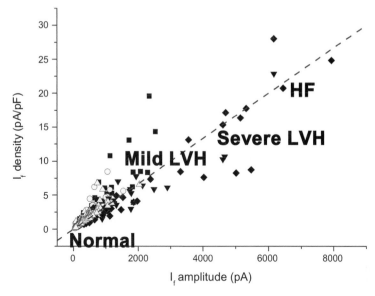

B. Man

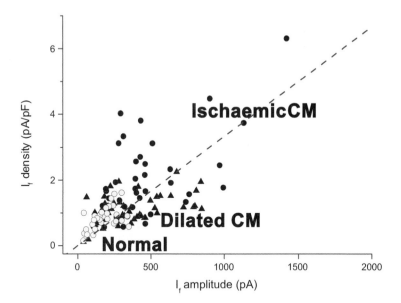

Fig. 6 Ventricular I_f expression is increased in cardiomyopathies. Each point represents I_f density versus I_f amplitude in ventricular cardiomyocytes from rat (A) or human (B) diseased hearts, and respective controls. In rats, maximal I_f overexpression was detected in cells from failing hearts (HF, black diamonds), greater than that measured in hearts with mild (black squares) or severe (black triangles) left ventricular hypertrophy (LVH); cells from control animals are indicated by open symbols. In humans, a higher I_f density was measured in cells from patients with ischaemic (black circles) than in those from patients dilated (black triangles) cardiomyopathy (CM), thus suggesting that the aetiology of heart disease may play a relevant role; cells from undiseased hearts are indicated by open circles.

as well as the SAN current – may represent a suitable target for bradycardic agents is an attractive hypothesis which deserves experimental and clinical evaluation. In this regard, it is interesting to note that abnormal automaticity is abolished[39] and I_f inhibited[40] by zatebradine in myocytes from rat hypertrophied heart.

The clinical availability of agents, which act by blocking specifically the f-channel,[41] will likely clarify the relevance of I_f overexpressed in the working myocardium and certainly assess the role of 'pure' heart rate reduction in the treatment of congestive heart failure.

Key points for clinical practice

- I_f, the so-called 'funny current', plays a fundamental role in spontaneous activity of the sinus node.

- Four subunits coded by hyperpolarisation-activated, cyclic nucleotide gated (HCN) channel genes co-assemble to form hyper-polarisation-activated f-channels, permeable to Na^+ and K^+ ions.

- Drugs which selectively block I_f reduce heart rate; a complete block of I_f reduces heart rate by 30–40% but does not stop the sinus node activity.

- Ivabradine is the only selective blocker of I_f channels which is clinically available; the effect of ivabradine is rate-dependent, *i.e.* the higher the heart rate, the greater is the drug effect.

- Clinical trials have documented that ivabradine has an anti-anginal efficacy comparable to that of atenolol and amlodipine.

- Experimental and clinical data are consistent with the view that heart rate reduction *per se* may be beneficial in heart failure.

- I_f is expressed in ventricular myocytes only in pathological conditions; its density is linearly related to the severity of the hypertrophy, being larger in heart failure.

- I_f may play a role in the enhanced susceptibility of the failing heart to fatal arrhythmias.

- On-going clinical trials will clarify the relevance of I_f over-expressed in the ventricular myocardium and the role of 'pure' heart rate reduction in the treatment of congestive heart failure.

References

1. Vassalle M. The relationship among cardiac pacemakers. Overdrive suppression. *Circ Res* 1977; **41**: 269–277.
2. DiFrancesco D. Funny channels in the control of cardiac rhythm and mode of action of selective blockers. *Pharmacol Res* 2006; **53**: 399–406.
3. Bogdanov KY, Vinogradova TM, Lakatta EG. Sinoatrial nodal cell ryanodine receptor and Na+–Ca2+ exchanger: molecular partners in pacemaker regulation. *Circ Res* 2001; **88**: 1254–1258.

4. Ludwig A, Zong X, Jeglitsch M, Hofmann F, Biel M. A family of hyperpolarization-activated mammalian cation channels. *Nature* 1998; **393**: 587–591.

5. Santoro B, Liu DT, Yao H *et al*. Identification of a gene encoding a hyperpolarization-activated pacemaker channel of brain. *Cell* 1998; **93**: 717–729.

6. Shi W, Wymore R, Yu H *et al*. Distribution and prevalence of hyperpolarization-activated cation channel (HCN) mRNA expression in cardiac tissues. *Circ Res* 1999; **85**: e1–e6.

7. Mannikko R, Elinder F, Larsson HP. Voltage-sensing mechanism is conserved among ion channels gated by opposite voltages. *Nature* 2002; **419**: 837–841.

8. DiFrancesco D. Dual allosteric modulation of pacemaker (f) channels by cAMP and voltage in rabbit SA node. *J Physiol (Lond)* 1999; **515**: 367–376.

9. Baruscotti M, Bucchi A, DiFrancesco D. Physiology and pharmacology of the cardiac pacemaker ('funny') current. *Pharmacol Therap* 2005; **107**: 59–79.

10. DiFrancesco D. Some properties of the UL-FS 49 block of the hyperpolarization-activated current (i(f)) in sino-atrial node myocytes. *Pflügers Arch* 1994; **427**: 64–70.

11. Goethals M, Raes A, Van Bogaert PP. Use-dependent block of the pacemaker current I$_f$ in rabbit sinoatrial node cells by zatebradine (UL-FS 49). On the mode of action of sinus node inhibitors. *Circulation* 1993; **88**: 2389–2401.

12. Bois P, Bescond J, Renaudon B, Lenfant J. Mode of action of bradycardic agent, S 16257, on ionic currents of rabbit sinoatrial node cells. *Br J Pharmacol* 1996; **118**: 1051–1057.

13. Bucchi A, Baruscotti M, DiFrancesco D. Current-dependent block of rabbit sino-atrial node I$_f$ channels by ivabradine. *J Gen Physiol* 2002; **120**: 1–13.

14. Valenzuela C, Delpon E, Franqueza L *et al*. Class III antiarrhythmic effects of zatebradine. Time-, state-, use-, and voltage-dependent block of hKv1.5 channels. *Circulation* 1996; **94**: 562–570.

15. Frishman WH, Pepine CJ, Weiss RJ, Baiker WM. Addition of zatebradine, a direct sinus node inhibitor, provides no greater exercise tolerance benefit in patients with angina taking extended-release nifedipine: results of a multicenter, randomized, double-blind, placebo-controlled, parallel-group study. *J Am Coll Cardiol* 1995; **26**: 305–312.

16. Pape HC. Queer current and pacemaker: the hyperpolarization-activated cation current in neurons. *Annu Rev Physiol* 1996; **58**: 299–327.

17. Borer JS, Fox K, Jaillon P, Lerebours G, for the Ivabradine Investigators Group. Antianginal and antiischemic effects of ivabradine, an I$_f$ inhibitor, in stable angina: a randomized, double-blind, multicentered, placebo-controlled trial. *Circulation* 2003; **107**: 817–823.

18. Tardif JC, Ford I, Tendera M, Bourassa MG, Fox K, for the INITIATIVE Investigators. Efficacy of ivabradine, a new selective I$_f$ inhibitor, compared with atenolol in patients with chronic stable angina. *Eur Heart J* 2005; **26**: 2529–2536.

19. Ruzyllo W, Ford I, Tendera M, Fox K. Antianginal and antiischaemic effects of the I$_f$ current inhibitor ivabradine compared to amlodipine as monotherapies in patients with chronic stable angina. Randomised, controlled, double-blind trial. *Eur Heart J* 2004; **25 (Suppl)**: 138.

20. Kjekshus J, Gullestad L. Heart rate as a therapeutic target in heart failure. *Eur Heart J Suppl* 1999; **1**: 64–69.

21. Swedberg K, Eneroth P, Kjekshus J, Wilhelmsen L. Hormones regulating cardiovascular function in patients with severe congestive heart failure and their relation to mortality. CONSENSUS Trial Study Group. *Circulation* 1990; **82**: 1730–1736.

22. Nul MD, Doval MD, Grancelli MD, Varini MD, Soifer MD. Heart rate is a marker of amiodarone mortality reduction in severe heart failure. *J Am Coll Cardiol* 1997; **29**: 1199–1205.

23. Lechat P, Hulot JS, Escolano S *et al*. Heart rate and cardiac rhythm relationships with bisoprolol benefit in chronic heart failure in CIBIS II Trial. *Circulation* 2001; **103**: 1428–1433.

24. Thackray SDR, Ghosh JM, Wright GA *et al*. The effect of altering heart rate on ventricular function in patients with heart failure treated with β-blockers. *Am Heart J* 2006; **152**: 710–713.

25. Mulder P, Barbier S, Chagraoui A *et al*. Long-term heart rate reduction induced by the selective I(f) current inhibitor ivabradine improves left ventricular function and intrinsic myocardial structure in congestive heart failure. *Circulation* 2004; **109**: 1674–1679.

26. Fox K, Ferrari R, Tendera M, Steg P, Ford I. Rationale and design of a randomized, double-blind, placebo-controlled trial of ivabradine in patients with stable coronary

artery disease and left ventricular dysfunction: the morBidity-mortality EvAlUation of the I_f inhibitor ivabradine in patients with coronary disease and left ventricULar dysfunction (BEAUTIFUL) study. *Am Heart J* 2006; **152**: 860–866.

27. Camm AJ. How does pure heart rate lowering impact on cardiac tolerability? *Eur Heart J Suppl* 2006; **8**: D9–D15.

28. Cerbai E, Pino R, Sartiani L, Mugelli A. Influence of postnatal-development on I_f occurrence and properties in neonatal rat ventricular myocytes. *Cardiovasc Res* 1999; **42**: 416–423.

29. Yasui K, Liu W, Opthof T *et al.* I_f current and spontaneous activity in mouse embryonic ventricular myocytes. *Circ Res* 2001; **88**: 536–542.

30. Sartini L, Bettiol E, Stilliyano F, Mugelli A, Cerbai E, Jaconi ME. Developmental changes in cardiomyocytes differentiated from human embryonic stem cells: a molecular and electrophysiological approach. *Stem Cells* 2007: In press (first published online January 25 2007)

31. Cerbai E, Barbieri M, Mugelli A. Characterization of the hyperpolarization-activated current, I(f), in ventricular myocytes isolated from hypertensive rats. *J Physiol (Lond)* 1994; **481**: 585–591.

32. Barbieri M, Varani K, Cerbai E *et al.* Electrophysiological basis for the enhanced cardiac arrhythmogenic effect of isoprenaline in aged spontaneously hypertensive rats. *J Mol Cell Cardiol* 1994; **26**: 849–860.

33. Cerbai E, Barbieri M, Mugelli A. Occurrence and properties of the hyperpolarization-activated current I_f in ventricular myocytes from normotensive and hypertensive rats during aging. *Circulation* 1996; **94**: 1674–-1681.

34. Sartiani L, De Paoli P, Stillitano F *et al.* Functional remodeling in post-myocardial infarcted rats: focus on beta-adrenoceptor subtypes. *J Mol Cell Cardiol* 2006; **40**: 258–266.

35. Cerbai E, Pino R, Porciatti F *et al.* Characterization of the hyperpolarization-activated current, I(f), in ventricular myocytes from human failing heart. *Circulation* 1997; **95**: 568–571.

36. Cerbai E, Sartiani L, DePaoli P *et al.* The properties of the pacemaker current I-F in human ventricular myocytes are modulated by cardiac disease. *J Mol Cell Cardiol* 2001; **33**: 441–448.

37. Hoppe UC, Jansen E, Sudkamp M, Beuckelmann DJ. Hyperpolarization-activated inward current in ventricular myocytes from normal and failing human hearts. *Circulation* 1998; **97**: 55–65.

38. Tomaselli G, Marban E. Electrophysiological remodeling in hypertrophy and heart failure. *Cardiovasc Res* 1999; **42**: 270–283.

39. Sridhar A, Dech SJ, Lacombe VA *et al.* Abnormal diastolic currents in ventricular myocytes from spontaneous hypertensive and heart failure (SHHF) rats. *Am J Physiol* 2006; **291**: H2192–H2198.

40. Romanelli MN, Cerbai E, Dei S *et al.* Design, synthesis and preliminary biological evaluation of zatebradine analogues as potential blockers of the hyperpolarization-activated current. *Bioorgan Med Chem* 2005; **13**: 1211–1220.

41. DiFrancesco D, Camm JA. Heart rate lowering by specific and selective I(f) current inhibition with ivabradine: a new therapeutic perspective in cardiovascular disease. *Drugs* 2004; **64**: 1757–1765.

Luigi A. Venetucci David A. Eisner

2

Intracellular calcium and cardiac disease

Calcium (Ca) plays a crucial role in linking the electrical excitation of the heart to contraction a process known as excitation-contraction coupling (EC coupling). It is now well established that the action potential produces a transient increase in cytosolic Ca concentration ($[Ca^{2+}]_i$) also known as the systolic Ca transient. This rise in $[Ca^{2+}]_i$ is responsible for the activation of the myofilaments and the generation of contraction. As shown in Figure 1, depolarisation of the cell membrane during the action potential (a) causes opening of the voltage-gated L-type Ca channels. A small amount of Ca enters the myocyte via these channels (b) and triggers further Ca release from the sarcoplasmic reticulum (SR) the main cellular Ca store (c), via a mechanism known as Ca-induced Ca-release (CICR), as reviewed by Bers.[1]. The channel responsible for this release is called the ryanodine receptor (RyR). This has the important property that the probability that it is open (and, therefore, allows calcium to leave into the cytoplasm) is increased by a local increase of cytoplasmic Ca concentration. The systolic Ca transient activates the myofilaments and contraction is generated (d). Relaxation is achieved by Ca removal from the cytosol. The majority of Ca is pumped back into the SR by the SR Ca-ATPase (SERCA) that uses the energy provided by ATP hydrolysis (e). The activity of SERCA is regulated not only by the cytoplasmic concentration of Ca but also by the accessory protein phospholamban. Unphosphorylated phospholamban inhibits SERCA and this inhibition is relieved by phosphorylation. A smaller amount of Ca is pumped out of the cell

Luigi A. Venetucci MB ChB MRCP PhD (for correspondence)
Lecturer in Cardiovascular Medicine, Unit of Cardiac Physiology, Core Technology Facility, University of Manchester, 46 Grafton Street, Manchester M13 9NT, UK
E-mail: lavenetucci@hotmail.com

David A. Eisner MA DPhil DMedSci
British Heart Foundation Professor of Cardiac Physiology, Unit of Cardiac Physiology, 3.18 Core Technology Facility, University of Manchester, 46 Grafton Street, Manchester M13 9NT, UK

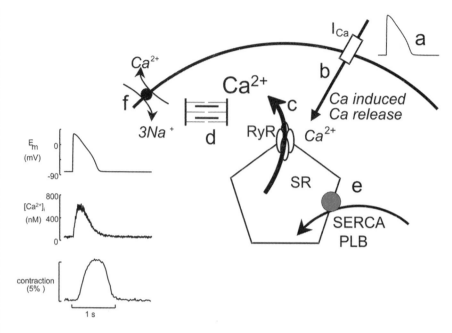

Fig. 1 Mechanisms involved in the control of contraction and calcium in cardiac cells. The main diagram shows the following events. (a) The surface membrane action potential. This opens the L-type Ca channel leading to a small influx of Ca (b). Some Ca binds to the RyR making it open and thereby releasing much more Ca into the SR (c). This Ca then activates the myofibrils (d). Relaxation occurs by Ca being reduced to diastolic levels by the combination of SERCA (e) which is controlled by the accessory protein phospholamban (PLB) and Na–Ca exchange (NCX), f. The inset shows recordings of (from top to bottom): membrane potential; $[Ca^{2+}]_i$; and cell length.

(f) by the Na/Ca exchanger (NCX) using the energy provided by 3 Na^+ ions entering the cell to pump one Ca^{2+} ion out. As a consequence of this stoichiometry, one net positive charge enters the cell each time a Ca^{2+} ion is pumped out; therefore, the NCX produces a depolarising current across the surface membrane of the cell.

CONTROL OF THE SYSTOLIC CALCIUM TRANSIENT

The main factors that determine the amplitude of the systolic Ca transient are: (i) the amount of Ca stored in the SR (SR Ca content); (ii) the amplitude of the Ca current; and (iii) β-adrenergic stimulation.

SARCOPLASMIC RETICULUM CA CONTENT

Increasing SR Ca content increases the amplitude of the systolic Ca transient and the corresponding contraction[2] by two different mechanisms:

1. The increased Ca concentration in the SR will increase the concentration gradient between SR and cytoplasm.

2. Experiments with RyRs incorporated into artificial lipid bilayers have demonstrated that increasing Ca on the luminal side increases the open probability.[3]

The net effect is that SR Ca content influences the amount of Ca released by each SR Ca release unit. SR Ca content depends not only on SR Ca transport pathways (RyR and SERCA), but also on cytoplasmic Ca concentration. Manoeuvres that increase Ca influx (Ca channels) or decrease Ca efflux will increase cytoplasmic and SR Ca content. Slowing the NCX, by increasing intracellular sodium, will increase SR Ca load and, as a result, the force of contraction. For example, the inotropic effects of digitalis are due to an increase in intracellular Na that, in turn, causes an increase in SR Ca content.

Ca CURRENT AMPLITUDE

The amplitude of the systolic Ca transient is tightly regulated by the L-type Ca current (I_{CaL}) (see Bers[1] for review) and increasing the amplitude of I_{CaL} results in a bigger Ca transient. The positive inotropic effects of increasing I_{CaL} are mediated by two different mechanisms:

1. An increase of the trigger for Ca release results in the recruitment of a greater number of Ca release units.
2. Greater Ca influx into the cell increases SR Ca content and thus the amplitude of the Ca transient.

'Ca antagonists', such as diltiazem and verapamil, inhibit I_{CaL} and reduce the amplitude of the Ca transient. The reduction in Ca transient amplitude is responsible for the negative inotropic negative effects of these drugs.

β-ADRENERGIC STIMULATION

This is the main regulator of cardiac contractility *in vivo* and accounts for much of the increase in contractility observed during exercise. Stimulation of the β-adrenergic receptor increases intracellular cAMP concentration via stimulation of the protein $G_{\alpha s}$. Levels of cAMP can also be increased by two compounds, milrinone and enosimone (drugs used as inotropic agents). These compounds inhibit phosphodiesterase, the enzyme responsible for cAMP degradation. cAMP activates protein kinase A and this, in turn, phosphorylates various intracellular substrates including the L-type channels, phospholamban/SERCA and RyR. Phosphorylation of the L-type channel increases I_{CaL} amplitude. Phospholamban is bound to SERCA and reduces SERCA activity by reducing its affinity for Ca. Phospholamban phosphorylation by PKA causes dissociation from SERCA and increased SERCA activity.[4] Stimulation of SERCA activity increases the rate of decay of the systolic Ca transient and this is partly responsible for the faster relaxation produced by β-adrenergic stimulation (lusitropic effect, see Fig. 2). The effects of β-adrenergic stimulation on RyR have been studied by several groups and are the subject of controversy. Marx *et al.*[5] proposed that β-adrenergic stimulation promotes PKA-mediated phosphorylation of RyR (at serine 2809). This phosphorylation causes the dissociation from RyR of FK506 binding protein 12.6 (FKBP 12.6), one of many accessory proteins. The consequence of this dissociation is an increase in RyR activity. These findings have been challenged by several groups (as reviewed by Bers *et al.*[6] and George *et al.*[7]). The net effect of β-adrenergic stimulation is an increase in the Ca transient amplitude, force of contraction and rate of relaxation (Fig. 2).

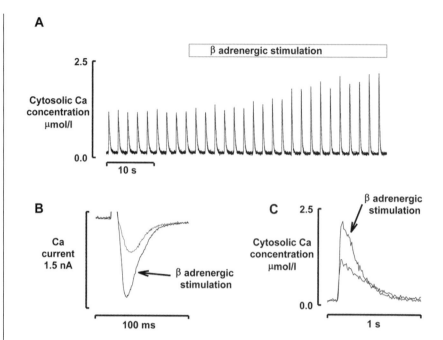

Fig. 2 The effects of β-adrenergic stimulation. (A) β-Adrenergic stimulation (with isoproterenol) produces an increase in the amplitude of the systolic Ca transient. This is due to a combination of the increase of the L-type Ca current (B) and phosphorylation of phospholamban leading of SERCA activity. This increased SERCA activity results in a faster decay of the Ca transient (C).

CALCIUM WAVES

As outlined above, Ca release from the SR occurs when the RyR is activated by influx on the L-type Ca current during an action potential. However, the SR can release Ca independently from an action potential even in the absence of a Ca current (Fig. 3). Waves of diastolic Ca release occur as Ca is released spontaneously from one part of the SR and then propagates as a wave along the cell.[8] Such Ca waves occur when SR Ca is elevated to a critical threshold level.[9] This threshold for waves can be changed by modulating RyR activity. Stimulation of RyR reduces wave threshold[10] and inhibition of RyR increases it.[11] Some of the calcium released into the cytosol during a Ca wave is pumped out of the cell by NCX thereby activating a depolarising membrane current.[1] Even before the waves and the resulting NCX current had been measured, their consequences were appreciated. Work done in the 1970s[12] showed that, under conditions where the SR is now known to be overloaded with calcium, the normal action potential was followed by a delayed after-depolarisation (DAD). A sufficiently large DAD can reach the action potential threshold and trigger an action potential. DADs were first shown to be produced by digitalis intoxication and suggested to be responsible for the ensuing triggered arrhythmias.[13] Subsequent work mainly on animal models has shown that DADs can also be responsible for arrhythmias in various clinical setting including ischaemia and reperfusion,[14] LQT-3[15] and right ventricular outflow tract VT.[16] Finally, there is a wealth of cellular studies demonstrating that

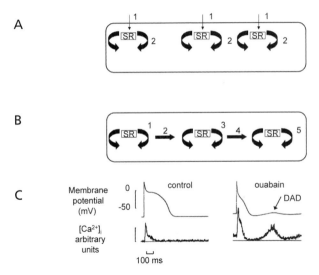

Fig. 3 Production of Ca waves in cardiac cells. (A) Normal e–c coupling. Ca enters via the L-type current (1) and releases Ca from the SR (2). (B) Ca waves. Ca is released spontaneously from one part of the SR (1) and Ca then diffuses to the next region (2) where further release (3) and diffusion (4) occur triggering further release (5). (C) Membrane potential and $[Ca^{2+}]_i$. As indicated, the records were obtained in control and after exposure to the digitalis like substance ouabain. [Records in (C) were reproduced from *Journal of General Physiology*, 1984: **83**: 395--415.[43] Copyright 1984 Rockefeller University Press.]

positive inotropic interventions that act by increasing intracellular Ca, such as β-agonists[17] and phosphodiesterase inhibitors, can produce DADs; it is likely, therefore, that the arrhythmias seen clinically also result from this mechanism.

CATECHOLAMINERIC POLYMORPHIC VENTRICULAR TACHYCARDIA

Leenhardt *et al.*[18] identified a cluster of patients who developed polymorphic ventricular tachycardia after physical or emotional stress. These patients had structurally normal hearts, normal resting ECG and a family history of juvenile sudden death. They called this condition catecholaminergic polymorphic ventricular tachycardia (CPVT) because, during physical or emotional stress, there is a profound catecholamine stimulation of the heart. They also observed that this tachycardia had similar morphology to the digitalis-induced tachycardia that was well known to be secondary to abnormal Ca handling and delayed after-depolarisations. They speculated that CPVT was secondary to abnormal Ca handling and delayed after-depolarisations. This hypothesis was confirmed a few years later when two genes responsible for CPVT were identified and both are involved in myocardial Ca handling. Two different forms of CPVT have been identified:[7] CPVT-1 which is autosomal dominant and CPVT-2 that is autosomal recessive.

CPVT-1

Priori et al.[19] have studied several families with CPVT-1 and discovered that in 50% of cases it is caused by mutations of RyR (locus 1q42-43). It is not clear

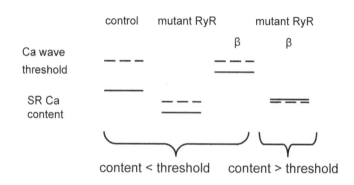

Fig. 4 The relationship between Ca wave threshold and SR content. In all panels the dashed lines show the threshold SR content required to produce waves and the solid lines the actual SR content. Four different conditions are illustrated. These show (from left to right). Control: the SR content is less than the threshold and therefore waves are not seen. Mutant RyR: here the threshold is reduced but, as a consequence of increased RyR opening, the SR content is also decreased and, therefore, waves are not seen. β-Adrenergic stimulation. Now the SR content is increased but to a level that is still less than the threshold so waves are still not seen. Mutant RyR and β-adrenergic stimulation. Now the threshold is less than the content and waves are seen.

which genes are responsible for the remaining 50% of cases. Tester et al.[20] suggested that mutations causing Andersen Tawil syndrome and LQT-5 (two forms of genetic long QT syndrome) can present with the clinical phenotype of CPVT and that these mutations account for the cases of CPVT that are not caused by CPVT. To date, 69 RyR mutations have been identified.[7] Several cellular studies have clarified the mechanisms responsible for CPVT. Liu et al.[21] have demonstrated that the mutation increases the incidence of DADs after β-adrenergic stimulation. Jiang et al.[22] suggested that the mutations predispose to the onset of Ca waves and DADs because they lower the SR threshold for Ca waves. We have, however, recently demonstrated that lowering the threshold for Ca waves in isolation is not sufficient to generate Ca waves and DADs.[23] Although the mutation lowers the SR threshold for Ca waves, the increased RyR activity will decrease SR content to below the threshold and Ca waves will not occur. During exercise, catecholamine stimulation increases SR content to the threshold for Ca waves and waves are seen (Fig. 4). Clinically, the first manifestation of CPVT, in most cases, is syncope triggered by exercise. The mean age of presentation of CPVT-1 is much lower for patients harbouring RyR mutation than for patients who have the clinical phenotype[19] of CPVT-1 but do not carry RyR mutation (8 ± 2 versus 20 ± 12). Three different VT patterns have been associated with CPVT: (i) bidirectional VT characterised by 180° alternating QRS axis on a beat-to-beat basis (Fig. 5A); (ii) polymorphic VT without a stable QRS axis alternans (Fig. 5B); and (iii) idiopathic VF. The best diagnostic tool is the exercise test (ETT). Priori et al.[19] reported that ETT causes ventricular arrhythmias in around 80% of patients who carry RyR mutations. In addition, they suggested that ETT is useful to risk stratify and titrate treatment. Holter monitoring can also be used for diagnosis and treatment titration.[19] Interestingly, infusion of the β-agonist isoprenaline induces arrhythmias in only 40% of patients and is not a reliable

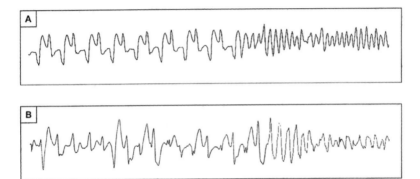

Fig. 5 Examples of bidirectional (A) and polymorphic (B) ventricular tachycardia degenerating into ventricular fibrillation in patients with CPVT. Taken from Priori et al.[19] with permission of the publisher. [Reproduced from Priori SG, Napolitano C, Memmi M et al. Clinical and molecular characterization of patients with catecholaminergic polymorphic ventricular tachycardia. *Circulation* 2002; **106**: 69–74. Copyright © 2002 Lippincott, Williams and Wilkins with permission.]

diagnostic tool. Similarly, programmed electrical stimulation fails to trigger arrhythmias in the majority of patients.

CPVT-2

This is autosomal recessive and is caused by mutations of calsequestrin (locus 1p23-21).[24] Calsequestrin is a protein that binds RyR on its lumen surface and has two main functions: (i) intra SR Ca buffer; and (ii) regulation of the sensitivity of RyR to free luminal Ca. Calsequestrin mutations increase the sensitivity of RyR to luminal Ca resulting in a lower SR threshold for Ca waves.[25] However, the lack of a large cohort of patients with CPVT-2 has not allowed a full characterisation of its clinical phenotype and a comparison with CPVT-1.

TREATMENT OF CPVT

The mainstay of treatment is β-blockade which achieves satisfactory arrhythmia control in around 60% of patients. Pharmacological treatment of CPVT would be revolutionised by an agent able to reduce RyR activity selectively. Wehrens et al.[26] suggested that JTV 519 (an agent that increases FKBP 12.6 binding to RyR) could be used to achieve this. Liu et al.[21] tested it on a mouse model of CPVT and failed to detect any efficacy in reducing arrhythmias after β-adrenergic stimulation. The use of an ICD is indicated when the pharmacological treatment does not achieve a satisfactory protection from arrhythmias.

HEART FAILURE

Heart failure is a clinical syndrome that occurs when the heart is unable to provide sufficient cardiac output to supply the metabolic demands of the organism. In the majority of cases, this is due to a decreased cardiac contractility. The disease progression is characterised by a progressive decline in contractile function and an increased incidence of fatal arrhythmias. The

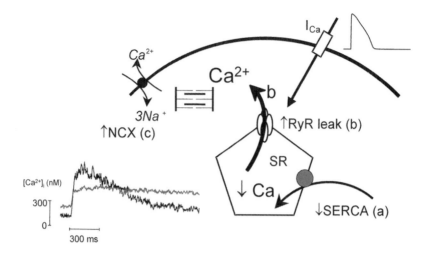

Fig. 6 Changes of Ca handling in heart failure. The inset shows Ca transients recorded from human ventricular myocytes from control (dark) and dilated cardiomyopathy (grey).[44] The main figures shows the major steps in e–c coupling that have been suggested to be affected in heart failure. These are: (a) decreased SERCA activity; (b) increased leak of Ca through the RyR; (c) increased NCX activity. Note that all these would results in a decrease of SR Ca content. [Reproduced from Beuckelmann DJ, Näbauer M, Erdmann E. Intracellular calcium handling in isolated ventricular myocytes from patients with terminal heart failure. *Circulation* 1992; **85**: 1046–1055. Copyright © 1992 Lippincott, Williams and Wilkins with permission.]

alterations of Ca handling apparatus in heart failure have been extensively studied both using animal models and human tissue from explanted hearts. In this section, we shall summarise the data available.

CA TRANSIENT AND SR CA CONTENT

Almost all models of heart failure have demonstrated a reduction in the amplitude of the Ca transient and the twitch contraction.[1] This reduction is more pronounced at fast heart rates.[27] The rate of decay of the Ca transient and, as a consequence, the rate of relaxation is substantially decreased in the majority of studies (Fig. 6). A substantial reduction in SR Ca content has consistently been demonstrated in all models.[27]

L-TYPE Ca CURRENT

The majority of the data regarding I_{CaL} amplitude and density suggest that there is no significant change during heart failure[27] and the prevailing opinion is that the reduced amplitude of the Ca transient is not produced by alterations in I_{CaL}.

RYANODINE RECEPTOR EXPRESSION AND FUNCTION IN HEART FAILURE

Sainte-Beuve *et al.*,[28] in 1997, described an increase in [³H]-ryanodine binding in failing hearts in the presence of normal RyR levels. On the basis of this observation, they suggested that, in heart failure, there is an altered channel activity. The idea of a change in the function of RyR in heart failure has been also suggested by Marx et al.[5] In their papers they show that, in failing human and animal hearts, increased adrenergic stimulation causes high levels of RyR phosphorylation (hyper-phosphorylation). As mentioned above, they suggested that this will cause dissociation of FKBP 12.6 and increased RyR opening. The increase in RyR activity causes diastolic Ca leak from the SR, and thence a decrease of both SR Ca and the Ca transient. In addition, they postulate that the diastolic Ca leak could cause the appearance of Ca waves that, in turn, would cause DADs and arrhythmias. These findings were confirmed by Yamamoto et al.,[29] who detected altered RyR FKBP 12.6 stoichiometry and abnormal RyR function in vesicles isolated from dogs with fast-pacing-induced heart failure. This hypothesis is very attractive but, at present, not entirely consistent with other studies.[6] Jiang et al.[30] failed to detect any hyper-phosphorylation in heart failure produced with fast-pacing. Li et al.[31] have demonstrated that adrenergically stimulated phosphorylation of RyR does not affect RyR activity. Carter et al.[32] have also suggested that, before β-adrenergic stimulation, RyR is already phosphorylated at 75% of its sites and that both increases or decreases in its phosphorylation levels produce a greater RyR activity. Recently, Ai et al.[33] have suggested that, in heart failure, there is an up-regulation of the Ca/calmodulin kinase II system and this is responsible for higher RyR phosphorylation and abnormal RyR function. The overall impression is that there is definitely abnormal RyR function in heart failure but it is not clear what causes it.

NA/CA EXCHANGER

Animal models and human studies have consistently demonstrated an increase in NCX expression and function in heart failure.[27] The up-regulated NCX competes more effectively against SERCA during relaxation; therefore, more Ca is pumped out of the cell and the SR is depleted of Ca.

SERCA EXPRESSION AND ACTIVITY

SERCA protein levels and function are reduced in most of the heart failure studies both from human and animal models.[34] Phospholamban (SERCA regulatory protein) levels seem to be preserved or reduced by a lesser amount compared to SERCA so that the phospholamban:SERCA ratio is increased and the level of pump inhibition by phospholamban is increased in heart failure.[27] The reduced SERCA on its own could account for the decrease in SR Ca content, the smaller Ca transient and the slower rate of decay of the Ca transient observed in heart failure. Interestingly, in human heart failure, the rate of decay of the Ca transient and relaxation are not always compromised.[35] The presence of impaired relaxation depends exclusively on the alterations of SERCA function.

In summary, the decreased Ca transient amplitude, force of contraction, SR Ca content and impaired relaxation observed in heart failure are due to a combination of factors including increased NCX activity, decreased SERCA function and possibly diastolic Ca leak due to increased RyR activity.

CALCIUM WAVES IN HEART FAILURE

Myocardial tridimensional mapping studies have demonstrated that, DADs or early after-depolarisations (EADs) are responsible for the genesis of many arrhythmias in heart failure.[36] The fact that waves are more likely to occur despite a decreased SR content could be explained by an increase of RyR open probability and consequent decrease of the SR threshold for Ca release.

CALCIUM HANDLING PROTEINS AS A THERAPEUTIC TARGET IN HEART FAILURE

The understanding of the Ca-handling abnormalities responsible for the decreased cardiac contractility in heart failure has stimulated a large body of research investigating the potential of Ca handling as a therapeutic target in heart failure. In this section, we shall summarise two main areas of research in this field – ryanodine receptor stabilisation, and enhancing SERCA function.

RYANODINE RECEPTOR STABILISATION

Reiken et al.[37] suggested that the beneficial effects of β-blockers in heart failure are due to the fact they reduce RyR phosphorylation and because of that normalise RyR activity. The unresolved issue is whether the improved RyR function is one of the main determinants of improved LV function or just an epiphenomenon associated with the improvement in LV function produced by these agents. This issue could only be solved by the development of an agent that selectively inhibits RyR. In 2003, Yano et al.[38] demonstrated that JTV 519 (an agent that increases binding of FKBP 12.6 to RyR and decreases its activity) protect against the development of pacing-induced heart failure. However, all the studies mentioned above have been carried out in animal models and, to date, no clinical trials have investigated the suitability of RyR inhibition as a treatment strategy in heart failure.

DECREASE IN SERCA FUNCTION

In heart failure there is a decreased SERCA function due to a reduction in expression of SERCA and/or to a change in the SERCA:phospholamban ratio. Theoretically, any manoeuvre that increases SERCA function could be used as a treatment strategy. The use of SERCA2a gene transfer to increase SERCA levels improved systolic and diastolic function and prolonged survival in a rat model of pressure overload heart failure.[39] An alternative strategy to increase SERCA function is to reduce the inhibition of phospholamban. Hoshijima et al.[40] generated a mutant phospholamban that is constitutively phosphorylated and has less inhibitory effects on SERCA. They demonstrated that transfection of the mutant phospholamban delays progression to heart failure in cardiomyopathic hamsters (a model of dilated cardiomyopathy). Phospholamban levels can also be decreased by using in vitro transfection of a missense sequence. This was tested in myocytes from heart failure patients and produced an increase in Ca uptake and cell shortening.[41] In summary, SERCA activity modulation seems a viable strategy to treat heart failure. The main limitations of all these studies are that they have used gene transfection. This is a good research tool but has a limited clinical application. To translate this strategy to the clinical level, a drug able to stimulate SERCA selectively is needed. Recently, MCC-135, an agent able to stimulate SERCA function directly, has been developed. Studies in diabetic rats with impaired relaxation have shown that MCC-135 stimulates SERCA and increases diastolic dysfunction. A study investigating the effect of MCC-135 in patients with heart failure has started[42] and the results are expected in the next few years.

CONCLUSIONS

It is clear that abnormalities in Ca handling play an important role in the pathophysiology of heart failure and some arrhythmias. A full understanding of Ca handling has identified some potential therapeutic targets. The next decade will see the development of many therapeutic agents that will revolutionise the treatment of these diseases.

Key points for clinical practice

- In cardiac muscle, the action potential initiates contraction by causing a transient increase in cytosolic calcium concentration also known as the systolic calcium transient. Most of this calcium is released from the sarcoplasmic reticulum.

- The force of contraction is mainly determined by the amplitude of the systolic calcium transient. Cardiac myocytes have a complex calcium handling system that allows them to modulate the amplitude of the calcium transient and the force of contraction.

- The sarcoplasmic reticulum can release calcium independently from an action potential. This process is called diastolic calcium release and has been linked with the genesis of arrhythmias in various clinical settings.

- Abnormalities in this calcium handling system have been linked to a genetic form of arrhythmias called catecholaminergic polymorphic ventricular tachycardia (CPVT).

- CPVT is characterised by the onset of polymorphic VT or bidirectional VT during exercise in patients with structurally normal heart and normal resting ECG.

- Heart failure causes profound changes in the cellular calcium handling system. These changes are responsible both for the decreased force of contraction and some of the arrhythmias that are associated with heart failure.

- Some calcium handling proteins have been identified as potential therapeutic targets for the treatment of heart failure and arrhythmias. Animal studies have confirmed the great potential of calcium handling as a therapeutic target in heart failure.

- Clinical trials have been set to test the efficacy of these therapeutic strategies.

ACKNOWLEDGEMENT

The authors are supported by the British Heart Foundation.

References

1. Bers DM. *Excitation-Contraction Coupling and Cardiac Contractile Force*, 2 edn. Dordrecht: Kluwer, 2001.
2. Eisner DA, Choi HS, Diaz ME, O'Neill SC, Trafford AW. Integrative analysis of calcium cycling in cardiac muscle. *Circ Res* 2000; **87**: 1087–1094.
3. Lukyanenko V, Györke I, Györke S. Regulation of calcium release by calcium inside the sarcoplasmic reticulum in ventricular myocytes. *Pflügers Arch* 1996; **432**: 1047–1054.
4. Tada M, Inui M. Regulation of calcium transport by the ATPase-phospholamban system. *J Mol Cell Cardiol* 1983; **15**: 565–575.
5. Marx SO, Reiken S, Hisamatsu Y *et al.* PKA phosphorylation dissociates FKBP12.6 from the calcium release channel (ryanodine receptor): defective regulation in failing hearts. *Cell* 2000; **101**: 365–376.
6. Bers DM, Eisner DA, Valdivia HH. Sarcoplasmic reticulum Ca^{2+} and heart failure: roles of diastolic leak and Ca^{2+} transport. *Circ Res* 2003; **93**: 487–490.
7. George CH, Jundi H, Thomas NL, Fry DL, Lai FA. Ryanodine receptors and ventricular arrhythmias: Emerging trends in mutations, mechanisms and therapies. *J Mol Cell Cardiol* 2007; **42**: 34–50.
8. Cheng H, Lederer MR, Lederer WJ, Cannell MB. Calcium sparks and $[Ca^{2+}]_i$ waves in cardiac myocytes. *Am J Physiol* 1996; **270**: C148–C159.
9. Diaz ME, Trafford AW, O'Neill SC, Eisner DA. Measurement of sarcoplasmic reticulum Ca^{2+} content and sarcolemmal Ca^{2+} fluxes in isolated rat ventricular myocytes during spontaneous Ca^{2+} release. *J Physiol (Lond)* 1997; **501**: 3–16.
10. Trafford AW, Sibbring GC, Diaz ME, Eisner DA. The effects of low concentrations of caffeine on spontaneous Ca release in isolated rat ventricular myocytes. *Cell Calcium* 2000; **28**: 269–276.
11. Overend CL, Eisner DA, O'Neill SC. The effect of tetracaine on spontaneous Ca release and sarcoplasmic reticulum calcium content in rat ventricular myocytes. *J Physiol (Lond)* 1997; **502**: 471–479.
12. Ferrier GR, Saunders JH, Mendez C. A cellular mechanism for the generation of ventricular arrhythmias by acetylstrophanthidin. *Circ Res* 1973; **32**: 600–609.
13. Rosen MR, Gelband H, Hoffman BF. Correlation between effects of ouabain on the canine electrocardiogram and transmembrane potentials of isolated Purkinje fibers. *Circulation* 1973; **47**: 65–72.
14. Karmazyn M, Gan XT, Humphreys RA, Yoshida H, Kusumoto K. The myocardial Na^+–H^+ exchange; structure, regulation and its role in heart disease. *Circ Res* 1999; **85**: 777–786.
15. Fredj S, Lindegger N, Sampson KJ, Carmeliet P, Kass RS. Altered Na^+ channels promote pause-induced spontaneous diastolic activity in long QT syndrome type 3 myocytes. *Circ Res* 2006; **99**: 1225–1232.
16. Lerman BB, Belardinelli L, West GA, Berne RM, DiMarco JP. Adenosine-sensitive ventricular tachycardia: evidence suggesting cyclic AMP-mediated triggered activity. *Circulation* 1986; **74**: 270–280.
17. Volders PG, Kulcsar A, Vos MA *et al.* Similarities between early and delayed after depolarizations induced by isoproterenol in canine ventricular myocytes. *Cardiovasc Res* 1997; **34**: 348–359.
18. Leenhardt A, Lucet V, Denjoy I, Grau F, Ngoc DD, Coumel P. Catecholaminergic polymorphic ventricular tachycardia in children : a 7-year follow-up of 21 patients. *Circulation* 1995; **91**: 1512–1519.
19. Priori SG, Napolitano C, Memmi M *et al.* Clinical and molecular characterization of patients with catecholaminergic polymorphic ventricular tachycardia. *Circulation* 2002; **106**: 69–74.
20. Tester DJ, Arya P, Will M *et al.* Genotypic heterogeneity and phenotypic mimicry among

unrelated patients referred for catecholaminergic polymorphic ventricular tachycardia genetic testing. *Heart Rhythm* 2006; **3**: 800–805.

21. Liu N, Colombi B, Memmi M *et al.* Arrhythmogenesis in catecholaminergic polymorphic ventricular tachycardia – insights from a RyR2 R4496C knock-in mouse model. *Circ Res* 2006; **99**: 292–298.

22. Jiang D, Xiao B, Yang D *et al.* RyR2 mutations linked to ventricular tachycardia and sudden death reduce the threshold for store-overload-induced Ca^{2+} release (SOICR). *Proc Natl Acad Sci USA* 2004; **101**: 13062–13067.

23. Venetucci L, Trafford AW, Eisner DA. Increasing ryanodine receptor open probability alone does not produce arrhythmogenic Ca waves: threshold Ca content is required. *Circ Res* 2007; **100**: 105–111.

24. Lahat H, Eldar M, Levy-Nissenbaum E *et al.* Autosomal recessive catecholamine- or exercise-induced polymorphic ventricular tachycardia – clinical features and assignment of the disease gene to chromosome 1p13-21. *Circulation* 2001; **103**: 2822–2827.

25. Terentyev D, Viatchenko-Karpinski S, Gyorke I, Volpe P, Williams SC, Gyorke S. Calsequestrin determines the functional size and stability of cardiac intracellular calcium stores: mechanism for hereditary arrhythmia. *Proc Natl Acad Sci USA* 2003; **100**: 11759–11764.

26. Wehrens XH, Lehnart SE, Reiken SR *et al.* Protection from cardiac arrhythmia through ryanodine receptor-stabilizing protein calstabin2. *Science* 2004; **304**: 292–296.

27. Hasenfuss G, Pieske B. Calcium cycling in congestive heart failure. *J Mol Cell Cardiol* 2002; **34**: 951–969.

28. Sainte-Beuve C, Allen PD, Dambrin G *et al.* Cardiac calcium release channel (ryanodine receptor) in control and cardiomyopathic human hearts: mRNA and protein contents are differentially regulated. *J Mol Cell Cardiol* 1997; **29**: 1237–1246.

29. Yamamoto T, Yano M, Kohno M *et al.* Abnormal Ca^{2+} release from cardiac sarcoplasmic reticulum in tachycardia-induced heart failure. *Cardiovasc Res* 1999; **44**: 146–155.

30. Jiang MT, Lokuta AJ, Farrell EF, Wolff MR, Haworth RA, Valdivia HH. Abnormal Ca^{2+} release, but normal ryanodine receptors, in canine and human heart failure. *Circ Res* 2002; **91**: 1015–1022.

31. Li Y, Kranias EG, Mignery GA, Bers DM. Protein kinase A phosphorylation of the ryanodine receptor does not affect calcium sparks in mouse ventricular myocytes. *Circ Res* 2002; **90**: 309–316.

32. Carter S, Colyer J, Sitsapesan R. Maximum phosphorylation of the cardiac ryanodine receptor at serine-2809 by protein kinase A produces unique modifications to channel gating and conductance not observed at lower levels of phosphorylation. *Circ Res* 2006; **98**: 1506–1513.

33. Ai X, Curran JW, Shannon TR, Bers DM, Pogwizd SM. Ca^{2+}/calmodulin-dependent protein kinase modulates cardiac ryanodine receptor phosphorylation and sarcoplasmic reticulum Ca^{2+} leak in heart failure. *Circ Res* 2005; **97**: 1314–1322.

34. Hasenfuss G. Alterations of calcium-regulatory proteins in heart failure. *Cardiovasc Res* 1998; **37**: 279–289.

35. Hasenfuss G, Schillinger W, Lehnart SE *et al.* Relationship between Na^+–Ca^{2+} exchanger protein levels and diastolic function of failing human myocardium. *Circulation* 1999; **99**: 641–648.

36. Pogwizd SM, Hoyt RH, Saffitz JE, Corr PB, Cox JL, Cain ME. Reentrant and focal mechanisms underlying ventricular tachycardia in the human heart. *Circulation* 1992; **86**: 1872–1887.

37. Reiken S, Gaburjakova M, Gaburjakova J *et al.* β-Adrenergic receptor blockers restore cardiac calcium release channel (ryanodine receptor) structure and function in heart failure. *Circulation* 2001; **104**: 2843–2848.

38. Yano M, Kobayashi S, Kohno M *et al.* FKBP12.6-mediated stabilization of calcium-release channel (ryanodine receptor) as a novel therapeutic strategy against heart failure. *Circulation* 2003; **107**: 477–484.

39. Del Monte F, Harding SE, Schmidt U *et al.* Restoration of contractile function in isolated cardiomyocytes from failing human hearts by gene transfer of SERCA2a. *Circulation* 1999; **100**: 2308–2311.

40. Hoshijima M, Ikeda Y, Iwanaga Y *et al.* Chronic suppression of heart-failure progression

by a pseudophosphorylated mutant of phospholamban via *in vivo* cardiac rAAV gene delivery. *Nat Med* 2002; **8**: 864–871.

41. del Monte F, Harding SE, Dec GW, Gwathmey JK, Hajjar RJ. Targeting phospholamban by gene transfer in human heart failure. *Circulation* 2002; **105**: 904–907.

42. Zile M, Gaasch W, Little W *et al*. A phase II, double-blind, randomized, placebo-controlled, dose comparative study of the efficacy, tolerability, and safety of MCC-135 in subjects with chronic heart failure, NYHA class II/III (MCC-135-GO1 study): rationale and design. *J Cardiac Fail* 2004; **10**: 193–199.

43. Wier WG, Hess P. Excitation-contraction coupling in cardiac Purkinje fibers. Effects of cardiotonic steroids on the intracellular (Ca^{2+}) transient, membrane potential, and contraction. *J Gen Physiol* 1984; **83**: 395–415.

44. Beuckelmann DJ, Näbauer M, Erdmann E. Intracellular calcium handling in isolated ventricular myocytes from patients with terminal heart failure. *Circulation* 1992; **85**: 1046–1055.

Mamas A. Mamas Ludwig Neyses

3

Cardiac metabolism: from bench to bedside Diabetic cardiomyopathy, a disease of cardiac metabolism?

Diabetes mellitus is the fastest growing metabolic disease in the developed and developing world and it is increasing at epidemic levels. The World Health Organization estimates there to be 150 million diabetic patients world-wide increasing to approximately 300 million patients in the next 20 years. Cardio-vascular complications are the leading causes of morbidity and mortality amongst patients with diabetes.[1] Indeed, it has been reported that 33% of diabetic patients requiring insulin will have died from cardiovascular disease by the age of 50 years.[2] A leading cardiovascular cause of death for diabetic patients is cardiac failure. The Framingham study demonstrated the increased incidence of congestive cardiac failure in diabetic males (2.4:1) and females (5:1) independent of age, hypertension, obesity, coronary artery disease and hyperlipidaemia.[3] Furthermore, there has often been observed an over-representation of patients with diabetes in a number of heart failure studies. Even though diabetes has a prevalence of about 5% in the community, diabetic patients make up to 30% of patients in a number of heart failure studies such as SOLVD (26%),[4] ATLAS (19%),[5] and V-HeFT II (20%).[6] Indeed, of the 11,327 heart failure patients enrolled in the pan-European EuroHeart survey, 30% of them where found to have diabetes.[7]

DIABETIC CARDIOMYOPATHY

It is over 30 years since Rubler *et al*.[8] described four diabetic patients with congestive cardiac failure, normal coronary arteries and no other aetiologies of

M. A. Mamas MA DPhil MRCP
Clinical Lecturer in Cardiology, Manchester Heart Centre, Manchester Royal Infirmary, Oxford Road, Manchester M13 9WL, UK.

Ludwig Neyses MD (for correspondence)
Professor of Medicine/Cardiology, Manchester Heart Centre, Manchester Royal Infirmary, Oxford Road, Manchester M13 9WL, UK
E-mail: ludwig.neyses@manchester.ac.uk

heart failure at post mortem and proposed that it was due to a diabetic cardiomyopathy. Since this initial description, numerous studies have been published on diabetic cardiomyopathy in humans and animals. Diabetic cardiomyopathy is a distinct clinical entity which is defined as the presence of a primary myocardial disease or 'cardiomyopathy' found in diabetic patients independent of hypertension, valvular and underlying coronary artery disease. Abnormalities in both systolic and diastolic performance have been demonstrated in diabetics in both human and animal studies.[9] An early manifestation of diabetic cardiomyopathy is that of diastolic dysfunction, often seen to develop before changes in systolic dysfunction are apparent. Diastolic dysfunction in diabetics was initially shown in data obtained by cardiac catheterisation. In normotensive, diabetic patients without coronary artery disease, Regan et al.[10] demonstrated an increase in left ventricular end diastolic pressure, and a decreased left ventricular end diastolic volume with a normal ejection fraction suggesting diastolic dysfunction. These observations have been extended with the use of echocardiography where diastolic dysfunction has been observed in diabetic patients free from coronary artery disease, hypertension or valvular disease. Various abnormalities in diastolic dysfunction such as prolonged isovolumic relaxation period, delayed mitral valve opening and impairment in rapid diastolic filling and reduced mitral E/A ratio have been characteristic findings. In the large majority of echocardiographic studies, abnormalities of diastolic function have been demonstrated in diabetic patients with intact systolic function.[11] Using Doppler echocardiography, Boyer et al.[12] reported that up to 75% of normotensive, asymptomatic, diabetic patients have diastolic dysfunction in the presence of a normal stress echocardiogram. In a further Doppler echocardiographic study of young asymptomatic diabetic patients with a mean age of 45 years, 47% were found to have diastolic dysfunction in the presence of a normal stress echocardiogram and normal echocardiogram at rest.[13] It appears that systolic dysfunction is a later manifestation of diabetic cardiomyopathy; for example, in the study of Raev,[14] diastolic dysfunction in asymptomatic, young diabetic patients occurred on average 8 years after the diagnosis of diabetes whereas systolic dysfunction occurred after a mean of 18 years. Furthermore, in this study of 157 patients only 30% of those with diastolic dysfunction had evidence of systolic dysfunction. A number of studies have documented the presence of systolic dysfunction.[9] Whilst the principal hallmark of systolic dysfunction is depressed left ventricular ejection fraction, recent work has shown that standard echocardiography may actually miss subtle left ventricular systolic dysfunction since circumferential left ventricular function is often assessed whereas longitudinal function is often overlooked.[15] Indeed, using this technique, 20–30% of diabetic patients with a 'normal' ejection fraction measured in one axis showed evidence of systolic dysfunction. In the context of diabetic cardiomyopathy, systolic dysfunction occurs late, often when patients have already developed significant diastolic dysfunction. In a prospective study of 1659 diabetic patients hospitalised with heart failure as defined by Framingham criterion, those with heart failure due to diabetic cardiomyopathy had a median survival of 3.56 years and a yearly mortality of around 15–20%.[16]

STRUCTURAL CHANGES IN DIABETIC CARDIOMYOPATHY

A number of studies in both human and animal models of diabetes have documented structural changes in parallel with functional changes observed in the heart in diabetic cardiomyopathy. In histopathological studies, it appears that the most prominent change in patients with diabetic cardiomyopathy is that of fibrosis, which may be perivascular, interstitial or both. As the cardiomyopathy progresses, there is an increased myocyte loss and replacement by fibrosis.[10] Similar observations were recorded from endomyocardial biopsies from the right ventricle in cardiac catheterisation studies of patients with diabetic cardiomyopathy. The degree of interstitial fibrosis in diabetic patients was significantly greater than controls.[17] Fibrosis in diabetic hearts has been correlated with diastolic dysfunction. Using techniques such as ultrasonic back-scatter, which is directly related to myocardial collagen content, Di Bello et al.[18] demonstrated that back-scatter was significantly greater from the septum and posterior wall in diabetic patients and that this was correlated with diastolic dysfunction.

These human study findings have been corroborated with the findings from animal studies. In a rat model of Type 2 diabetes, diastolic dysfunction on echocardiography was associated with extracellular fibrosis. Indeed, the collagen area/visual field in left ventricular wall and the collagen content to dry tissue weight of the heart was greater in the diabetic animals compared to that of controls.[19] These increased fibrotic changes in the myocardium in diabetic cardiomyopathy may, in part, explain the function changes in diastolic function observed clinically.

MECHANISMS OF DIABETIC CARDIOMYOPATHY

The development of diabetic cardiomyopathy is likely to be multifactorial and many underlying mechanisms have been postulated. There appears to be a growing body of evidence that changes in cardiac metabolism and substrate utilisation may, in part, contribute to the underlying pathophysiological mechanisms of diabetic cardiomyopathy.

CARDIAC METABOLISM

Under physiological conditions, the myocardium is able to utilise multiple substrates including fatty acids, carbohydrates, amino acids and ketone bodies.[20] Carbohydrates and fatty acids are the main substrates whose metabolism provides the energy requirements of the heart. Under physiological conditions, 70% of the energy requirements of the heart are obtained from fatty acids and the remaining 30% from glucose. The heart is able to switch its substrate selection rapidly to accommodate different physiological and pathophysiological states and ensure continuous ATP generation to maintain cardiac function.

GLUCOSE METABOLISM

Physiologically, glucose is the major carbohydrate metabolised by the heart. Glucose is taken up into the myocardium by two membrane-bound, transporter systems, GLUT-1 and GLUT-4. GLUT-1 is localised in the sarcolemma and is involved in the basal transport of glucose across the cell membrane under 'resting' conditions. GLUT-4 is the dominant transport system and is localised in intracellular vesicles. Insulin binding to the sarcolemmal insulin receptor mediates a signalling cascade in which GLUT-4 is translocated from an intracellular compartment to the sarcolemma for transport of glucose into the myocardium. Insulin is also able to regulate GLUT-4 indirectly through up-regulation of GLUT-4 gene expression. Once glucose has crossed the cell membrane, it is broken down by a series of reactions, glycolysis, to pyruvate (Fig. 1). The main rate-limiting enzyme in glycolysis is phosphofructokinase-1 (PFK-1) which catalyses the conversion of fructose-6-phosphate to fructose 1,6-biphosphate. PFK-1 is activated by fructose 2,6-biphosphate which is synthesised by phosphofructokinase-2 (PFK-2), an enzyme activated by insulin. In aerobic metabolism, glycolysis contributes to around 10% of ATP generated. After glycolysis, pyruvate is transported into mitochondria and decarboxylated to acetyl-CoA by the enzyme complex pyruvate dehydrogenase (PDH). Acetyl-CoA then enters the tricarboxylic acid cycle (TCA or Krebs' cycle) where it is catabolised to CO_2 and H_2O in a series of reactions with the formation of ATP and reducing equivalents NADH and $FADH_2$; these are re-oxidised by the electron transport chain, resulting in the production of further molecules of ATP.

FATTY ACID METABOLISM

Fatty acid metabolism is the major source of energy in the heart and contributes around 70% of the ATP generated in the myocardium in aerobic metabolism. Fatty acids are obtained from either albumin-bound fatty acids or triglyceride-rich lipoproteins. Lipoproteins are hydrolysed to release fatty

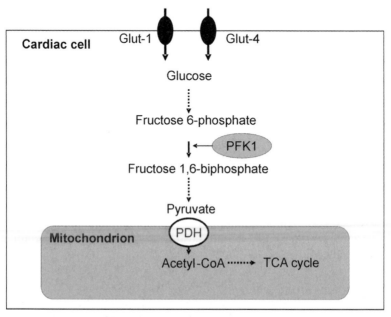

Fig. 1 Schematic representation of glucose metabolism occurring in a cardiac cell and within the mitochondrion. PFK-1. phosphofructokinase-1; PDH, pyruvate dehydrogenase.

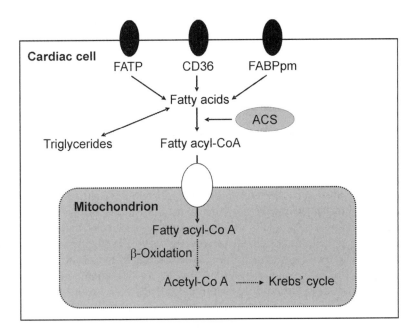

Fig. 2 Schematic representation of fatty acid metabolism occurring in a cardiac cell and within the mitochondrion. ACS, acyl-CoA synthase.

acids by the enzyme lipoprotein lipase (LPL) which is expressed in cardiac myocytes and found on their cell surface. Fatty acids released in this manner are then transported across the sarcolemma via three membrane transporters – CD36, fatty acid transport protein (FATP) and fatty acid binding protein plasma membrane (FABPpm). Once inside the cell, fatty acids are esterified to fatty acyl-CoA derivatives by the enzyme acyl-CoA synthase (ACS). Fatty acyl-CoA can then be transported into the mitochondria for β-oxidation into acetyl-CoA which enters the TCA cycle as in glucose metabolism or can be used for intracellular synthesis of triglycerides (Fig. 2). ACS not only catalyses esterification of fatty acids but has a central role in controlling fatty acid homeostasis. Studies have shown that ACS is associated with the fatty acid transporters FATP and CD36 and can influence fatty acid uptake, thereby altering metabolic flux. Under normal conditions, about 70–90% of fatty acids which enter the myocyte are oxidised to form ATP whereas 10–30% are converted to triglycerides. Fatty acids can regulate their own metabolism through effects at the transcriptional level by actions on PPARs (cardiac peroxisome proliferator-activated receptors). PPARs are a group of ligand-activated transcription factors, which are activated by a number of ligands including fatty acids. Once activated, they form complexes with retinoid X receptors, bind to promoter regions and enhance transcription of a number of proteins which control fatty acid metabolism. PPAR has three isoforms – PPAR-α, PPAR-β and PPAR-γ – although it appears that only PPAR-α and PPAR-β have an important role in fatty acid regulation in the heart, promoting expression of genes that regulate fatty acid metabolism at various steps including fatty acid uptake (LPL, CD36 and FABP), fatty acid esterification

(ACS) and fatty acid oxidation. Overexpression of PPAR-α receptors augments fatty acid uptake and oxidation whereas PPAR-α knock-out animals switch substrate metabolism from fatty acids to glucose.

ALTERATION OF CARDIAC METABOLISM IN DIABETES

Diabetes is first and foremost a disorder of abnormal insulin regulation either due to an abnormal insulin secretion and or impaired insulin action. About 10% of diabetic adults exhibit insulin deficiency (Type 1 diabetes) and the remainder exhibit some form of target tissue insulin resistance (Type 2 diabetes). Insulin and, therefore, diabetes in which there is an insulin deficiency or resistance influences cardiac metabolism in a number of ways. Insulin has an important role in the cardiac uptake of glucose. Insulin binds to extracellular sarcolemmal cell surface receptors and activates a signalling cascade which results in the translocation of the transmembrane glucose transporter GLUT-4 from intracellular vesicles to the sarcolemma, thereby facilitating transmembrane transport of glucose into the myocytes. In diabetes (in which there is insulin deficiency or resistance), glucose transport into the myocardium is, therefore, reduced, whereas fatty acid transport across the cell membrane (which is not insulin regulated) results in increased fatty acid delivery to the cardiac myocyte because of the increased circulating fatty acids. Insulin inhibits the release of fatty acids from adipose tissue; hence, in the diabetic state, this inhibition of fatty acid release from adipose tissue is lost and so serum fatty acids increase. This increase in intracellular fatty acid levels further inhibits glucose metabolism through inhibition of glycolysis and glucose oxidation at a number of key sites. Fatty acids inhibit glycolysis through inhibition of the glucokinase enzyme pathway and glucose oxidation via inhibition of the Krebs' (TCA) cycle through inhibition of pyruvate dehydrogenase. With increased intracellular fatty acid levels, the myocardium adapts to utilisation of fatty acids. Activation of PPAR-α, PPAR-β and PPAR-γ by the increase in intracellular fatty acids results in an increase in transcription of enzymes involved in fatty acid metabolism, thereby further increasing metabolic flux through this pathway.

DEFECTS IN CARBOHYDRATE METABOLISM IN DIABETES

A major restriction to utilisation of glucose by the diabetic heart is the slow rate of glucose transport into the myocardium across the sarcolemmal membrane due to cellular depletion of the main glucose transporters in the heart GLUT-1 and GLUT-4.[21] Under physiological conditions, it is well documented that insulin binding to the sarcolemmal insulin receptor mediates a signalling cascade in which GLUT-4 is translocated from an intracellular compartment to the sarcolemma. In the fasting state, only 15% of GLUT-4 can be isolated from the sarcolemma whereas, following insulin exposure, this rapidly rises to well over 80%.[22] This process is further inhibited in the presence of free fatty acids. In diabetes, a condition of cellular insulin resistance and/or insulin deficiency, GLUT-4 translocation to the membrane would be reduced and so the ability of the myocardium to utilise glucose would be impaired. Indeed, using FDG-PET scanning to assess myocardial glucose utilisation in diabetic patients, Ohtake et al.[23] documented a reduction of both glucose uptake into the myocardium and glucose utilisation in diabetic myocardium. Using a mouse genetic model of diabetes (db/db model) which exhibits hyperglycaemia, insulin resistance and hyperinsulinaemia and exhibits a diabetic cardiomyopathy, Belke et al.[24] showed that the rate of glycolysis from exogenous glucose was only 48% of control values; this was associated with both systolic and diastolic dysfunction in isolated mouse working heart preparations, similar to those observed clinically in diabetic cardiomyopathy. Using transgenic db/db mice which overexpressed GLUT-4, they demonstrated a normalisation of glycolysis and of cardiac function,[24] providing indirect evidence that changes in glucose uptake in the myocardium may, in part, contribute to the cardiomyopathy seen in diabetic patients.

A second method by which utilisation of glucose may be impaired in the diabetic myocardium is the inhibitory effect of fatty acids on various sites in glycolysis and glucose oxidation as described previously. For example, fatty acids elevated in diabetes have an inhibitory action on the pyruvate dehydrogenase complex, a key enzyme in the Krebs' cycle. This will reduce metabolic flux through the Krebs' cycle and so result in the reduction of NADH production, a key molecule involved in the oxidative phosphorylation pathway and the production of ATP. ATP is the universal energy store in cells and hydrolysis of ATP produces energy which drives a number of cellular processes including cell contraction. A reduction in ATP synthesis through such an inhibitory effect of fatty acids could impair cardiac function. In experimental studies, it has been demonstrated that diabetic animals with minimal hypertriglyceridaemia are resistant to the development of a diabetic cardiomyopathy.[25]

DEFECTS IN FATTY ACID METABOLISM IN DIABETES

Fatty acid transport in the myocardium is facilitated by specific transporters as described earlier. In many animal models of diabetes, such as streptozotocin (STZ)-induced diabetes (STZ is a pancreatic islet cell toxin), there is an increase in plasma membrane fatty acid transporters including CD36 and FABPpm resulting from increased protein expression.[26] In Zucker fatty diabetic rats, it appears that, although there is no change in total protein content, there is relocation of the fatty acid transporters from intracellular vesicles to the plasma membrane hence increasing transport capacity.[27] This increased capacity for the transport of fatty acids into the myocardium, in addition to increased circulating plasma fatty acids, will serve to increase flux through fatty acid metabolic pathways. Furthermore, activation of the PPAR-α receptor, which up-regulates the expression of fatty acid metabolism enzymes, has also been demonstrated in almost all animal models of diabetes;[28,29] this would further increase metabolic flux through fatty acid metabolism.

Interestingly, in transgenic mice which overexpress cardiac PPAR-α, a similar metabolic phenotype in the heart is observed to that seen in diabetic hearts. In addition, systolic dysfunction and ventricular hypertrophy are observed in these hearts, indicating that, in the absence of systemic metabolic changes, alterations to cardiac metabolism per se can alter cardiac contractile dysfunction.[29]

This provides indirect evidence that changes in fatty acid metabolism may, in part, contribute to development of diabetic cardiomyopathy.

When compared with glucose, oxidation of fatty acids requires more oxygen molecules per ATP produced (2.58 versus 2.33 ATP molecules per oxygen atom); therefore, cardiac efficiency (ratio of cardiac work to myocardial oxygen consumption) changes depending on which substrate is utilised. A decrease in cardiac efficiency is observed in cardiac function in diabetes in human[30] and animal models of diabetes.[31] This reduction in cardiac efficiency makes the myocardium especially vulnerable to damage following increased workload and ischaemia and may represent a mechanism for the cardiomyopathy seen in diabetic patients. A number of studies has also suggested that increased intracellular fatty acid levels during diabetes induce lipotoxicity and contribute to the development of cardiomyopathy. Studies with transgenic mice have demonstrated that elevation of intracellular fatty acids results in lipotoxicity in the absence of any systemic metabolic disturbance. For example, cardiac overexpression of lipoprotein lipase or FATP1 significantly increases intracellular fatty acids, with lipid storage and lipotoxic cardiomyopathy with contractile dysfunction, in the absence of systemic metabolic disturbances.[32,33] Furthermore, increasing fatty acid utilisation as an energy substrate by cardiac overexpression of PPAR-α or ACS also causes cardiac contractile dysfunction and a lipotoxicity cardiomyopathy similar to that seen in diabetes.[34] Cellular mechanisms which mediate cardiac lipotoxicity are not well characterised, but are thought to involve reactive oxygen species (ROS) which cause myocyte cell damage and augment apoptosis.[35]

CORRELATION OF METABOLIC CHANGES WITH LV DYSFUNCTION

Using streptozotocin, a pancreatic toxin which induces diabetes experimentally, Kita et al.[36] demonstrated a strong correlation between contractile dysfunction in rat isolated papillary muscles and blood glucose levels. In clinical studies, Hausdorf et al.[37] followed 36 children with Type 1 diabetes and demonstrated that the severity of diastolic dysfunction, evaluated by computer-assisted analysis of M-mode echocardiograms (time interval between minimal cavity dimension and mitral valve opening), was related to the mean value of HbA1c over the prior 2 years. Similarly, in a study of 50 Type 1 diabetic children with a mean age of 13 years and a mean diabetic duration of 5.9 years, a significant delay in LV filling was reported[38] and there was a correlation between poor glycaemic control and greater impairment of LV filling. In a further study including both Type 1 and Type 2 diabetic patients, a correlation between diastolic dysfunction and glycaemic control as assessed by HbA1c was reported.[39]

CORRELATION OF LV DYSFUNCTION WITH GLYCAEMIC CONTROL

The response of cardiac dysfunction to hypoglycaemic therapy supports the correlation between metabolic changes and cardiac dysfunction in diabetic cardiomyopathy. Using diabetic dogs with marked hyperglycaemia, Pogotsa et *al.*[40] demonstrated that treatment of the animals with insulin was associated with reversal of systolic and diastolic cardiac dysfunction. These observations have been repeated in a number of other studies using a variety of different animal models of diabetes. Using diabetic rats, Stroedter *et al.*[41] showed that the decline in cardiac output in diabetic cardiomyopathy was associated with a 36% decrease in glucose utilisation mediated, in part, through a reduction of glucose uptake into the myocardium. Both islet cell transplantation and insulin treatment were associated with a complete reversal of both metabolic and cardiac changes observed. Similar observations have been recorded clinically in humans although often there is only an improvement in haemodynamic parameters rather than a complete reversal as seen in animal experiments. This may, in part, reflect the longer chronicity of the diabetes in clinical studies than that in experimental studies, which is generally in the magnitude of days or weeks. Shapiro *et al.*[42] studied 69 Type II diabetics before and after hypoglycaemic therapy using both systolic time intervals and M-mode echocardiography. The pre-ejection period/LV ejection time ratio (an inverse measure of contractility, *i.e.* a higher ratio is associated with a decrease in contractility) was increased in the untreated group, and this ratio correlated well with blood glucose concentration. Treatment resulted in a fall in pre-ejection period/LV ejection time ratio in 54 patients with a modestly increased initial ratio but no response in the remaining 15 patients with a markedly elevated initial ratio after 4 months of therapy. Isovolumetric relaxation (reflecting diastolic dysfunction) was prolonged in diabetics, but it was not affected by hypoglycaemic therapy. In another study of 15 Type I diabetic subjects, systolic time intervals were evaluated at rest and after exercise during poor and good metabolic control, obtained by means of insulin therapy. Resting systolic time intervals were normal during poor and good metabolic control although, after exercise, a greater increase in pre-ejection period/LV ejection time ratio was found during poor control, and a smaller increase in the ratio occurred during good metabolic control, suggesting that good diabetic control is associated with the improvement in LV function.[43]

Glycaemic control can benefit cardiac metabolism and performance in the diabetic patient with heart failure by decreasing myocardial free fatty acid oxidation and increasing glucose utilisation. In a small study of 10 patients with New York Heart Association (NYHA) functional class 3 and 4 heart failure, dichloroacetate (a pyruvate dehydrogenase stimulator) was shown to increase stroke volume and left ventricular performance by reducing myocardial free fatty utilisation and increasing glucose oxidation and lactate extraction.[44]

Improvement in diabetic control is not always associated with improvement in LV dysfunction. For example, Hiramatsu *et al.*[45] studied 246 non-insulin-dependent Type 2 diabetic patients using Doppler echocardiography and demonstrated significant diastolic dysfunction compared to age-matched controls. Of the 246 patients, 48 were randomly selected and treated with insulin for 6 months, Doppler echocardiography was repeated and it was found that only 28 patients showed any evidence in improvement of diastolic parameters. In the study of Gough *et al.*,[46] LV diastolic function was assessed with pulsed wave Doppler mitral flow velocities in 20 normotensive patients with a new diagnosis of Type 2 diabetes mellitus. The E/A ratio (used to assess diastolic function) was significantly reduced in the diabetic group but despite improvements in glycaemic control over 3 months (HbA1c 9.9% to 7.4%), maintained at 6 months (HbA1c 7.0%), there were no changes in the E/A ratio. In the largest, prospective, randomised study to date, in which intensive versus standard glycaemic control was compared in 153 male Type 2 diabetic patients, there was no significant difference in LV systolic or diastolic function as assessed by radionucleotide ventriculography in the two treatment groups.[47]

CONCLUSIONS

Heart failure is one of the most important causes of cardiovascular morbidity and mortality in diabetic patients. There are significant changes in cardiac metabolism during diabetes with a switch from glucose metabolism to fatty acid metabolism. Both clinical and animal experiments support the view that some of these changes in cardiac metabolism may, in part, contribute to the pathophysiology of diabetic cardiomyopathy. Optimisation of diabetic control and hence prevention of the deleterious changes in cardiac metabolism has been shown to improve cardiac function although the effects are variable. Clearly, the effects of good glycaemic control on cardiac function in diabetic cardiomyopathy warrants further investigation. Cardiac metabolism may represent a novel therapeutic target for the future development of novel drug therapies for the treatment of diabetic cardiomyopathy.

Key points for clinical practice

- Diabetes mellitus is the fastest growing metabolic disease world-wide. The commonest cause of morbidity and mortality in diabetes is cardiovascular disease, often heart failure.

- Diabetic cardiomyopathy is a distinct clinical entity in which a cardiomyopathy is observed in diabetic patients in the absence of underlying coronary artery disease, hypertension or valvular heart disease. It is characterised, initially, by diastolic dysfunction; systolic dysfunction appears to occur as a later phenomenon.

- Of myocardial energy requirements, 70% is obtained from fatty acids and the remaining 30% from glucose. The heart is able to metabolise a number of substrates to meet its energy requirements.

- Glucose is transported into the myocardium by specific carrier systems, undergoes glycolysis and further oxidation by the Krebs' cycle resulting in the generation of ATP. Reducing equivalents (NADH and $FADH_2$) enter the electron transport chain with further generation of ATP.

- Fatty acids are transported across the cell membrane by three carrier systems and are esterified by acyl-CoA synthase and transported into mitochondrion where β-oxidation into acetyl-CoA and entry into the Krebs' cycle occurs. Cardiac peroxisome proliferator-activated receptors (PPARs) are important regulators of fatty acid metabolism.

Key points for clinical practice *(continued)*

- Changes in cardiac metabolism occur in diabetes with a switch from glucose metabolism to fatty acid metabolism occurring through a number of mechanisms.

- Changes in carbohydrate metabolism are seen in animal and human studies occurring through a number of different mechanisms. Transgenic animal model work has shown interruption of these processes can inhibit development of diabetic cardiomyopathy.

- Increased fatty acid availability and utilisation occurring through enhanced fatty acid transport across cell membranes and activation of PPAR transcription pathways may contribute to impaired cardiac function by a number of mechanisms including decreased cardiac efficiency for substrate utilisation and lipotoxicity.

- Good glycaemic and metabolic control has been demonstrated to result in an improvement in cardiac function in diabetic cardiomyopathy both clinically and experimentally in a number of studies; other studies have shown contradictory results. Further, randomised, control trials are required to address this issue.

References

1. Stamler J, Vaccaro O, Neaton JD, Wentworth D. Diabetes, other risk factors, and 12-yr cardiovascular mortality for men screened in the Multiple Risk Factor Intervention Trial. *Diabetes Care* 1993; **16**: 434–444.
2. Timmis A. Diabetic heart disease: clinical considerations. *Heart* 2001; **85**: 463–469.
3. Kannel WB, Hjortland M, Castelli WP. Role of diabetes in congestive heart failure: the Framingham Study. *Am J Cardiol* 1976; **34**: 29–34.
4. Shindler DM, Kostis JB, Yusuf S *et al*. Diabetes mellitus, a predictor of morbidity and mortality in the Studies of Left Ventricular Dysfunction (SOLVD) Trials and Registry. *Am J Cardiol* 1996; **77**: 1017–1020.
5. Ryden L, Armstrong PW, Cleland JG *et al*. Efficacy and safety of high-dose lisinopril in chronic heart failure patients at high cardiovascular risk, including those with diabetes mellitus. Results from the ATLAS trial. *Eur Heart J* 2000; **21**: 1967–1978.
6. Cohn JN. Lessons from V-HeFT: questions for V-HeFT II and the future therapy of heart failure. *Herz* 1991; **16**: 267–271.
7. Cleland JG, Swedberg K, Follath F *et al.*; Study Group on Diagnosis of the Working Group on Heart Failure of the European Society of Cardiology. The EuroHeart Failure survey programme – a survey on the quality of care among patients with heart failure in Europe. Part 1: patient characteristics and diagnosis. *Eur Heart J* 2003; **24**: 442–463.
8. Rubler S, Dlugash J, Yuceoglu YZ, Kumral T, Branwood AW, Grishman A. New type of cardiomyopathy associated with diabetic glomerulosclerosis. *Am J Cardiol* 1972; **30**: 595–602.
9. Fang ZY, Prins JB, Marwick TH. Diabetic cardiomyopathy: evidence, mechanisms, and therapeutic implications. *Endocr Rev* 2004; **25**: 543–567.
10. Regan TJ, Lyons MM, Ahmed SS *et al*. Evidence for cardiomyopathy in familial diabetes mellitus. *J Clin Invest* 1977; **60**: 884–899.
11. Cosson S, Kevorkian JP. Left ventricular diastolic dysfunction: an early sign of diabetic cardiomyopathy? *Diabetes Metab* 2003; **29**: 455–466.
12. Boyer JK, Thanigaraj S, Schechtman KB *et al*. Prevalence of ventricular diastolic dysfunction in asymptomatic, normotensive patients with diabetes mellitus. *Am J Cardiol* 2004; **93**: 870–875.

13. Zabalgoitia M, Ismaeil MF, Anderson L et al. Prevalence of diastolic dysfunction in normotensive, asymptomatic patients with well-controlled type 2 diabetes mellitus. Am J Cardiol 2001; 87: 320–323.

14. Raev DC. Which LV function is impaired earlier in the evolution of diabetic cardiomyopathy? An echocardiographic study of young type I diabetic patients. Diabetes Care 1994; 17: 633–639.

15. Petrie MC, Caruana L, Berry C, McMurray JJV. Diastolic heart failure caused by subtle left ventricular systolic dysfunction? Heart 2002; 87: 29–31.

16. Varela-Roman A, Grigorian L, Barge E, Mazon P, Rigueiro P, Gonzalez-Juanatey JR. Influence of diabetes on the survival of patients hospitalized with heart failure: a 12-year study. Eur J Heart Fail 2005; 7: 859–864.

17. Nunoda S, Genda A, Sugihara N, Nakayama A, Mizuno S, Takeda R. Quantitative approach to the histopathology of the biopsied right ventricular myocardium in patients with diabetes mellitus. Heart Vessels 1985; 1: 43–47.

18. Di Bello V, Talarico L, Picano E et al. Increased echodensity of myocardial wall in the diabetic heart: an ultrasound tissue characterization study. J Am Coll Cardiol 1995; 25: 1408–1415.

19. Mizushige K, Yao L, Noma T et al. Alteration in left ventricular diastolic filling and accumulation of myocardial collagen at insulin-resistant prediabetic stage of a type II diabetic rat model. Circulation 2000; 101: 899–907.

20. Avogaro A, Nosadini R, Doria A et al. Myocardial metabolism in insulin-deficient diabetic humans without coronary artery disease. Am J Physiol 1990; 258: E606–E618.

21. Garvey WT, Hardin D, Juhaszova M, Dominguez JH. Effects of diabetes on myocardial glucose transport system in rats: implications for diabetic cardiomyopathy. Am J Physiol 1993; 264: H837–H844.

22. Czech MP, Corvera S. Signaling mechanisms that regulate glucose transport. J Biol Chem 1999; 274: 1865–1868.

23. Ohtake T, Yokoyama I, Watanabe T et al. Myocardial glucose metabolism in noninsulin-dependent diabetes mellitus patients evaluated by FDG-PET. J Nucl Med 1995; 36: 456–463.

24. Belke DD, Larsen TS, Gibbs EM, Severson DL. Glucose metabolism in perfused mouse hearts overexpressing human GLUT-4 glucose transporter. Am J Physiol 2001; 280: E420–E427.

25. Rodrigues B, Cam MC, Kong J, Goyal RK, McNeill JH. Strain differences in susceptibility to streptozotocin-induced diabetes: effects on hypertriglyceridemia and cardiomyopathy. Cardiovasc Res 1997; 34:199–205.

26. Luiken JJ, Arumugam Y, Bell RC et al. Changes in fatty acid transport and transporters are related to the severity of insulin deficiency. Am J Physiol 2002; 283: E612–E621.

27. Coort SL, Luiken JJ, van der Vusse GJ, Bonen A, Glatz JF. Increased FAT (fatty acid translocase)/CD36-mediated long-chain fatty acid uptake in cardiac myocytes from obese Zucker rats. Biochem Soc Trans 2004; 32: 83–85.

28. Buchanan J, Mazumder PK, Hu P et al. Reduced cardiac efficiency and altered substrate metabolism precedes the onset of hyperglycemia and contractile dysfunction in two mouse models of insulin resistance and obesity. Endocrinology 2005; 146: 5341–5349.

29. Finck BN, Lehman JJ, Leone TC et al. The cardiac phenotype induced by PPARalpha overexpression mimics that caused by diabetes mellitus. J Clin Invest 2002; 109: 121–130.

30. Doria A, Nosadini R, Avogaro A, Fioretto P, Crepaldi G. Myocardial metabolism in type 1 diabetic patients without coronary artery disease. Diabet Med 1991; 8: S104–S107.

31. How OJ, Aasum E, Severson DL, Chan WY, Essop MF, Larsen TS. Increased myocardial oxygen consumption reduces cardiac efficiency in diabetic mice. Diabetes 2006; 55: 466–473.

32. Chiu HC, Kovacs A, Blanton RM et al. Transgenic expression of fatty acid transport protein 1 in the heart causes lipotoxic cardiomyopathy. Circ Res 2005; 96: 225–233.

33. Yagyu H, Chen G, Yokoyama M et al. Lipoprotein lipase (LpL) on the surface of cardiomyocytes increases lipid uptake and produces a cardiomyopathy. J Clin Invest 2003; 111: 419–426.

34. Chiu HC, Kovacs A, Ford DA et al. Novel mouse model of lipotoxic cardiomyopathy. J Clin Invest 2001; 107: 813–822.

35. Zhou YT, Grayburn P, Karim A et al. Lipotoxic heart disease in obese rats: implications

for human obesity. *Proc Natl Acad Sci USA* 2000; **97**: 1784–1789.

36. Kita Y, Shimizu M, Sugihara N *et al.* Correlation between histopathological changes and mechanical dysfunction in diabetic rat hearts. *Diabetes Res Clin Pract* 1991; **11**: 177–188.

37. Hausdorf G, Rieger U, Koepp P. Cardiomyopathy in childhood diabetes mellitus: incidence, time of onset, and relation to metabolic control. *Int J Cardiol* 1988; **19**: 225–236.

38. Cerutti F, Vigo A, Sacchetti C *et al.* Evaluation of left ventricular diastolic function in insulin dependent diabetic children by M-mode and Doppler echocardiography. *Panminerva Med* 1994; **36**: 109–114.

39. Astorri E, Fiorina P, Contini GA *et al.* Isolated and preclinical impairment of left ventricular filling in insulin-dependent and non-insulin-dependent diabetic patients. *Clin Cardiol* 1997; **20**: 536–540.

40. Pogatsa G, Bihari-Varga M, Szinay G. Effect of diabetes therapy on the myocardium in experimental diabetes. *Acta Diabetol Lat* 1979; **16**: 129–138.

41. Stroedter D, Schmidt T, Bretzel RG, Federlin K. Glucose metabolism and left ventricular dysfunction are normalized by insulin and islet transplantation in mild diabetes in the rat. *Acta Diabetol* 1995; **32**: 235–243.

42. Shapiro LM, Leatherdale BA, Coyne ME, Fletcher RF, Mackinnon J. Prospective study of heart disease in untreated maturity onset diabetics. *Br Heart J* 1980; **44**: 342–348.

43. Cerasola G, Donatelli M, Cottone S *et al.* Effects of dynamic exercise and metabolic control on left ventricular performance in insulin-dependent diabetes mellitus. *Acta Diabetol Lat* 1987; **24**: 263–270.

44. Bersin RM, Wolfe C, Kwasman M *et al.* Improved hemodynamic function and mechanical efficiency in congestive heart failure with sodium dichloroacetate. *J Am Coll Cardiol* 1994; **23**: 1617–1624.

45. Hiramatsu K, Ohara N, Shigematsu S *et al.* LV filling abnormalities in non-insulin-dependent diabetes mellitus and improvement by a short-term glycemic control. *Am J Cardiol* 1992; **70**: 1185–1189.

46. Gough SC, Smyllie J, Barker M, Berkin KE, Rice PJ, Grant PJ. Diastolic dysfunction is not related to changes in glycaemic control over 6 months in type 2 (non-insulin-dependent) diabetes mellitus: a cross-sectional study. *Acta Diabetol* 1995; **32**: 110–115.

47. Pitale SU, Abraira C, Emanuele NV *et al.* Two years of intensive glycemic control and LV function in the Veterans Affairs Cooperative Study in Type 2 Diabetes Mellitus (VA CSDM). *Diabetes Care* 2000; **23**: 1316–1320.

Vaikom S. Mahadevan Bernard Clarke

4

Interventions in the adult patient with congenital heart disease

With the advances which have been made in paediatric cardiology and cardiac surgery, the majority of children born in the Western world with congenital heart disease are expected to survive into adulthood. This has created the speciality of adult congenital heart disease (ACHD) also known as grown-up congenital heart disease (GUCH). Over the past decade, there have been a number of transcatheter interventional procedures developed specifically to treat adults with congenital heart disease. Some of these have supplanted cardiac surgery and others offer the option of postponing further cardiac surgery in a patient with multiple previous surgical procedures. The purpose of this chapter is to provide a brief overview of the more commonly performed transcatheter interventional procedures in adults with congenital heart disease.

DEVICE CLOSURE OF DEFECTS

ATRIAL SEPTAL DEFECTS

Device closure of defects in the interatrial septum is one of the more commonly performed congenital interventions in adults. Since the first reported transcatheter occlusion of a secundum atrial septal defect (ASD) nearly three decades ago,[1] a number of studies have shown transcatheter closure to be safe and as efficacious as surgical intervention, but with less morbidity.[2] Patients

Vaikom S. Mahadevan MD MRCP (for correspondence)
Consultant Cardiologist and Interventionist in Adult Congenital Heart Disease, Manchester Heart Centre, Manchester Royal Infirmary, Oxford Road, Manchester M13 9WL, UK
E-mail: vaikom.mahadevan@cmmc.nhs.uk

Bernard Clarke BSc(Hons) MD FRCP(Lond.) FRCP(Edin) FESC FACC
Consultant Cardiologist, Manchester Heart Centre, Manchester Royal Infirmary, Oxford Road, Manchester M13 9WL, UK
E-mail: bernard.clarke@man.ac.uk

often present in adult life since many, and especially those with smaller defects, can remain relatively asymptomatic until later in life. While some may be discovered incidentally, they may also present with dyspnoea and palpitations due to atrial arrhythmias.[3] These arrhythmias initially are paroxysmal but, untreated, they can become established. If right ventricular (RV) enlargement is present, the defect should be considered for closure regardless of the presence or absence of symptoms.[4]

The diagnosis is established using transthoracic and transoesophageal (TOE) echocardiography and attention should be paid to the following details: (i) the size and position of the defect; (ii) the direction of the shunt; (iii) the presence or absence of margins of the defect; (iv) the drainage of the pulmonary veins; (v) an estimation of the pulmonary arterial pressure; and (vi) the presence of any other cardiac abnormalities.

Only secundum-type defects measuring not greater than 38 mm on balloon sizing are suitable for closure including residual leaks in this position following previous surgical repair. Multiple defects are also suitable for closure.[5] Deficiency of the aortic rim is not a contra-indication for device closure of these defects.

The procedure is performed under fluoroscopic and echocardiographic guidance. Intracardiac echocardiography is increasingly used for this purpose and avoids the need for general anaesthesia, which is required when TOE guidance is used. The size of the defect is measured using a sizing balloon and an appropriate device is chosen based on the measurement.[6] The Amplatzer Septal Occluder™ (ASO; AGA Medical Inc., Golden Valley, MN, USA) is the most widely used device and has been shown to have excellent closure rates in the intermediate term.[7] The procedural risks include device embolisation, thrombus formation and infection.[6] The risk of erosion into the aorta in a recent series was low at 0.1%.[8] It has been suggested that a deficient aortic rim and oversizing of the device could increase this risk.[8]

Transcatheter closure has been shown to result in improvement of right ventricular (RV) size, pressures and volume[9,10] with improved functional capacity for the patient.[11] Right heart remodelling seems to occur even in those aged greater than 60 years undergoing device closure of ASD.[12]

Follow-up care includes treatment with an antiplatelet agent for at least a 6-month period. Endocarditis prophylaxis is advised for the same period. Long-term follow-up (to detect erosions) is required in all, and especially in those with large devices.

PATENT FORAMEN OVALE

This is a common condition seen in nearly 25% of the adult population.[13] Whilst in the vast majority it is of no consequence, in some patients it may require closure. There is a known association between the presence of a patent foramen ovale (PFO) and atrial septal aneurysm with cryptogenic stroke.[14] It is thought that the presence of a PFO predisposes to recurrent cerebral ischaemic events.[15] The commonest current indication for closure of these defects is the evidence of a cryptogenic cerebral (stroke) or other vascular event in a patient with no other risk factors. In this situation, it is presumed that such patients (with a patent foramen ovale) may have had a paradoxical embolus arising from the venous system and entering the systemic circulation via this defect. Patients undergoing device closure of PFO for paradoxical embolism subsequently have a low frequency of recurrent systemic embolic events.[16,17]

The diagnosis of PFO is confirmed by echocardiography with the injection of bubble contrast and the demonstration of its appearance across the interatrial septum, either at rest or during a Valsalva manoeuvre. Transcranial Doppler examination can also be used as an added diagnostic tool to detect shunting.[18] Additional investigations to be undertaken in these patients include: (i) CT or MR brain imaging; (ii) exclusion of carotid and disease of other cerebral vessels for patients with stroke; and (iii) exclusion of coagulation abnormalities. Long-term studies are in progress to compare the protective benefit of device closure against long-term anticoagulation in patients with PFO and stroke.

PFO closure and migraine

One of the more recent indications for which closure is considered is for migraine. There are initial indications that migraine with aura may decrease following closure of PFO with a device.[19] In the recent MIST trial,[19a] 42% in the device closure arm and 23% in the control arm had a 50% reduction in headache days, which was significant. However, the primary end-point of cessation of migraine headaches was not reached. It is reasonable to summarise that while initial data are encouraging, further study results are required prior to considering PFO device closure as a definitive treatment for migraine.

These procedures can be performed either under local anaesthesia with fluoroscopic guidance or under a general anaesthetic with fluoroscopic and TOE guidance. There are various devices to close these defects including the 'umbrella devices', which are made of Dacron with arms made of Nitinol. The most recent development has been the introduction of the BioSTAR® (NMT Medical, USA) device where instead of Dacron, a bio-absorbable acellular porcine intestinal collagen layer matrix material (Organogenesis, MA, USA) is used. The initial results have shown closure rates of 92% at 30 days and 96% at 6 months.[20]

Procedural risks for device closure of PFO are low but include the risk of device embolisation and atrial arrhythmias. Follow-up care includes use of antiplatelet agents for 3–6 months and echocardiography with a contrast study to ensure complete abolition of the shunt across the defect.

VENTRICULAR SEPTAL DEFECTS

Device closure of ventricular septal defects is more commonly performed in children than in adults. The availability of a specific device for perimembranous defects has meant that both these and muscular type of defects can be considered for device closure. Indications for consideration of device closure in an adult for these defects include evidence of: (i) a significant left-to-right shunt with a Qp:Qs ≥ 2:1; and (ii) ventricular volume overload as shown by left heart dilatation and recurrent endocarditis. The presence of significant pulmonary hypertension, as evidenced by pulmonary pressures greater than two-thirds systemic pressure, requires careful further assessment prior to considering closure. In a recently reported series of 33 adult patients, complete closure was obtained in 55% immediately after the procedure and there was a residual shunt in only 5% on follow-up at 6 months with no cases of complete heart block.[21] In a recent paediatric series, the success rate for deployment of a perimembranous device was 93%, and 2% developed complete heart block requiring a pace maker.[22] Other risks include new or increased aortic regurgitation, device embolisation and involvement of the AV valves.

RELIEF OF OBSTRUCTION

STENTING OF AORTIC COARCTATION

Untreated aortic coarctation has a poor outcome with a mean survival of 35 years and mortality of 75% by 50 years of age.[23] Coarctations are usually distal to the origin of the left subclavian artery and may be associated with hypoplasia of the transverse aortic arch. A pressure gradient of ≥ 20 mmHg between the arm and leg is considered to be significant.[24] Patients often present with hypertension and its presence, particularly in young patients with no other evident cause, should prompt a search for this condition.

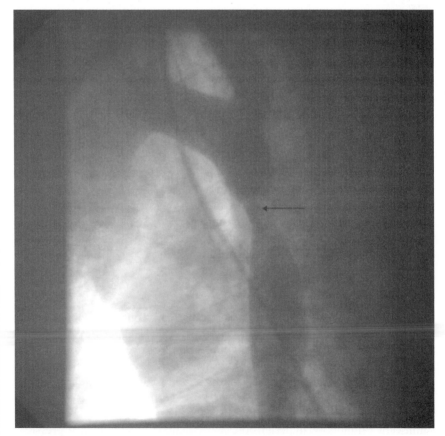

Fig. 1 Tight aortic coarctation (arrow) in a young adult.

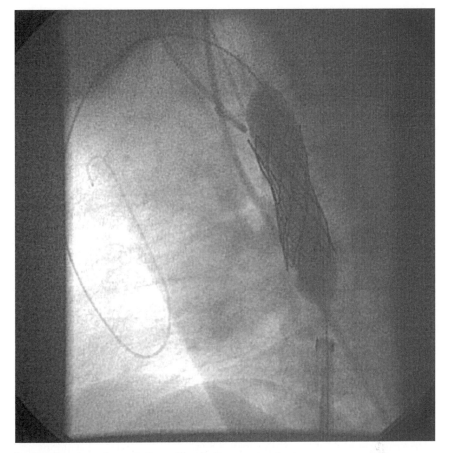

Fig. 2 Dilatation of coarctation with a balloon and a stent.

Diagnosis is by clinical examination, echocardiography and contrast CT or MRI scanning of the aorta. With modern imaging, there is a decreasing need for angiography for diagnostic purposes in this condition.

Transcatheter treatment with balloon dilatation and stenting has been in use for a number of years. More recently, most adults are treated by primary stenting, a procedure which has been shown to be highly effective in gradient reduction, with beneficial effects on the control of hypertension. In a recent series, patients treated with stenting had a fall in systolic upper limb blood pressure from 142 ± 14 mmHg to 133 ± 15 mmHg at 6 weeks and to 125 ± 12 mmHg ($P < 0.05$) at 1 year.[25]

The technique involves obtaining access via the femoral artery and crossing the coarctation retrogradely. A large sized sheath (12-Fr) is required to deploy a stent (Figs 1–3). In some centres, access is also obtained simultaneously via the radial artery and a catheter positioned proximal to the coarctation adjacent to the left subclavian artery. It is well worth obtaining an angiogram immediately after stent deployment (prior to removing the deflated balloon). This saves valuable time in the event of there being an endovascular leak. The NumedCP® stent is one of the most widely used stents. It is made of platinum and is compatible with cardiac MR scanning. The major procedural risk is

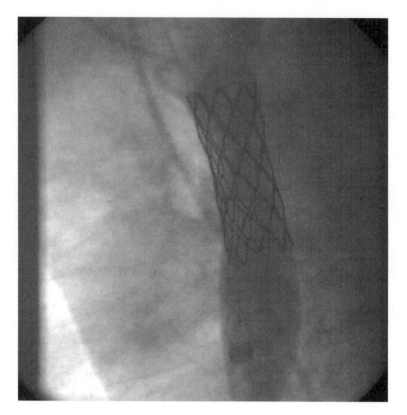

Fig. 3 Stent *in situ* with complete relief of stenosis.

aortic rupture and endovascular leak. Older age, oversizing of balloons and post dilatation may possibly predispose to such a complication.[26] While the use of covered stents may potentially reduce this complication, it has been reported even with their use.[27]

Long-term follow-up is required for all these patients, even if there has been a very successful outcome with stenting. Aneurysms of the stented region have been reported on follow-up.[25,28] The long-term significance of these is unclear at present and continued surveillance is required.

PULMONARY ARTERY STENOSIS

Pulmonary artery stenosis often involves the point of bifurcation of the main pulmonary and frequently extends into one or both branches. Adults with previously corrected Fallot's tetrology may develop distal pulmonary stenosis in later life and treatment of such stenosis with percutaneous intervention may result in improvement in pulmonary regurgitation.[29] Stent placement requires the use of a large-sized sheath (11-Fr) and the balloon size to deploy the stent is based on the diameter of the adjacent normal pulmonary artery segment (Figs 4 and 5).

Stent placement in pulmonary arteries increases vessel diameters significantly with concomitant fall in gradients.[30] Restenosis can occur in the stented segments and these can be redilated successfully.[31,32]

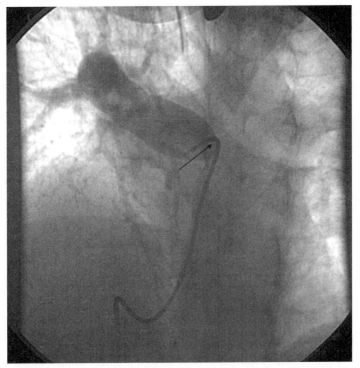

Fig. 4 Severe ostial stenosis of left pulmonary artery (arrow) in a patient with three previous cardiac surgical procedures.

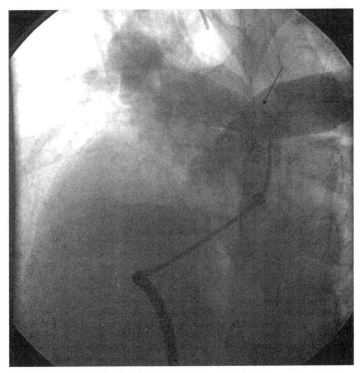

Fig. 5 Stent across ostium of left pulmonary artery (arrow) with relief of stenosis.

PULMONARY VALVE STENOSIS

Pulmonary valve stenosis is a congenital condition which may require intervention in adult life. The valve may be either thin and domed with a narrow orifice or may be dysplastic with thickened cusps. The severity of the stenosis is classified by the peak systolic gradient.[33] Patients with moderate (50–79 mmHg) and severe (> 80 mmHg) gradients should be considered for intervention. Infudibular right ventricular outflow tract obstruction is muscular and not amenable to transcatheter intervention.

The right ventricular outflow and the main pulmonary artery should be visualised angiographically and the pulmonary annulus measured. The recommended balloon:annulus ratio is 1.2–1.4 in a valve with typical morphology.[34]

The outcome following pulmonary valve balloon dilatation is usually quite good. In one series of 87 adults undergoing this procedure, the peak gradient fell significantly from 105 ± 39 mmHg to 34 ± 26 mmHg post procedure and the benefits were maintained on intermediate follow-up.[35] While pulmonary regurgitation can occur, it is often mild and usually well tolerated. Results following balloon dilatation of dyplastic valves are less satisfactory[34] and surgery may be required.

AORTIC VALVE STENOSIS

This is usually seen in the setting of a bicuspid aortic valve. The young adult with congenital aortic stenosis is more amenable to balloon valvuloplasty than the elderly with calcified valves.

Most valves can be crossed retrogradely. Brief, rapid pacing of the right ventricle with a temporary pacing wire can be used in the younger patients as an alternative to adenosine to prevent balloon displacement during inflation.[36] The balloon size is chosen to be slightly smaller than the annular diameter to decrease the risk of significant aortic regurgitation. The achieved reduction in the gradient varies but often the technique is effective as a palliative procedure so as to delay an eventual surgical procedure.

RIGHT VENTRICLE TO PULMONARY ARTERY CONDUITS

Right ventricle to pulmonary artery conduits can develop progressive stenosis with resultant increase in right ventricular pressures. In patients with discrete lesions, it may be possible to achieve a good result with stenting (Figs 6 and 7). Diffuse narrowing of the conduit usually does not respond quite as well to stenting. A large-sized sheath (11-Fr) is required for this procedure. With the use of suture-based closure devices such as Perclose®, immediate haemostasis can be obtained across femoral venous access sites even in the presence of anticoagulation.[37]

In a series of 221 patients, of whom a majority were in the 5–18-year age group, stenting of the conduits decreased RV–PA peak gradients significantly from 59 ± 19 mmHg to 27 ± 14 mmHg with a median freedom from conduit surgery of 3.9 years in those older than 5 years of age.[38] However, stent fractures are not uncommon in this situation and careful follow-up is needed.

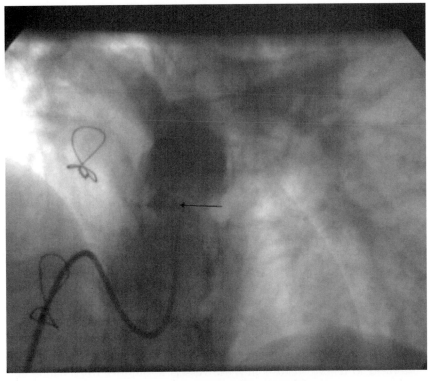

Fig. 6 Severe stenosis (arrow) of a very calcified RV–PA conduit.

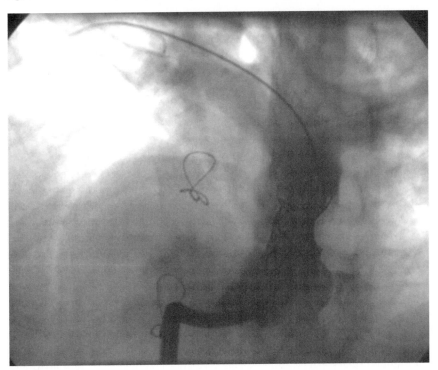

Fig. 7 Post stenting of conduit stenosis, with severe calcification outside the conduit.

STENOSIS OF MUSTARD AND SENNING BAFFLES

Systemic venous pathway obstruction is common in patients with a previous Mustard's operation. It can occur in up to 15% of patients on follow-up[39] and should be treated if symptomatic. Stenosis of the superior limb of the systemic venous baffle is more common than that of the inferior limb. Patients are often asymptomatic because of venous run-off through the azygous system; in this situation, intervention may not be necessary. Intervention is required in symptomatic patients with fullness or flushing around the head or arm with SVC baffle obstruction or in those with stenosis in whom a permanent pacemaker lead is being implanted. These usually respond quite well to stenting.

AORTO-PULMONARY COLLATERAL VESSELS

These are usually seen in the setting of pulmonary atresia. These collaterals can be a significant source of left-to-right shunting and can complicate cardiac surgery. These collaterals can be embolised either with coils or the Amplatzer® vascular plug just prior to surgery. In some patients with Eisenmenger's syndrome, aorto-pulmonary or broncho-pulmonary collaterals can give rise to haemoptysis and in intractable cases, embolisation of these vessels can be considered.[40]

In certain patients who are not candidates for curative surgery and who develop increasing cyanosis, stenting of these vessels[41] and shunts[42] can be performed to relieve stenosis in these vessels to improve oxygenation and, hence, systemic saturation.

OCCLUSION OF ABNORMAL COMMUNICATIONS

PATENT DUCTUS ARTERIOSUS

Occlusion of patent ductus arteriosus (PDA) in adults is undertaken for haemodynamic reasons and for elimination of the ductus as a substrate for infective endocarditis. Currently, the practice is to advise closure of all clinically apparent ducts in adults.[4,43] Patients with significant pulmonary hypertension secondary to a duct need careful evaluation prior to considering closure.

While coils are quite useful in children, in adults the ducts tend to be larger; in this situation, the Amplatzer® ductal occluder is a more suitable device with a lower risk of embolisation. Usually, the procedure is performed using a femoral venous approach under a local anaesthetic and the duct is entered at its insertion point in the pulmonary artery. Occasionally, arterial access may be required to enter the duct from the aortic end. The closure rate is reported to be between 95–100% at 6 months in various series.[44]

CORONARY ARTERY FISTULA

While small fistulae incidentally seen during coronary angiography are unlikely to be of haemodynamic consequence, larger fistula often arising from the right coronary artery and entering a cardiac chamber (the right atrium or ventricle) may need closure (Fig. 8). The larger ones may produce a significant

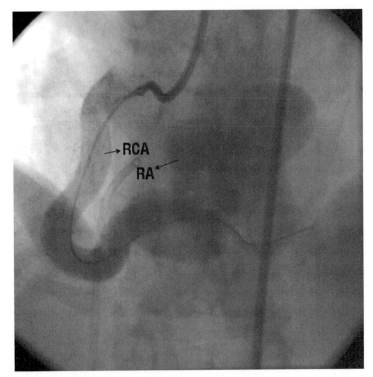

Fig. 8 Large coronary fistula from RCA to RA.

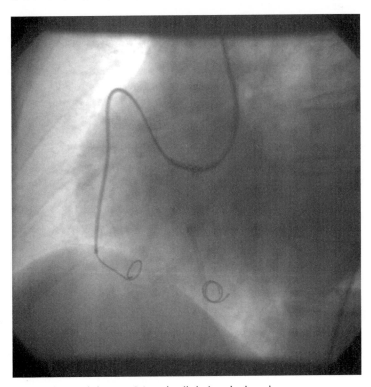

Fig. 9 Catheter advanced deep to RA and coils being deployed.

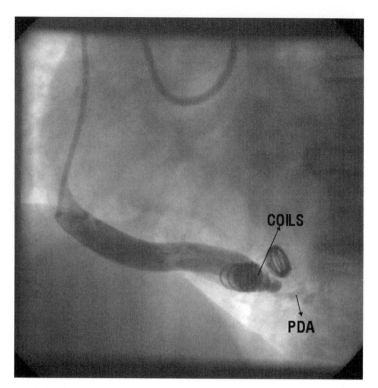

Fig. 10 Occlusion of fistula with coils with preservation of posterior descending branch (PDA) of RCA.

shunt with volume overload, or myocardial ischaemia due to steal phenomenon. The decision concerning closure needs to be made on an individual patient basis.

Closure involves occluding the fistula proximal to its entry into the connecting chamber while preserving the functional branches of the coronary tree. It can be quite a challenging procedure (particularly in the case of a fistula arising from the left coronary artery) because of the acute angle between the fistula and the parent coronary artery. Coils have been used and it is necessary to advance the delivery catheter sufficiently into the communication prior to delivery of coils (Figs 9 and 10). Occlusion rates are high.[45] The Amplatzer® vascular plug has also been used for this purpose.[46]

PULMONARY AV FISTULA

These can occur as a congenital condition or can occur in patients who have had a classical Glenn shunt (SVC–RPA connection)[47] and can be embolised successfully to improve systemic saturations.

EMERGING THERAPIES

PERCUTANEOUS VALVE IMPLANTATION

Percutaneous pulmonary valve implantation is being performed as a palliation or alternative to further surgery in patients with previous surgery to the RV outflow and presenting with RV outflow obstruction or significant pulmonary regurgitation. It consists of a bovine jugular venous valve mounted on a stent[48] and is deployed using a large-sized venous sheath. There is evidence of significant reduction in pulmonary regurgitant fraction, RV end diastolic volume[49] and significant fall in RV outflow gradient and RV systolic pressure in patients with predominant RV outflow obstruction[50] following implantation of this valve.

Aortic valves are being implanted percutaneously in elderly patients with severe aortic stenosis who are deemed at very high risk for aortic valve replacement. There are valves designed for antegrade and retrograde delivery. These procedures are experimental at the present time.

PARAVALVULAR LEAKS

Device closure of paravalvular leaks in the mitral and aortic position have been performed in patients who have a significant leak with haemodynamic consequences and who are considered to be at very high risk for further surgery. The Amplatzer® duct occluder has been commonly used, although various other devices have been used for this purpose. It is usually performed in patients with prosthetic valves although it can be performed in patients with bioprosthetic valves as well. Mitral paravalvar leaks are particularly challenging. Using a transeptal approach, the leak is accessed with a wire, which is snared from the aorta and exteriorised via the femoral artery to form an arterio-venous loop via the leak.[51] TOE guidance is required along with fluoroscopy to ensure the wire has crossed through the defect and not the valve orifice itself. An appropriate size device is then deployed across the defect and released if satisfactory positioning is obtained.

Key points for clinical practice

- Device closure is the preferred treatment for all suitable secundum atrial septal defects.

- All patients with a crytogenic stroke should be investigated for the presence of patent foramen ovale and referred for closure if present.

- Native and re-coarctation in adults should be considered for stenting as the first-line treatment.

- Pulmonary balloon valvuloplasty in the young often has a very good outcome and avoids the need for surgery.

- Patients with discrete stenosis of right ventricular–pulmonary artery conduits should be considered for stenting.

- Device occlusion of a patent ductus arteriosus is a highly successful procedure in adults.

- Moderate- and large-sized coronary fistula should be considered for transcatheter embolisation.

(continued on next page)

Key points for clinical practice *(continued)*

- Patients with significant paravalvular leaks who are at high risk for further surgery should be considered for transcatheter device closure.

- Adult congenital intervention procedures are complex and should be performed only in specialist centres with necessary surgical back up, by physicians with appropriate expertise.

References

1. King TD, Thompson SL, Steiner C, Mills NL. Secundum atrial septal defect. Nonoperative closure during cardiac catheterization. *JAMA* 1976; **235**: 2506–2509.

2. Cowley CG, Lloyd TR, Bove EL *et al.* Comparison of results of closure of secundum atrial septal defect by surgery versus Amplatzer septal occluder. *Am J Cardiol* 2001; **88**: 589–591.

3. Rigby M. Atrial septal defects. In: Gatzoulis WD, Daubeney PEF. (eds). Diagnosis and management of adult congenital heart disease. London: Churchill Livingstone, 2003; 164.

4. Therrien J, Gatzoulis M, Graham T, Webb GW. Canadian Cardiovascular Society Consensus Conference 2001 Update: recommendations for the management of adults with congenital heart disease – Part 1. *Can J Cardiol* 2001; **17**: 940–959.

5. Mahadevan VS, Gomperts N, Haberer K *et al.* Procedural and clinical outcomes in adults undergoing transcatheter closure of atrial septal defects with multiple devices. *Eur Heart J* 2005; **26 (Abstract Suppl)**: 557.

6. Amin Z. Transcatheter closure of secundum atrial septal defects. *Catheter Cardiovasc Intervent* 2006; **68**: 778–787.

7. Fischer G, Stieh J, Uebing A *et al.* Experience with transcatheter closure of secundum atrial septal defects using the Amplatzer septal occluder: a single centre study in 236 consecutive patients. *Heart* 2003; **89**: 199–204.

8. Amin Z, Hijazi ZM, John L *et al.* Erosion of Amplatzer septal occluder device after closure of secundum atrial septal defects: review of registry of complications and recommendations to minimize future risk. *Catheter Cardiovasc Intervent* 2004; **63**: 496–502.

9. Veldtman GR, Razack V, Siu S *et al.* Right ventricular form and function after percutaneous atrial septal defect device closure. *J Am Coll Cardiol* 2001; **37**: 2108–2113.

10. Kort HW, Balzer DT, Johnson MC. Resolution of right heart enlargement after closure of secundum atrial septal defect with transcatheter technique. *J Am Coll Cardiol* 2001; **38**: 1528–1532.

11. Brochu MC, Baril JF, Dore A, Juneau M, De Guise P, Mercier LA. Improvement in exercise capacity in asymptomatic and mildly symptomatic adults after atrial septal defect percutaneous closure. *Circulation* 2002; **106**: 1821–1826.

12. Swan L, Verma C, Yip J *et al.* Transcatheter device closure of atrial septal defects in the elderly: technical considerations and short-term outcomes. *Int J Cardiol* 2006; **107**: 207–210.

13. Meissner I, Khandheria BK, Heit JA *et al.* Patent foramen ovale: innocent or guilty? Evidence from a prospective population-based study. *J Am Coll Cardiol* 2006; **47**: 440–445.

14. Cabanes L, Mas JL, Cohen A *et al.* Atrial septal aneurysm and patent foramen ovale as risk factors for cryptogenic stroke in patients less than 55 years of age: a study using trans-esophageal echocardiography. *Stroke* 1993; **24**: 1865–1873.

15. Cujec B, Mainra R, Johnson DH. Prevention of recurrent cerebral ischemic events in patients with patent foramen ovale and crytogenic strokes of transient ischemic attacks. *Can J Cardiol* 1999; **15**: 57–64.

16. Windecker S, Wahl A, Chatterjee T *et al.* Percutaneous closure of patent foramen ovale in patients with paradoxical embolism: long-term risk of recurrent thromboembolic events. *Circulation* 2000; **101**: 893–898.

17. Martin F, Sanchez PL, Doherty E *et al.* Percutaneous transcatheter closure of patent foramen ovale in patients with paradoxical embolism. *Circulation* 2002; **27**: 1121–1126.

18. Spencer MP, Moehring MA, Jesurum J *et al*. Power m-mode transcranial Doppler for diagnosis of patent foramen ovale and assessing transcatheter closure. *J Neuroimaging* 2004; **14**: 342–349.

19. Giardini A, Donti A, Fromigari R *et al*. Transcatheter patent foramen ovale closure mitigates aura migraine headaches abolishing spontaneous right-to-left shunting. *Am Heart J* 2006; **151**: 922.

19a. MIST Trial. http://www.migraine-mist.org/_Content/PDFs/MIST_presentation.pdf (03/04/07)

20. Mullen MJ, Hildick-Smith D, De Giovannio JV *et al*. BioSTAR Evaluation STudy (BEST), a prospective, multicenter, phase I clinical trial to evaluate the feasibility, efficacy and safety of the BioSTAR bioabsorable septal repair implant for the closure of atrial-level shunts. *Circulation* 2006; **114**: 1962–1967.

21. Chessa M, Carrozza M, Butera G *et al*. The impact of interventional cardiology for the management of adults with congenital heart defects. *Catheter Cardiovasc Intervent* 2006; **67**: 258–264.

22. Holzer R, de Giovanni J, Walsh KP *et al*. Transcatheter closure of perimembranous ventricular septal defects using the Amplatzer membranous VSD occluder: immediate and midterm results of an international registry. *Catheter Cardiovasc Intervent* 2006; **68**: 620–628.

23. Campbell M. Natural history of coarctation of aorta. *Br Heart J* 1970; **32**: 633–640.

24. Ledesma M, Alva C, Gomez FD, Sanchez-Soberanis A. Results of stenting for aortic coarctation. *Am J Cardiol* 2001; **88**: 460–461.

25. Mahadevan VS, Vondermuhll IF, Mullen MJ. Endovascular aortic coarctation stenting in adolescents and adults: angiographic and hemodynamic outcomes. *Catheter Cardiovasc Intervent* 2006; **67**: 268–275.

26. Mahadevan VS, Mullen MJ. Endovascular management of aortic coarctation. *Int J Cardiol* 2004; **97**: 75–78.

27. Collins N, Mahadevan VS, Horlick E. Aortic rupture following a covered stent for coarctation: delayed recognition. *Catheter Cardiovasc Intervent* 2006; **68**: 653–655.

28. Harrison DA, McLaughlin PR, Lazzam C *et al*. Endovascular stents in the management of coarctation of the aorta in the adolescent and adult: one year follow up. *Heart* 2001; **85**: 561–566.

29. Chaturvedi RR, Kilner P, White PH. Increased airway pressure and simulated branch pulmonary stenosis increase pulmonary regurgitation after repair of Tetrology of Fallot: real-time analysis using conductance catheter technique. *Circulation* 1997; **95**: 643–649.

30. Spadoni I, Giusti S, Bertolaccini P *et al*. Long-term follow-up of stents implanted to relieve peripheral pulmonary arterial stenosis: hemodynamic findings and results of lung perfusion scanning. *Cardiol Young* 1999; **9**: 585–591.

31. Ing FF, Grifka RG, Nihill MR, Mullins CE. Repeat dilation of intravascular stents in congenital heart defects. *Circulation* 1995; **92**: 893–897.

32. Duke C, Rosenthal E, Qureshi SA. The efficacy and safety of stent redilatation in congenital heart disease. *Heart* 2003; **89**: 905–912.

33. Therrien J, Gatzoulis M, Graham T, Webb G. Canadian Cardiovascular Society Consensus Conference 2001 Update: recommendations for the management of adults with congenital heart disease – Part II. *Can J Cardiol* 2001; **18**: 1029–1050.

34. McCrindle BW. Independent predictors of long-term results after balloon pulmonary valvuloplasty. Valvuloplasty and Angioplasty of Congenital Anomalies (VACA) Registry Investigators. *Circulation* 1994; **89**: 1751–1779.

35. Fawzy ME, Awad M, Galal O *et al*. Long-term results of pulmonary balloon valvulotomy in adult patients. *J Heart Valve Dis* 2001; **10**: 812–818.

36. Daehnert I, Rotzsch C, Wiener M, Schneider P. Rapid right ventricular pacing is an alternative to adenosine in catheter interventional procedures for congenital heart disease. *Heart* 2004; **90**: 1047–1050.

37. Mahadevan VS, Jimeno SS, Benson LN *et al*. Pre-closure of femoral venous access sites used for large sized sheath insertion with the Perclose™ device in adults undergoing cardiac intervention. *Heart* 2006; [E-pub ahead of print].

38. Peng LF, McElhinney DB, Nugent AW *et al*. Endovascular stenting of obstructed right ventricle-to-pulmonary artery conduits: a 15-year experience. *Circulation* 2006; **113**: 2598–2605.

39. Moons P, Gewillig M, Sluysmans T *et al*. Long term outcome up to 30 years after the Mustard or Senning operation: a nationwide multicentre study in Belgium. *Heart* 2004; **90**: 307–313.

40. Broberg C, Ujita M, Babu-Narayan S *et al*. Massive pulmonary artery thrombosis with haemoptysis in adults with Eisenmenger's syndrome: a clinical dilemma. *Heart* 2004; **90**: e63.

41. Brown SC, Mertens L, Dumoulin M, Gewillig M. Percutaneous treatment of stenosed major aortopulmonary collaterals with balloon dilatation and stenting: what can be achieved? *Heart* 1998; **79**: 24–28.

42. El-Said HG, Clapp S, Fagan TE *et al*. Stenting of stenosed aortopulmonary collaterals and shunts for palliation of pulmonary atresia/ventricular septal defect. *Catheter Cardiovasc Intervent* 2000; **49**: 430–436.

43. Rao PS. Transcatheter occlusion of patent ductus arteriosus: which method to use and which ductus to close. *Am Heart J* 1996; **132**: 905–909.

44. Hornung TS, Benson L, McLaughlin PR. Catheter interventions in adult patients with congenital heart disease. *Curr Cardiol Report* 2002; **4**: 54–62.

45. Trehan V, Yusuf J, Mukhopadhyay S *et al*. Transcatheter closure of coronary artery fistulas. *Indian Heart J* 2004; **56**: 132–139.

46. Behera SK, Danon S, Levi DS, Moore JW. Transcatheter closure of coronary artery fistulae using the Amplatzer duct occluder. *Catheter Cardiovasc Intervent* 2006; **68**: 242–248.

47. Kopf GS, Laks H, Stansel HC *et al*. Thirty-year follow-up of superior vena cava-pulmonary artery (Glenn) shunts. *J Thorac Cardiovasc Surg* 1990; **100**: 662–670.

48. Bonhoeffer P, Boudjemline Y, Saliba Z *et al*. Percutaneous replacement of pulmonary valve in a right-ventricle to pulmonary-artery prosthetic conduit with valve dysfunction. *Lancet* 2000; **356**: 1403–1405.

49. Khambadkone S, Coats L, Taylor A *et al*. Percutaneous pulmonary valve implantation in humans: results in 59 consecutive patients. *Circulation* 2005; **23**: 1189–1197.

50. Coats L, Khambadkone S, Derrick G *et al*. Physiological and clinical consequences of relief of right ventricular outflow tract obstruction late after repair of congenital heart defects. *Circulation* 2006; **113**: 2037–2044.

51. Pate GE, Thompson CR, Munt BI, Webb JG. Techniques for percutaneous closure of prosthetic paravalvular leaks. *Catheter Cardiovasc Intervent* 2006; **67**: 158–166.

Ihab Diab Clifford Garratt

5

The congenital long QT syndrome: does the underlying genotype matter?

The congenital long QT syndrome (LQTS) is an inherited disease of cardiac repolarisation that predisposes some affected individuals to serious cardiac arrhythmias and sudden cardiac death. LQTS affects about 1 in 5000 of newborns.[1] It is caused by a number of abnormalities in the genes that encode cardiac ion channels and related proteins, giving rise to the different phenotypic variants of the syndrome. Our understanding of the underlying causes of this syndrome have increased significantly in the last few years; in this paper, we aim to address the clinical relevance of the different underlying genetic causes of the syndrome.

MOLECULAR MECHANISMS OF QT PROLONGATION AND INCREASED RISK OF SUDDEN DEATH

The characteristic abnormality in LQTS is prolongation of cardiac repolarisation manifest as a long QT interval on the surface ECG. The duration of the QT interval in normal individuals is dependent on the duration of the action potentials occurring in normal cardiac myocytes. The duration of the action potential, in turn, is governed by the fine balance of inward and outward currents that occur in a specific sequence as the myocytes are activated electrically (depolarised) and recover (repolarisation). As repolarisation of normal cardiac myocytes is dominated by sudden activation of outward potassium currents (including the slow and rapid components of

Ihab Diab MB BS MSc MD
Clinical Electrophysiology Fellow, Manchester Heart Centre, Manchester Royal Infirmary, Oxford Road, Manchester M13 9WL, UK

Clifford Garratt DM FRCP FESC (for correspondence)
Professor of Cardiology, Manchester Heart Centre, Manchester Royal Infirmary, Oxford Road, Manchester M13 9WL, UK
E-mail: clifford.garratt@cmmc.nhs.uk

the delayed rectifier potassium currents, I_{Ks} and I_{Kr}), the duration of the normal action potential is heavily dependent on these currents and it comes as no surprise that inherited defects in potassium channel function ('loss of function' effect) can delay repolarisation and prolong both the action potential and the QT interval. It has, however, become clear that action potential duration is also dependent, to some extent, on preceding ionic events, in particular the inward sodium current that is associated with myocyte depolarisation. An inherited abnormality resulting is supranormal amounts of inward sodium current ('gain of function' effect) can result in a similar prolongation of action potential duration and consequent clinical characteristics.

The characteristic arrhythmias associated with LQTS (*torsades de pointes* [TdP], polymorphic ventricular tachycardia and ventricular fibrillation [VF]) are the mechanisms by which these patients are at risk of sudden death. Despite over two decades of detailed investigation, the exact mechanism of polymorphic VT in the setting of the congenital LQTS is not known. A number of lines of investigation have shown that there is an increased dispersion of ventricular repolarisation in affected patients, due to particularly prolonged repolarisation of myocytes in some regions of the heart. This may be a substrate for the generation of re-entrant waves of electrical activation, possibly in the form of 'spiral waves' drifting rapidly through the ventricles. A related hypothesis is that early or late after-depolarisations may occur and lead to ventricular arrhythmias as a consequence of triggered activity (Fig. 1). After-depolarisations are known to occur in cardiac myocytes under similar circumstances to those that exist in myocytes from patients with LQTS, *i.e.* prolonged action potential duration and a resultant increase in intracellular calcium concentration.

DIFFERENT TYPES OF CONGENITAL LQTS

Two phenotypic variants of LQTS were initially identified. The Jervell Lange–Nielsen syndrome (JLN) was described in 1957,[2] showing autosomal recessive inheritance and associated sensorineural deafness. The Romano–Ward syndrome (RW) was described in 1960, showing autosomal dominant inheritance and normal hearing.[3,4] We now know that the Romano–Ward syndrome is the common form of the syndrome and is due to heterozygous mutations in a wide range of different genes (LQT1–9, see below). The Jervell Lange–Nielsen syndrome occurs when homozygous mutations occur (or more rarely two different heterozygous mutations) in the *KCNQ1* and *KCNE1* genes coding for potassium channels present in both the cardiac muscle and the inner ear; this

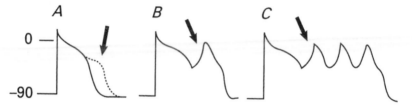

Fig. 1 Early after-depolarisations. Prolongation of the action potential (A) leads to oscillations of the membrane potential at the end of the plateau (B) and triggering of tachycardia (C). [From: Wit AL, Rosen MR. Cellular electrophysiology of cardiac arrhythmias. *Modern Concepts Cardiovasc Dis* 1981; **50**: 7–11 with permission.]

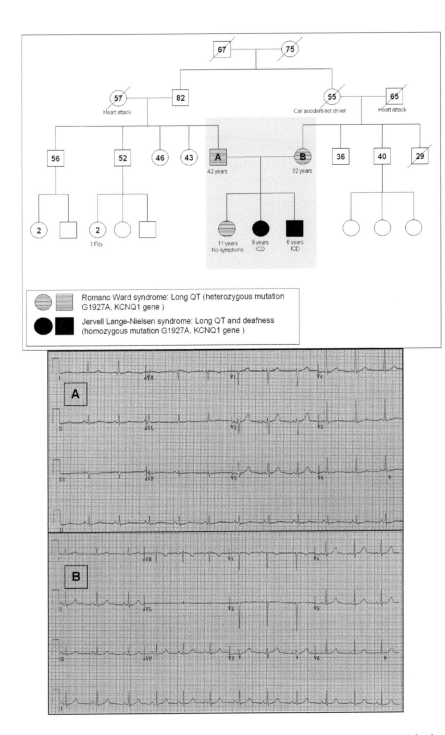

Fig. 2 Example of Romano–Ward and Jervell Lange–Nielsen syndromes. Parent A had evidence of QT prologation on the 12-lead ECG but parent B did not. Two of their three children had a homozygous mutation (Jervell Lange-Neilsen syndrome) with marked prolonged QT intervals and recurrent syncope and required implantation of ICDs. Their other child had a heterozygous mutation (Romano-Ward syndrome), borderline QT prolongation and asymptomatic.

syndrome has a much more severe phenotype in terms of length of the QT interval, ventricular arrhythmias and risk of sudden death (Fig. 2).

SUBTYPES OF THE ROMANO–WARD SYNDROME

LQT1 is caused by an anomaly of the *KCNQ1* gene on chromosome 11 which codes for the α-subunit of the potassium channel conducting the slow and catecholamine sensitive component of the rectifier current (I_{Ks}). It is the most prevalent type of LQTS and accounts for 40% of all LQTS patients in whom the genetic basis is known.

LQT2 is caused by an anomaly of the *KCNH2* gene on chromosome 7 which codes for the α-subunit of the potassium channel (HERG) conducting the rapid component of the rectifier current (I_{Kr}). It is the second most prevalent type of LQTS and accounts for 35% of all genotyped LQTS patients.

LQT3 is caused by an anomaly of the *SCN5A* gene on chromosome 3 that codes for the protein of the sodium channel causing a gain in function anomaly and leading to an increased late inward sodium current (I_{Na}) and prolongation of repolarisation and the action potential. It accounts for up to 10% of all genotyped patients.

LQT4 is a rare abnormality of a gene on chromosome 4 that does not code for an ion channel protein, but for a scaffolding protein known as ankyrin B. This protein anchors the Na^+/K^+ ATPase and the Na^+/Ca^{2+} exchanger and its abnormalities cause a build-up of Na^+ ions inside the cell and a compensatory increase in Ca^{2+}.[5]

LQT5 is caused by an anomaly of the *KCNE1* gene on chromosome 21 which codes for the β-subunit (MinK) of the potassium channel conducting I_{Ks}. It accounts for < 1% of all LQTS patients genotyped.

LQT6 is caused by an anomaly of the *KCNE2* gene on chromosome 21 which codes for the β-subunit of the potassium channel conducting I_{Kr} (MIRP). It accounts for < 1% of all LQTS patients genotyped.

LQT7 (Andersen syndrome) is due to loss-of-function mutations of the *KCNJ2* gene causing abnormalities in the inward rectifying potassium current. LQT was the primary cardiac manifestation, present in 71% of *KCNJ2* mutation carriers, with ventricular arrhythmias present in 64%. Periodic paralysis is seen in 62%. Characteristic physical features including low-set ears, micrognathia, and clinodactyly.[6]

LQT8 (Timothy syndrome) is caused by gain-of-function mutations in the *CACNA1C* gene coding for the L-type calcium ion channels with nearly complete loss of voltage-dependent L-type calcium channel inactivation during the plateau.

In the past few months, two further genetic types have been added to the list of LQTS syndromes. **LQT9** has been linked to the gene coding for caveolin-3. This is a membrane structural protein which forms caveolae in which the voltage-gated sodium channel sits. Defects of these proteins cause a syndrome similar to LQT3 in which there is a 'gain-of-function' with an increase in the late sodium current causing impairment and prolongation of repolarisation.[7] **LQT10** is a novel mutation described in December 2006 in the gene *SCN4B* coding for an auxiliary subunit of the pore-forming, voltage-gated, sodium channel causing functional and clinical effect similar to LQT3.[8]

GENOTYPE–PHENOTYPE RELATIONSHIPS

Specific clinical characteristics have been described for some of the genetic types especially LQT1, LQT2 and LQT3 which together constitute the great majority of all genotyped LQTS patients.

RELEVANCE OF GENOTYPE TO TRIGGERS OF CARDIAC EVENTS

Sudden cardiac death is reported to occur in 14% of untreated patients with LQTS and is usually related to adrenergic stimulation. In LQT1, cardiac events (syncope, cardiac arrest and sudden death) are known to occur in the setting of physical exertion, and are especially related to swimming. In a series of 670 patients with LQTS, 62% of events in LQT1 occurred during exercise. LQT2 arrhythmias are classically associated with sudden auditory stimuli like alarms, bells, telephone rings, *etc.*, and also with postpartum syncope. LQT3 is most known for death or syncope during sleep.[9–11]

EFFECT OF GENOTYPE ON PROGNOSIS (UNTREATED)

The largest study examining the effect of genotype on LQTS prognosis is that of Priori *et al*.[12] This was an analysis based on an observational registry of 647 genotyped patients (386 individuals from 104 LQT1 families, 206 individuals from 68 LQT2 families and 55 individuals from 21 LQT3 families). Over a mean observation period of 28 years, 13% of all patients had cardiac arrest or died

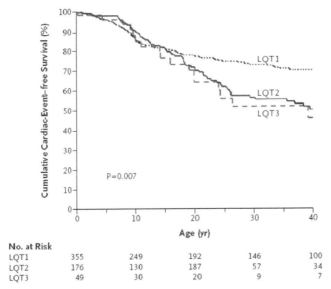

Fig. 3 LQT1–3 and cumulative cardiac events. (Reproduced from Priori *et al*[12] with permission – copyright © 2003 Massachusetts Medical Society)

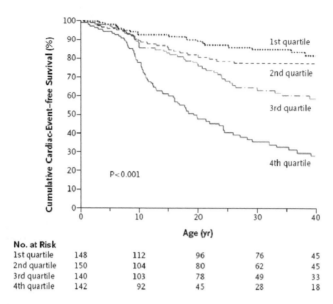

No. at Risk

1st quartile	148	112	96	76	45
2nd quartile	150	104	80	62	45
3rd quartile	140	103	78	49	33
4th quartile	142	92	45	28	18

Fig. 4 Relationship between quartiles based on QT duration and cumulative cardiac events. The 4th Quartile consists of individuals with a QT interval greater than 500 ms. (Reproduced from Priori et al[12] with permission – copyright © 2003 Massachusetts Medical Society)

suddenly prior to the initiation of therapy. There were statistically significant differences in the rates of cardiac arrest/sudden death depending upon the underlying genotype; 10% of those with LQT1, 20% of those with LQT2 and 16% of those with LQT3. Similar differences were seen when the analysis was extended to include syncope as well as cardiac arrest/sudden death, the equivalent figures being 30%, 46% and 42% (Fig. 3). Genotype and QTc were both independent predictors of cardiac events (syncope/cardiac arrest/ sudden death); patients with a QTc (measured from lead II) greater than 500 ms were at particularly high risk (Fig. 4). The authors performed a further sub-analysis of the data, creating 12 categories of patient based on genetic locus, age and QTc, creating a scheme for risk stratification amongst patients with LQTS (Table 1). In this scheme, the highest risk group (with a > 50% risk of cardiac events over the 28-year period) were those with either LQT1 or LQT2 combined with a QTc > 500 ms and males with LQT3. The study found that, in patients with LQT3, sex was a more important predictor of events than QTc, although they did comment that this result should be treated with some caution given the relatively low number of patients with LQT3.

EFFECT OF GENOTYPE ON RESPONSE TO β-BLOCKADE

Ever since the early recognition that arrhythmias associated with the LQTS are triggered by adrenergic stimulation in the majority of cases, anti-adrenergic medication (β-blockade) has been the main therapeutic approach. Non-randomised studies have provided evidence of such a powerful protective effect of propranolol and nadolol, in particular, that randomised studies have been considered inappropriate. After a first episode of syncope in LQTS

Table 1 Risk of cardiac arrest or sudden death before the age of 40 years. (Reproduced from Priori *et al*[12] with permission – copyright © 2003 Massachusetts Medical Society)

	Male			Female		
	LQT1	LQT2	LQT3	LQT1	LQT2	LQT3
QTc ≥ 500 ms	High	High	High	High	High	Inter-mediate
QTc < 500 ms	Low	Low	Inter-mediate	Low	Inter-mediate	Inter-mediate

High risk ≥ 50%; intermediate risk 30–50%; low risk < 30% over 28 years.

patients, the mortality at 15 years was 9% in patients on anti-adrenergic treatment (β-blockers and/or sympathetic denervation) versus 53% in patients not on such treatment.[13] Priori *et al*.[14] have published an analysis of cardiac events (syncope, ventricular tachycardia/*torsades de pointes*, cardiac arrest, sudden cardiac death) amongst a series of genotyped LQTS patients receiving β-blockade and treated for an average of 5 years. Using this extended definition (*i.e.* including VT/*torsades de pointes*), they demonstrated a statistically significant effect of genotype, with events occurring during β-blockade therapy in 10% of 187 LQT1 patients, 23% of 120 LQT2 patients and 32% of 28 LQT3 patients. As with the previous study, a QTc of > 500 ms (on therapy) was an important additional independent predictor of risk, as was occurrence of a first cardiac event before the age of 7 years. When cardiac arrest and sudden cardiac deaths were considered alone, LQT2 and LQT3 patients remained at increased risk compared with those with LQT1 (8% versus 1%). There were 4 sudden cardiac deaths in the group as a whole (1 LQT1 and 3 LQT3).

It is of interest that the arrhythmias associated with LQT3 (classically occurring during sleep rather than adrenergic stimulation) are perhaps the least responsive to β-blockade. In an experimental study utilising pharmacologically induced LQT1, LQT2 and LQT3 in canine LV wedge preparations, isoproterenol facilitated the occurrence of spontaneous or stimulation-induced TdP in LQT1 and LQT2 models and propranolol was effective in completely inhibiting this facilitation. However, in LQT3 isoproterenol had a protective effect and suppressed both spontaneous and stimulation induced TdP. This protective effect was reversed by propranolol causing an increased incidence of TdP.[15]

WHAT IS THE CLINICAL ROLE OF GENETIC TESTING IN THE LQTS?

The most important factors with regard to recommendations concerning genetic testing in specific conditions are: (i) the diagnostic yield of the test, particularly when there is significant genetic heterogeneity (defects in many different genes causing the condition); (ii) implications for patient life-style, clinical management or prognosis; and (iii) implications for screening of family members. In a patient with a definite clinical diagnosis of the Romano–Ward form of the congenital long QT syndrome (Schwartz and Moss score ≥ 4),[16] the

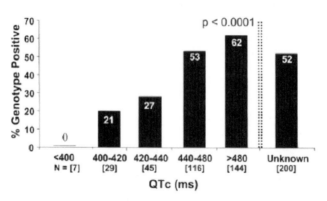

Fig. 5 Effect of corrected QT interval (QTc). The yield ranged from 0% when the subject's QTc was < 400 ms to 62% when the QTc was > 480 ms ($P < 0.0001$). [Reproduced from: Tester DJ, Will ML, Haglund CM, Ackerman MJ. Effect of clinical phenotype on yield of long QT syndrome genetic testing. *J Am Coll Cardiol* 2006; **47**: 764–768. Copyright © 2006 Elsevier with permission.]

sensitivity of genetic testing for pooled data from the five commonest LQTS-associated channel genotypes (LQT1,2,3,5,6) is high (Fig. 5; approximately 60%[17]); as can be seen from the discussion above, a positive result has considerable relevance for clinical management and prognosis. The triggers for lethal and non-lethal cardiac events differ depending upon genotype and knowledge of genotype allows specific life-style advice to be given to the patient. The most commonly prescribed treatment, oral β-blockade, differs in its efficacy according to genotype and may be ineffective in patients with LQT3. Prognosis varies according to genotype both in asymptomatic patients and those taking β-blockade. The benefit gained from successful genotyping of such a patient is not limited to that individual. Once the genetic basis for the condition has been determined, genetic testing is likely to be much more effective and cost-effective than clinical methods of screening family members. As in a number of other conditions for which a scoring system of 'diagnostic' clinical features has been proposed, clinically-derived false positives and negative diagnoses are common. For all of these reasons, an extremely strong case can be made for genetic testing of patients presenting with features typical of the congenital long QT syndrome.

This having been said, it is clear that, when a family history is absent or when clinical features are uncertain or 'borderline' according to clinical scoring methods, there is a significant fall-off in the yield of genetic testing from 60% to about 30%. Given the fact that a negative genetic test does not exclude the diagnosis, it is likely that genetic testing will be unhelpful from a diagnostic point of view in the majority of such cases. Consequently, it seems prudent to restrict such diagnostic testing to clinical environments in which expert clinical and detailed family assessment is available.

The above discussion on the role of genetic testing refers to the Romano–Ward (heterozygous) form of the syndrome. More specific forms of the syndrome are the result of gene mutations that have been particularly well characterised, and genetic testing has particular value in these cases. The Jervell Lange–Neilsen syndrome is caused by homozygous or compound heterozygous mutations in two genes (*KCNQ1* and *KCNE1*) in at least 80% of cases. Consequently, genetic testing is rapid and has a high yield. In addition, it confers prognostic information relevant to important management decisions as patients with *KCNQ1* mutations have an almost 6-fold greater risk of arrhythmic events.[18]

Timothy syndrome is characterised by a long QT interval, malignant arrhythmias, webbing of fingers and toes, congenital cardiac abnormalities and autism.[19] As all patients share the same mutation in the *CACNA1c* gene, genetic testing is very fast, cheap and sensitive. The diagnosis carries important prognostic information and is relevant in terms of reproductive counselling.

Andersen syndrome is characterised by a long QT interval, ventricular arrhythmias, periodic paralysis and skeletal developmental abnormalities.[20] It is caused by mutations in *KCNJ2*, which encodes the inward rectifier K$^+$ channel Kir2.1. Genetic testing has very high yields and is important for reproductive counselling.

Key points for clinical practice

- The LQTS is a heterogeneous group of ion channelopathies (LQT4 is not, strictly speaking, a 'channelopathy') that cause prolongation of cardiac repolarisation and in some cases predispose to sudden death.

- Ten gene defects have been described up till now caused by numerous mutations. LQT1, LQT2 and LQT3, together, constitute the majority of cases.

- No gene defects have been identified in 25% of LQTS patients.

- ECG manifestations, clinical triggers of cardiac events and response to adrenaline provocation may vary between different types of LQTS.

- The most important predictors of first cardiac events in LQTS remain a QTc > 500 ms and the genotype.

- β-Blockers may not be an effective treatment for patients with LQT3.

- Genetic testing is indicated in a patient with a definite clinical diagnosis of congenital LQTS.

References

1. Vincent GM, Timothy K, Zhang L. Congenital long QT syndrome. *Card Electrophysiol Rev* 2002; **6**: 57–60.
2. Jervell A, Lange-Nielsen F. Congenital deaf-mutism, functional heart disease with prolongation of the Q-T interval and sudden death. *Am Heart J* 1957; **54**: 59–68.
3. Ward OC. A new familial cardiac syndrome in children. *J Irish Med Assoc* 1964; **54**: 103–106.
4. Romano C, Gemme G, Pongiglione R. Aritmie cardiache rare dell'eta pediatrica. *Clin Pediatr* 1963; **45**: 656–683.

5. Mohler PJ, Schott J-J, Gramolini AO *et al*. Ankyrin-B mutation causes type 4 long-QT cardiac arrhythmia and sudden cardiac death. *Nature* 2003; **421**: 634–639.

6. Tristani-Firouzi M, Jensen JL, Donaldson MR *et al*. Functional and clinical characterization of *KCNJ2* mutations associated with LQT7 (Andersen syndrome) *J Clin Invest* 2002; **110**: 381–388.

7. Vatta M, Ackerman MJ, Ye B *et al*. Mutant caveolin-3 induces persistent late sodium current and is associated with long-QT syndrome. *Circulation* 2006; **114**: 2104–2112.

8. Domingo A, Kaku T, Tester D *et al*. AB16-6 sodium channel B4 subunit mutation causes congenital long QT syndrome. *Heart Rhythm* 2006; 3: S34–S34.

9. Schwartz PJ, Priori SG, Spazzolini C *et al*. Genotype–phenotype correlation in the long-QT syndrome: gene-specific triggers for life threatening arrhythmias. *Circulation* 2001; **103**: 89–95.

10. Wilde AA, Jongblood RJ, Doevendans PA *et al*. Auditory stimuli as a trigger for arrhythmic events differentiate HERG-related (LQTS2) patients from KvLQT1-related patients (LQTS1). *J Am Coll Cardiol* 1999; **33**: 327–332.

11. Moss AJ, Robinson JL, Gessman L *et al*. Comparison of clinical and genetic variables of cardiac events associated with loud noise vs. swimming among subjects with the long QT syndrome. *Am J Cardiol* 1999; **84**: 876–879.

12. Priori SG, Schwartz PJ, Napolitano C *et al*. Risk stratification in the long-QT syndrome. *N Engl J Med* 2003; **348**: 1866–1874.

13. Schwartz PJ, Locati E. The idiopathic long QT syndrome. Pathogenic mechanisms and therapy. *Eur Heart J* 1985; **6 (Suppl D)**: 103–114.

14. Priori SG, Napolitano C, Schwartz PJ *et al*. Association of long QT syndrome loci and cardiac events among patients treated with beta-blockers. *JAMA* 2004; **292**: 1341–1344.

15. Shimizu W, Antzelevitch C. Differential effects of beta-adrenergic agonists and antagonists in LQT1, LQT2 and long QT3 models of the long QT syndrome. *J Am Coll Cardiol* 2000; **35**: 778–786.

16. Schwartz PJ, Moss AJ, Vincent GM, Crampton RS. Diagnostic criteria for the long QT syndrome. An update. *Circulation* 1993; **88**: 782–784.

17. Ackerman MJ. Genetic testing for risk stratification in hypertrophic cardiomyopathy and long QT syndrome: fact or fiction? *Curr Opin Cardiol* 2005; **20**: 175–181.

18. Schwartz PJ, Spazzolini C, Crotti L *et al*. The Jervell and Lange-Nielsen syndrome: natural history, molecular basis, and clinical outcome. *Circulation* 2006; **113**: 783–790.

19. Splawski I, Timothy KW, Sharpe LM *et al*. Ca(V)1.2 calcium channel dysfunction causes a multisystem disorder including arrhythmia and autism. *Cell* 2004; **119**: 19–31.

20. Tristani-Firouzi M, Jensen JL, Donaldson MR *et al*. Functional and clinical characterisation of *KCNJ2* mutations associated with LQT7 (Andersen syndrome). *J Clin Invest* 2002; **110**: 381–388.

Sarah Vause Bernard Clarke Derek J Rowlands

6

Heart disease in pregnancy

Cardiac disease is now the second most common cause of maternal death (after psychiatric causes) and is more common than the most frequent 'direct' cause of maternal death, thrombo-embolism. The *2000–2002 Confidential Enquiries into Maternal Deaths*[1] reported a total of 44 deaths from heart disease related to pregnancy. This was an increase from the previous triennium in relation to which 35 deaths were reported.[2] Many cardiologists see only a small number of pregnant women with heart disease each year, but they are likely to be consulted by their obstetric colleagues when pregnant patients under their care are known, or suspected, to have heart disease. It is essential therefore, to clarify the important facts and principles in relation to the inevitable cross-disciplinary problems.

The Confidential Enquiry highlighted the fact that a degree of substandard care was present in 40% of the deaths. The main criticisms of the care related to:

1. Lack of prompt access to a frank discussion concerning the risks of pregnancy in relation to the cardiac status (with resulting failure to explore the option of termination of pregnancy).

2. Inappropriate use of family members as interpreters (when family members are used as interpreters, they are often too biased in favour of the patient's desire to become pregnant to relay accurately all the perceived risks as conveyed by the medical team).

Sarah Vause MD MRCOG
Consultant in Fetal and Maternal Medicine, Department of Obstetrics, St Mary's Hospital, Hathersage Road, Manchester M13 0JH, UK

Bernard Clarke BSc MD FRCP(Lond.) FRCP(Edin) FESC FACC (for correspondence)
Consultant Cardiologist, Manchester Heart Centre, Manchester Royal Infirmary, Oxford Road, Manchester M13 9WL, UK
E-mail: bernard.clarke@manchester.ac.uk

Derek J. Rowlands BSc MD FRCP FACC FESC
Consultant Cardiologist, Alexandra Hospital, The Beeches Consulting Centre, Mill Lane, Cheadle, Cheshire SK8 2PY, UK. E-mail: djr@djr12ecg.demon.co.uk

3. Lack of recognition of relevant features in the history, the clinical signs or the symptoms.

4. Lack of multidisciplinary collaboration.

5. Suboptimal management of cardiac arrest in obstetric patients.

EPIDEMIOLOGY

CONGENITAL HEART DISEASE

Patients with congenital heart disease (CHD) form the greatest workload in a cardiac antenatal clinic. The population of adults with CHD is growing rapidly both in numbers and in the complexity of disease. In the year 2000, there were an estimated 133,000 adults with CHD in the UK, 10,000 of whom had complex disease. This population is expected to grow to 166,000 by 2010 with a 50% increase in those with complex conditions. Half of this population is female, the majority of whom, in adulthood, are well enough to contemplate pregnancy

ACQUIRED HEART DISEASE

Although women with congenital heart disease form the greater part of the workload in an obstetric cardiac clinic, the majority of women who die from heart disease in pregnancy have acquired heart disease. The number of maternal deaths from acquired heart disease has increased steadily over the last 20 years (Fig. 1).[1]

CHANGES IN CARDIOVASCULAR PHYSIOLOGY IN RELATION TO PREGNANCY, DELIVERY AND THE PUERPERIUM

Major physiological changes occur in the maternal cardiovascular system in association with pregnancy, predominantly as a result of the need to increase delivery of oxygenated blood to the fetus.

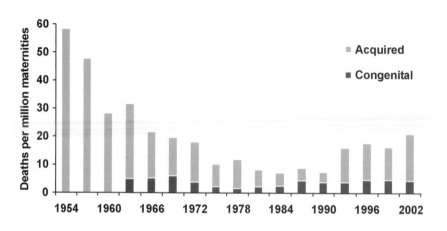

Fig. 1 Maternal deaths from congenital and acquired heart disease.

PREGNANCY

Changes in maternal haemodynamics during pregnancy

The main cardiovascular changes of pregnancy are:[3]

1. The circulating blood volume increases appreciably during pregnancy. The increase is measurable by the sixth week, rises rapidly until about the twentieth week and increases more slowly thereafter. The extent of the blood volume expansion varies between 20% and 100%.

2. The heart rate increases (typically by about 10–20 beats/min).

3. The stroke volume increases in early pregnancy.

4. The cardiac output increases by a total of about 50%. Half of the total increase occurs by 8 weeks' gestation. In the early part of pregnancy, the increase is predominantly stroke-volume related. In the later part of pregnancy, the heart rate increment makes a greater contribution.

5. The systemic vascular resistance (strictly impedance) falls (typically a 20–30% reduction occurs by the 8 weeks of gestation).

6. The blood pressure falls during the first trimester, reaching a nadir in mid pregnancy often rising to pre-pregnancy levels late in the third trimester.

7. There are minor changes in the electrocardiogram (ECG): (i) the frontal plane QRS axis moves to the left but usually remains within the normal range; (ii) small q-waves and inverted T- and P-waves may appear in lead III purely as a consequence of the axis shift; and (iii) slight ST segment depression and T-wave inversion in the inferior and lateral leads has been noted.

8. Atrial or ventricular premature beats are more frequent during pregnancy.

9. There is an increase in blood coagulability related partly to an increase in many clotting factors (including factors VII, VIII, X and von Willibrand factor) and partly to a reduction in fibrinolytic potential. This should particularly be borne in mind in relation to the management of women at known risk of thrombo-embolism (*e.g.* those with cardiomyopathy, cyanotic heart disease, atrial fibrillation, prosthetic valves) and those at risk of paradoxical embolism (*e.g.* those with ASD or any right to left shunt).

10. There is a mild dilutional anaemia.

As a result of these major haemodynamic changes, 90% of pregnant women will have an ejection systolic murmur; the vast majority of these will not have murmurs when not pregnant. The physical signs in the cardiovascular system will be those of a hyperdynamic circulation, with an increase in the heart rate, an increase in the pulse pressure (difference between the systolic and diastolic pressures) and an increase in the pulse volume (the clinical equivalent of the stroke volume).

Impact of multiple pregnancies

All the observed physiological changes noted above are more pronounced in women with multiple pregnancies. If a woman with heart disease is undergoing IVF treatment, only one embryo should be replaced to reduce the risk of multiple pregnancy.

Impact of pregnancy on haemodynamic status of women with heart disease

Whilst women with normal cardiac function tolerate the haemodynamic changes well, women with cardiac disease may decompensate during pregnancy. It should be realised, however, that the impact of pregnancy on the maternal circulation is not uniform across the spectrum of maternal cardiac problems. Pregnancy is a low afterload condition because of reduced peripheral vascular resistance. It follows that regurgitant valve lesions are well tolerated in pregnancy. (It should be remembered that a very important part of the practical management of these valve conditions in the non-pregnant state is the use of vasodilator drugs). Mitral incompetence and aortic incompetence are generally very well tolerated in pregnancy unless they are sufficiently severe to cause left ventricular dysfunction.

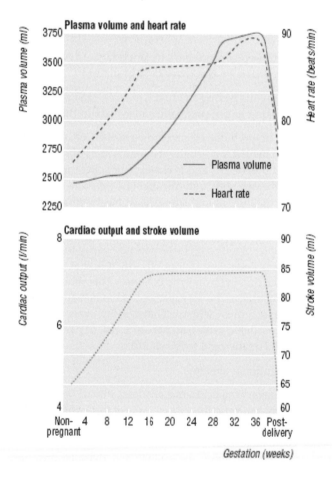

Fig. 2 Cardiovascular changes during pregnancy (adapted from Thorne,[4] with permission). Plasma volume and cardiac output increase steadily until the end of the second trimester, when cardiac output reaches a plateau at 30–50% above prepregnancy levels. Obstructive heart lesions (such as aortic or mitral valve stenosis), which limit cardiac output, are particularly compromised during pregnancy. The increase in blood volume may precipitate heart failure. Cyanosis often worsens during pregnancy as pregnancy-related systemic vasodilation may lead to increased right-to-left shunting.

Supine hypotensive syndrome of pregnancy

It is well known that profound hypotension can occur in late pregnancy following the adoption of the supine position. It is rapidly relieved when this position is abandoned and it is predominantly related to a dramatic reduction in venous return to the heart as a result of inferior vena caval compression.

LABOUR AND DELIVERY

Cardiac output and oxygen consumption increase significantly during labour. Uterine contractions, voluntary 'pushing', pain and anxiety, all contribute to these changes. Systolic, diastolic and mean blood pressure all increase during contractions.

IMMEDIATE POST PARTUM PERIOD

Immediately after delivery, as the placenta is expelled, this process is accompanied by an auto-transfusion of approximately 500 ml of blood from the contracting uterus into the maternal circulation. This auto-transfusion produces a substantial and rapid increase in the venous return within the maternal circulation as a result of which both the heart rate and cardiac output peak in the immediate post partum period, despite the blood loss. Within 2 weeks after delivery, cardiac output falls considerably towards non-pregnant levels.

The greatest haemodynamic load and, therefore, the greatest cardiovascular risks occur at the times when cardiac output is high or is changing rapidly. Early pregnancy, the second stage of labour and immediately post partum are the times of greatest change (Fig. 2).[4]

GENERAL PRINCIPLES CONCERNING THE MANAGEMENT OF PREGNANCY IN A WOMAN WITH HEART DISEASE

PRE-CONCEPTUAL CARE

Ideally, the maternity care of a woman with heart disease should begin preconceptually. In practice, this opportunity is frequently missed.

Heart disease is, of course, no bar to sexual activity. In the UK, 10% of babies are born to teenagers. A proactive approach to the preconception counselling of girls known to have heart disease should, therefore, be started in adolescence (at age 12–15 years, depending on individual maturity) and this should clearly include advice on safe and effective contraception.[5] Such advice may help to prevent accidental and, in the case of some cardiac problems, dangerous pregnancies. It should also enable young women to come to terms with their future child-bearing potential, with an awareness of the risks involved and the strategies available to minimise those risks.

Many young women with heart disease have never given any serious thought to the possible risks of pregnancy. Others may have unduly pessimistic or unduly optimistic expectations in relation to pregnancy. The preconceptual appointment is an opportunity to provide women with a realistic estimate of the maternal and fetal risks involved. Pre-conceptual counselling should be driven by the aim of promoting the autonomy of the woman, thereby enabling her to determine her personal priorities and support her decision making.

The discussion during the preconceptual consultation should include:

1. The small possibility of recurrence of cardiac abnormalities in the fetus.

2. The availability of prenatal testing for fetal abnormalities and the implications of the results.

3. The suggested clinical management (cardiac and obstetric) during pregnancy.

4. The chance that the baby may need to be delivered prematurely, because of worsening maternal cardiac function during the pregnancy. Premature delivery, before 28 weeks' gestation, is associated with a significant risk of handicap in the baby.

5. The probability that the maternal risks might change with time. Women whose cardiac function is likely to worsen with time should be advised that, if they are wanting to embark on pregnancy, it would be better to do this sooner rather than later.

6. Other women, for whom effective intervention is planned (*e.g.* valve surgery) should be advised to delay pregnancy until after treatment unless the treatment proposed might increase the maternal risks during pregnancy.

7. Women whose prospective valve surgery is likely to involve valve replacement face a particularly difficult dilemma. If it is deemed safe for them to have pregnancy prior to surgery, then an early commitment to this course would seem advisable. If the risks of pregnancy prior to valve surgery are considered unacceptable, the woman may (in the case of aortic valve replacement) have to choose between having a biological or a non-biological prosthestic valve. The first option would eliminate concerns about anticoagulation during pregnancy but would make a re-replacement (with its accompanying mortality and morbidity risks) inevitable 10–15 years later.

8. The long-term maternal outlook and life expectancy.

9. Contraception.

The preconceptual consultation also provides the ideal opportunity to minimise risks and to assess and optimise cardiac function and general health before pregnancy. This may include:

1. General preconceptual advice regarding folic acid supplements, smoking cessation and dental care.

2. Treatment of underlying medical conditions (*e.g.* hypertension, diabetes).

3. Detailed review of the cardiac status to assess the probable risks of pregnancy and to optimise the cardiac management.

4. Review of any current medication with alteration, where necessary, to avoid the continuing use of teratogenic agents (*e.g.* warfarin, ACE inhibitors, *etc.*).

One very important aspect of the preconceptual appointment is to ensure that the woman knows how to access services when she does becomes pregnant and that she is aware of the need to access services as soon as possible once pregnancy is confirmed.

ACCESS TO MULTIDISCIPLINARY SPECIALIST CARE

The *Confidential Enquiry into Maternal Deaths* emphasised the need for multidisciplinary specialist care.[1] Recognised networks for the provision of such care for women with heart disease and appropriate referral pathways should be established locally to facilitate the early provision of specialist multidisciplinary care to women with pre-existing heart disease, or for women whose heart disease is diagnosed for the first time during pregnancy.

Awareness of, and ease of access to, services for the termination of pregnancy is also important for women with heart disease who find themselves unexpectedly pregnant and who choose not to continue with the pregnancy.

For women with heart disease, in whom pregnancy is felt to pose a significant health risk, the initial consultation should include an open and frank discussion of all the risks. The option of termination of pregnancy should be explained in a non-judgmental way. If the doctor and the woman do not speak the same language, family members must not be relied upon to act as interpreters. It is recognised that, in their desire to support the woman having a baby, they may not accurately convey information about risks.[1]

RISKS POSED BY HEART DISEASE IN PREGNANCY

MATERNAL RISKS

A group from Toronto has suggested and validated a scoring system for predicting the chance of a women having cardiac complications in pregnancy.[6] This information may be of value to someone considering embarking on pregnancy, and attending for preconceptual care. In the scoring system, a woman scores 1 for each of the following: (i) cyanosis ($SaO_2 < 90\%$) or poor functional class (NYHA > 2); (ii) left heart obstruction; (iii) systemic ventricle ejection fraction < 40%; and (iv) prior CVS event (pulmonary oedema, arrhythmia, CVA/TIA). The risk is then calculated from the total score (Table 1).

FETAL RISKS

The vast majority of pregnant women naturally have concerns about the well being of their fetus. This is clearly a vital issue even though it is generally accepted that, throughout the pregnancy, the medical staff should prioritise the needs of the mother over those of the fetus.

The fetus can be affected by: (i) recurrence of a structural anomaly currently present in the mother; (ii) a genetically determined congenital abnormality; (iii) teratogenesis related to drug therapy; and (iv) poor oxygen transfer across the placenta.

Risk of structural abnormality being passed to the fetus
Women with congenital heart disease have a 5–6% risk of having a fetus with congenital heart disease.[7] Although nuchal lucency measurement has been

Table 1 Prediction of risk of cardiac complications during pregnancy (Sui *et al.*[6])

Score (number of risk factors present)	Chance of cardiac complications in pregnancy
0	5%
1	27%
>1	75%

advocated as a screening test for congenital heart defects, the level of risk in women who themselves have congenital heart disease is such that fetal echocardiography should be offered to all, irrespective of the nuchal lucency measurement. In some hospitals, fetal echo can be done at 14–16 weeks, but in most hospitals is offered around 20 weeks' gestation.

Risk of genetic abnormality in the fetus

The risk of congenital heart abnormalities in the fetus is higher if the mother carries the 22q deletion, as there is then a 1:2 chance of the fetus inheriting the deletion. A fetus which has inherited the 22q deletion has approximately a 10% chance of having congenital heart disease.[8] (Not 100%, as the gene has variable expression). Although the deletion can be diagnosed on amniocentesis, the woman must be made aware that, even if the deletion is found, there is a 90% chance that the fetus will have a normal heart. Screening by fetal echo may, therefore, be more appropriate and this approach would, of course, avoid the risk of an amniocentesis procedure related miscarriage.

When the mother (or father) has Marfan's syndrome, there is a 50% chance that the child will inherit the condition, although the degree of cardiac involvement is variable.[9] Long-term follow-up, often co-ordinated by a clinical geneticist, should be instituted for the offspring of such parents.

Women with other inherited conditions, such as some cardiomyopathies or long QT syndrome, will need specialised counselling regarding their options for prenatal diagnosis.

Teratogenic risks of maternal medications

It is widely recognised that pregnant women should avoid taking any medication which is not strictly essential. Women with heart disease may need to remain on medication for their own well-being but it is essential to recognise that they may be taking medications known to have teratogenic properties (*e.g.* warfarin or ACE inhibitors). Where this is the case, safer alternatives should be used, preferably before conception since the risks are greatest in early pregnancy. Some medications also carry the risk of harming the fetus later in pregnancy, for example warfarin (by causing intracranial haemorrhage), or amiodarone (by causing thyroid dysfunction).

EFFECT OF CARDIAC DISEASE ON THE PLACENTA

With the more severe forms of maternal cardiac disease, increased rates of fetal and neonatal morbidity and mortality are found. Severe cardiac disease may

Table 2 Live-birth rates associated with various maternal oxygen saturation and haemoglobin levels[12]

SaO$_2$ (%)	Live-birth rate (%)	Hb (g/dl)	Live-birth rate (%)
> 90	92	< 16	71
85–90	45	17–19	45
< 85	12	> 20	8

result in reduced placental perfusion, a condition which increases the number of growth-restricted fetuses.[10]

Maternal hypoxia is associated with alterations in placental growth factors, angiogenesis and apoptosis within the placenta (Table 2).[11] The rate of pre-term delivery is increased and iatrogenic pre-term delivery to curtail the pregnancy because of worsening maternal condition may be indicated in women with severe cardiac disease. The well-being of the mother should always be the priority over that of the fetus.

MONITORING BY THE MULTIDISCIPLINARY TEAM

Fundamental to the appropriate care of women with heart disease during pregnancy is an early evaluation of the nature and severity of the cardiac condition and the level of risk that it poses to pregnancy. Clearly, this should be done as early in pregnancy as possible.

Women perceived to be at intermediate and high-risk, by virtue of their cardiac status, require tertiary level care by a multidisciplinary team experienced in the management of such conditions. Conditions thought to be trivial or mild should be re-evaluated in case they have been misdiagnosed or the condition has progressed since the last assessment. When, after careful assessment, the woman is genuinely thought to be at low risk of complications, she can be re-assured and any tendency to over-treatment counteracted.

The obstetrician has the role of 'care co-ordinator' and has overall responsibility for both the mother and her fetus. Obstetricians do not have the particular expertise of the cardiologist, but they do have a particular understanding of both the physiological changes to the woman brought about by her pregnancy and of fetal growth and well-being. Obstetricians are also accustomed to making judgements involving the well-being of both the mother and her fetus, and helping to decide when and how a baby should be delivered. They are also in a position to detect pathology of pregnancy which may adversely affect cardiac function, for example pre-eclampsia.

The cardiologist plays a crucial role by clarifying the diagnosis, defining both any interventional procedures which have been performed and also the current cardiac anatomy and function. Obstetricians and anaesthetists often need, and appreciate, a review of the relevant anatomical and physiological issues in order to understand the potential complications and to plan appropriate care.

Individual plans for care need to be developed. These will vary according to the severity of the mother's cardiac condition, its stability, the need for on-going adjustment of therapy, functional status and any intercurrent co-pathology.

Women with cardiac disease can be divided into those who are at low risk of having maternal or fetal complications, and those who are at moderate or high risk. In women with low-risk lesions, unnecessary investigation and intervention should be avoided, and the woman should deliver in her own local hospital. Development of multidisciplinary care networks, with clear pathways for advice and referral, should facilitate more women delivering locally.

CARDIAC RISKS (OF MATERNAL OR FETAL COMPLICATIONS) POSED BY SPECIFIC CONDITIONS

Cardiac lesions posing trivial or minimal risk

1. Small ventricular septal defects.
2. Repaired ventricular septal defects with normal cardiac function.
3. Trivial mitral valve prolapse.

Cardiac lesions posing low risk

1. Corrected Tetralogy of Fallot.
2. Bioprosthetic valve replacement.
3. Patent ductus arteriosus.
4. Mitral stenosis with minimal limitation of maternal physical activity.
5. Mild or moderate mitral incompetence.
6. Mild or moderate aortic incompetence.

Cardiac lesions posing moderate risk

1. Haemodynamically significant mitral stenosis.
2. Aortic stenosis.
3. Uncorrected Tetralogy of Fallot.
4. Marfan's syndrome.
5. Aortic co-arctation.
6. Artificial valve replacement.

Cardiac lesions posing high risk

1. Eisenmenger syndrome.
2. Pulmonary hypertension.
3. Aortic co-arctation with valvular involvement.
4. Any patient in functional class III or IV, whatever the underlaying conditions.

Women with moderate- or high-risk lesions should deliver in a maternal cardiac centre and be managed by a multidisciplinary team. Individual care plans for the pregnancy and delivery then need to be formulated. These need to be disseminated widely to all members of the multidisciplinary team and to relevant ward areas, and a copy should be carried by the woman herself. Such care plans should include clear documentation of: (i) the cardiac diagnosis; (ii) current functional status; (iii) a plan for management during labour, delivery and post partum; (iv) contingency plans for complications such as preterm labour, post partum haemorrhage; (v) drugs which are contra-indicated and suggested alternatives; (vi) contact numbers for advice; and (vii) planned post-natal follow-up.

Arrangements for continuing cardiac follow-up in the post-natal period should be made during the pregnancy. At the time of a woman's discharge from hospital with her new-born baby, it is likely that these arrangements will be forgotten and the woman lost to follow-up, unless the post-natal appointment has already been made.

INTERACTION BETWEEN THE UNDERLYING CARDIAC PATHOLOGY AND PREGNANCY

The strength of multidisciplinary management lies in the teams being aware of the interactions between the pregnancy and the underlying cardiac condition. Some examples are given below but this list is not, of course, exhaustive.

PRE-ECLAMPSIA

This is a multisystem disease which is characterised by raised blood pressure, proteinuria and increased capillary permeability. There can be marked fluid shifts from the intravascular compartment to the interstitial compartment which can predispose to pulmonary oedema. In a woman with a left heart lesion this would compound her existing pathology. Under these circum- stances there may only be a deceptively modest rise in blood pressure. Testing the urine for proteinuria may be the most useful investigation. It is also important to remember that a urea of 5 mmol/l is high for pregnancy.

BLEEDING

This is an inherent risk in pregnancy, particularly during labour and in the immediate post partum period. In women with univentricular circulations or left outflow tract obstruction, even a modest haemorrhage could compromise their cardiac output significantly. Strategies for managing this include accurate and prompt fluid replacement with invasive monitoring, low-dose syntocinon infusions, misoprostol (a uterotonic prostaglandin with minimal cardiovascular side effects), and compression sutures (B Lynch suture).

HYPOTENSION SECONDARY TO REGIONAL ANALGESIA/ANAESTHESIA

This can cause problems similar to those encountered during bleeding. Left lateral tilt (a simple manoeuvre which is often forgotten) is very helpful in reducing aortocaval compression and, thereby, facilitating an adequate venous return. This manoeuvre may, by itself, be sufficient (by permitting adequate filling of the right side of the heart) to prevent clinically significant hypotension. Gentle incremental induction of regional blockade (to minimise vasodilatation), titration of a vasoconstrictor such as ephedrine or phenyl- ephrine (to increase the systemic vascular resistance) and the careful, but appropriate, use of intravenous fluids (to maintain adequate filling of the right side of the heart) can all help to alleviate the problem.

SLOW PROGRESS IN SECOND STAGE OF LABOUR

Slow progress during the second stage may result in a woman 'pushing' for a prolonged time. This increases heart rate, cardiac output and blood pressure. The increase in heart rate reduces the total diastolic filling time per minute. Reduction in the diastolic filling time (because of the heart rate increase) would be particularly disadvantageous in patients with tight mitral stenosis and hypertrophic obstructive cardiomyopathy. 'Pushing' also produces peaks of hypertension (by repeated Valsalva manoeuvres) which would be very undesirable in women with Marfan's syndrome or myocardial ischaemia. The need for a short, active second stage should be highlighted in the woman's notes and care plan. Regional analgesia may facilitate a longer passive second stage, allowing the fetal head to descend through the maternal pelvis, and reducing the need for active pushing. Early resort to instrumental vaginal delivery may be appropriate.

PRETERM LABOUR

This is unpredictable and frequently treated by drugs which have cardiovascular side effects such as nifedipine, indomethacin and β-agonists. The care plan should clearly specify which drugs are contra-indicated and list appropriate alternatives. Atosiban is a selective oxytocin receptor antagonist which has been shown to be as effective as β-agonists, but with a better cardiac safety profile. It appears to have little or no effect on maternal heart rate, contractility or blood pressure and is, therefore, probably the tocolytic of choice for women with heart disease.

THE QUESTION OF ANTIBIOTIC PROPHYLAXIS IN RELATION TO DELIVERY

Infective endocarditis (IE) is a serious condition associated with significant morbidity and mortality, even when treated optimally. Procedures used for prophylaxis against this condition are based almost entirely on a combination of circumstantial evidence and studies on prophylaxis in animal models of endocardial infection. There are no prospective studies to show the effectiveness of antibiotic prophylaxis in preventing IE. It is highly unlikely that there will ever be any randomised, controlled trials because of the large number of patients required and the formidable ethical issues involved. Despite this, most clinicians recommend antibiotic prophylaxis in some clinical situations and numerous sets of guidelines exist.

Whether or not antibiotic prophylaxis is recommended in any given situation depends, in general, on two factors. First is the likelihood of significant bacteraemia in relation to the medical event or procedure in respect of which the prophylaxis is being considered; second, is the degree of susceptibility of the cardiac condition to endocardial infection.

In this chapter, the only 'procedures' being considered are vaginal and abdominal delivery. The American College of Cardiology/American Heart Association joint guidelines[14] and the European Society of Cardiology guidelines[15] do not recommend antibiotic prophylaxis in relation to either of these procedures and the incidence of IE after childbirth is low (0.03–0.14 per 1000 deliveries[16]). For these reasons, antibiotic prophylaxis is not generally given in relation to vaginal delivery. Recent reports, however, have indicated a higher rate of bacteraemia after labour and delivery compared with the earlier presumed low rates of bacteraemia on vaginal and abdominal delivery on which the guidelines were based.[17] These recent reports referred to 14% bacteraemia after labour or rupture of membranes,[18] 19% of 235 blood cultures during delivery being positive,[19] and bacteraemia in 9.4% in women with and 5% in women without pre-labour rupture of membranes.[20] Furthermore, in a review of IE complicating 68 pregnancies, the calculated maternal and fetal mortality rates were 22% and 15%, respectively.[21] These figures have lead Elkayam and Bitar,[17] and others,[22,23] to give prophylactic antibiotic treatment for labour routinely in patients with valve disease. Elkayam and Bitar[17] recommend ampicillin 2.0 g intramuscularly or intravenously plus gentamicin 1.5 mg/kg (and not more than 120 mg) at the initiation of labour or within 30 min of caesarean section, followed by ampicillin (1.0 g intramuscularly or intravenously) or amoxicillin (1.0 g orally) 6 h later. For patients allergic to penicillin, they recommend vancomycin 1.0 g intravenously over 1–2 h. The British Society for Antimicrobial Chemotherapy has recently issued guidelines for the prevention of endocarditis. It is worth noting that, in the initial 'Draft for consultation', it recommended prophylactic antibiotics, in respect of patients with valve disease, both for vaginal and for caesarian delivery, but in the formal report, published in April 2006, prophylaxis was recommended for caesarian delivery but not for vaginal delivery.[24]

In relation to the cardiac condition, it should be noted that not all cardiac structural abnormalities are equally susceptible to IE. Some conditions virtually never predispose to IE; in relation to these conditions, the question of antibiotic prophylaxis does not arise – in other conditions, the risks are appreciably higher.

Cardiac conditions carrying an extremely low risk of IE[15]

1. Ischaemic heart disease without valve lesions.
2. Previous coronary artery surgery.
3. Previous percutaneous intervention.
4. Atrial septal defect (secundum variety) before or after closure.
5. Closed ventricular septal defects and ducts, without left-sided valve abnormalities.
6. Isolated pulmonary stenosis.
7. Unrepaired Ebstein's abnormality.
8. Patients with a murmur but no structural disease on echocardiographic evaluation.
9. Patients with mitral valve prolapse or thickening but with no regurgitation or calcification.

In the European Society Guidelines on Prevention, Diagnosis and Treatment of Infective Endocarditis, patients who have had Fontan type or Mustard operations are listed under those not requiring antibiotic prophylaxis.[15] In this publication, reference is made to Li and Somerville[25] who refer to the fact that, in their 18-year database: 'no case of infective endocarditis was detected in 100 patients with Fontan and 45 with Mustard operation'. These authors, however, then add: 'but this is not enough evidence to advise abstaining from prophylaxis'. It would, therefore, seem prudent to offer antibiotic prophylaxis to such patients.

Cardiac conditions carrying the highest risk of IE

1. Prosthetic heart valves.
2. Complex congenital cyanotic heart disease.
3. Patients with previous infective endocarditis.
4. Patients with surgically constructed systemic or pulmonary conduits.

Cardiac conditions carrying an intermediate risk of IE

1. Acquired valvular heart disease.
2. Hypertrophic cardiomyopathy.
3. Mitral valve prolapse with regurgitation.
4. Non-cyanotic congenital heart disease (other than secundum ASD or isolated pulmonary stenosis).

It is difficult to summarise this complex topic. There is no clear evidence that prophylactic administration of antibiotics will prevent endocarditis following uncomplicated vaginal delivery. However, the need for clinical discretion is paramount, particularly as the current guidelines are (inevitably) not based on the results of controlled trials. As pointed out by Ashrafian and Bogle,[26] in their balanced comment on the recently published British Society for Antimicrobial Chemotherapy guidelines, absence of evidence does not reflect evidence of absence.

Suggested approach to the question of antibiotic prophylaxis

The following proposals appear reasonable. Definitive recommendations cannot be made because of the inadequate database. Careful clinical judgement in this area remains paramount.

1. Prophylactic antibiotics are generally given in relation to operative delivery to all women with those cardiac lesions carrying intermediate or high risk.

2. For women with pre-existing cardiac disease deemed to be at low risk, the administration of antibiotics is unnecessary.

3. The threshold for the use of antibiotics should be lower if there is any suspicion of chorio-amnionitis.

4. Antibiotic cover should be given, in relation to vaginal or abdominal delivery, to all those with high-risk cardiac lesions. Although unproven, it seems likely that this policy will reduce the small, but very important, group who suffer the catastrophic consequences of endocarditis with its associated mortality and morbidity.[27]

Each case requires careful assessment by the cardiologist and obstetrician and, where appropriate (for example in cases of previous drug allergy or intolerance), the involvement of the bacteriologist, Decisions should be made well in advance of anticipated delivery and specific instructions relating to antibiotic prophylaxis should be written in the care plan.

Preterm, prelabour rupture of membranes poses a particular problem as there may be a desire to prolong the pregnancy in the fetal interests but this puts the woman at risk of infection, possibly for several weeks. Close monitoring for signs of infection, antibiotic prophylaxis, and discussion on an individual basis taking into account the level of risk of endocarditis and fetal gestation are important.

SPECIFIC CARDIAC PROBLEMS DURING PREGNANCY

THE COMMON CARDIAC CAUSES OF MATERNAL DEATH

Cardiologists will encounter a different spectrum of disease in the pregnant population compared with what they can expect in their routine clinics. Some conditions are more common in young women, whilst others present specific problems in relation to pregnancy.

The following four conditions will be discussed as these are the most common causes of maternal death from cardiac disease (Fig. 3):[1] (i) pulmonary hypertension; (ii) ischaemic heart disease and coronary artery dissection; (iii) aortic disease; and (iv) cardiomyopathy.

Pulmonary hypertension
Congenital heart disease accounts for 20% of all cardiac deaths. Almost half of the deaths from congenital heart disease are due to pulmonary hypertension, reflecting the 30–50% maternal mortality rate associated with severe

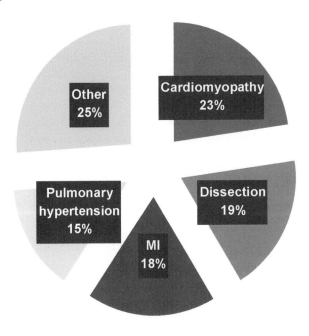

Fig. 3 The common cardiac causes of maternal death.

pulmonary vascular disease.[28,29] In view of the high maternal mortality, women with pulmonary hypertension should be advised against pregnancy, given clear contraceptive advice and offered termination should they become pregnant. If, however, a woman who is fully informed of the risks chooses to continue her pregnancy, early treatment with new pulmonary vascular therapy may improve the outlook although the benefit at the present time is both uncertain and limited.

Echocardiographic studies in women at risk of developing pulmonary hypertension from congenital heart disease should be repeated during pregnancy. In women with Eisenmenger syndrome, right-to-left shunting increases during pregnancy because of systemic vasodilatation. This both decreases pulmonary blood flow and also increases arterial desaturation, which is often clinically obvious as an increase in maternal cyanosis. The placenta, of course, receives a desaturated arterial supply.

Cyanosis is a risk factor both for a poor fetal and maternal outcome. Women with pulmonary hypertension frequently need to be delivered prematurely because of deteriorating fetal or maternal condition. It is, therefore, vital that women with pulmonary hypertension are managed in centres with the appropriate support from physicians, intensivists, obstetricians and neonatologists.

Several series have shown that the most common time for women with pulmonary hypertension to die is in the first week post partum.[30] This seems likely to be related to the haemodynamic changes occurring around the time of delivery. The disadvantageous haemodynamic situation will almost certainly be aggravated if the delivery is delayed until the woman is in extremis. Sometimes there may be a (potentially fatal) relaxation of monitoring in the post partum period. The team need to be aware that the immediate post partum period is a time of increased, rather than reduced, risk. Increased, rather than relaxed, vigilance is needed at this time.

Ischaemic heart disease

The prevalence of coronary artery disease in women is increasing owing to a variety of factors, including changing life-styles, diet, smoking and delaying child-bearing. It is likely that the incidence of ischaemic heart disease in pregnancy will rise. The peak incidence of myocardial infarction in pregnancy is in the third trimester, in parous women, over 33 years old.[31] The diagnosis is confirmed by the characteristic ECG changes and increase in cardiac enzyme levels. Cardiac troponin I is unaffected by normal pregnancy, labour, and delivery; therefore, it is the investigation of choice in the diagnosis of acute coronary syndrome.

In respect of women with known (pre-existing) ischaemic heart disease, some will be on treatment with clopidogrel and may be taking it during pregnancy. Although no fetotoxic effects have been reported, data are limited. Clopidogrel does, however, have a long-lasting effect on platelet function, which is not reversible by platelet transfusion. This results in the woman having an uncorrectable bleeding tendency. Consideration should, therefore, be given to discontinuing clopidogrel or changing to an alternative therapy well before the anticipated time of delivery.

Coronary artery dissection

Although this condition is rare in the non-pregnant population, it has been shown to cause 16% of myocardial infarctions during pregnancy and is the primary cause of infarction in the postpartum period.[1,31] There should be a low threshold for angiography when myocardial infarction occurs in pregnancy or the puerperium since this allows the possibility of intervention with percutaneous transluminal coronary angioplasty. Whilst this involves exposing the fetus to a small dose of radiation (0.02–0.1 mSv), under the circumstances the benefits to the mother outweigh the risk to the fetus.

Aortic aneurysm dissection

Of the disorders affecting the aorta during pregnancy Marfan's syndrome and Ehlers Danlos Type IV are the most important. Approximately 80% of women with Marfan's syndrome have some cardiac involvement, the majority having mitral valve prolapse.[29] Aortic dissection is most common in the third trimester and peripartum and this is probably related to the haemodynamic changes.

Women with Marfan's syndrome should have regular echocardiographic assessment during pregnancy. Women with an aortic root less than 40 mm should be re-assured that the risk of dissection is around 1%. Women with an aortic root above 40 mm should be made aware of the increased risk of an adverse outcome. This risk increases: (i) with absolute aortic size; (ii) if there is a rapid rate of change of aortic dimension; or (iii) in the presence of a positive family history. The European Society of Cardiology recommends that delivery by caesarean section should be considered for women with an aortic root of over 45 mm.[29]

Women with Ehlers Danlos Type IV are known to be at risk of aortic dissection even if the aortic root is of normal size.

Cardiomyopathy

There are different types of cardiomyopathy – peripartum, dilated, hypertrophic – all of which can be encountered in pregnancy.

Peripartum cardiomyopathy. This typically presents either as a woman approaches term or in the first few weeks after delivery, although it can occur up to 5 months' post partum.[32] Whilst it is commoner in older women, obese women, black or hypertensive women, it can present in women with no risk factors and who have previously been well. Unexplained breathlessness, tachycardia, gross oedema or supraventricular tachycardia should prompt echocardiography. There is a high recurrence risk in future pregnancies.

Dilated cardiomyopathy. If this is diagnosed, the question of the use of anticoagulation needs to be addressed. In mild cases (with only mildly or moderately reduced left ventricular ejection fraction and in the presence of sinus rhythm), it could well be judged that the risks (to mother and fetus) of using any form of anticoagulation might outweigh the benefits. When there is severe depression of left ventricular function, particularly when there is also an arrhythmia (most commonly atrial fibrillation), treatment with low molecular weight heparin should be instigated.

Hypertrophic cardiomyopathy (HOCM). This is an autosomal dominant condition which shows 'anticipation' (*i.e.* gets worse in each subsequent generation). Usually, pregnancy is reasonably well tolerated unless there is severe diastolic dysfunction.[29] Several features may jeopardise the chances of a favourable outcome.

1. *Bleeding* – The left ventricular hypertrophy impairs left ventricular filling and further reduction in cardiac filling as a result of haemorrhage is not well tolerated. Blood loss should be minimised as far as possible and blood replacement should be prompt and complete.

2. *Tachycardia* – Tachycardia produces a much greater reduction in the duration of diastole than of systole in each heart beat. It follows that the total diastolic time per minute (and, therefore, the total ventricular filling time per minute) falls and this issue is critical since left ventricular filling is impaired by the ventricular hypertrophy, which reduces the myocardial compliance. β-Blockers, by reducing the heart rate, prolong the relative duration of diastole and facilitate adequate ventricular filling.

3. *Vasodilatation* – This is disadvantageous whenever there is a significant obstructive element in the circulation (particularly in relation to obstructive cardiomyopathy but also in relation to tight aortic stenosis). Drugs with a powerful vasodilator action should be avoided. For example, nifedipine should not be used as a tocolytic agent in these women.

4. *Arrhythmias* – Atrial fibrillation is the commonest haemodynamically significant arrhythmia in this condition. In a patient with severe HOCM, the onset of atrial fibrillation may result in acute, severe haemodynamic deterioration requiring immediate DC cardioversion. Ventricular tachycardia can also occur in this condition and will also require DC cardioversion.

PREGNANCY IN PATIENTS WITH NON-BIOLOGICAL PROSTHETIC HEART VALVES

The importance of preconceptual counselling

The management of pregnancy in patients with non-biological prosthetic heart valves presents a very major problem in relation to the question of anticoagulation. Pre-conception counselling is particularly important in this area.

If possible, women should consider having any desired pregnancies in advance of valve replacement. If valve replacement is necessary before pregnancy, consideration should be given to the use of a biological prosthetic valve. This approach has the obvious advantage that it eliminates concerns about anticoagulation during pregnancy. However, the patient must realise that, whilst non-biological prosthetic valves are expected to last for the life-time of the recipient, biological valves have a finite life-span. In general, biological prosthetic valves require re-replacement after 10–15 years. There have been a number of reports giving a strong indication that accelerated structural valve deterioration (SVD) occurs during pregnancy. This would imply the possible need for re-replacement even earlier. Other reports, however, have failed to support these findings and the case for accelerated SVD in pregnancy is not considered proven (or disproved). The issue has been reviewed by Elkayam and Bitar.[34]

The mortality rate of elective re-replacement of a prosthetic valve is likely to be greater than that of the initial replacement procedure and, even with the probable 10–15-year life-span of the biological valve, the re-replacement procedure is likely to occur at a time when the woman has a young or teenage child. This may seem a relatively minor matter at the pre-pregnancy discussion, but it will assume much greater importance later and it should be brought into the initial discussion.

Patients who elect to have, or who already have, non-biological prosthetic valves

Patients with non-biological prosthetic valves (usually mitral and/or aortic) need life-long warfarin anticoagulation and must maintain the prothrombin time (expressed as the international normalised ratio [INR]) at all times within limits clearly defined for each individual case.

As indicated earlier, pregnancy is accompanied by an increase in blood coagulability and a decrease in fibrinolytic potential. Despite anticoagulation, the risks of valve thrombosis (potentially fatal) and of arterial thrombo-embolism (potentially with major consequences) are higher during pregnancy than at other times. Elkayam and Bitar[33] refer to reports describing thrombo-embolic events in 7–23% (average 13%) of patients (half with valve thrombosis). Such complications are more likely with older generations of non-biological prosthetic valves, with valves in the mitral, rather than the aortic, position, in patients with atrial fibrillation and in those with left ventricular dysfunction; these reports may give an unduly pessimistic view of the current risks facing most patients. What is clear, however, is that valve thrombosis is always a very serious complication, which is likely to be fatal if not rectified. The treatment options for this complication include heparin, thrombolysis and valve surgery. Valve surgery during pregnancy carries a high risk of fetal loss.[35] Guidelines issued in 1997 suggested thrombolysis as the first-line treatment of choice (despite natural concern about the use of thrombolytic agents during pregnancy) for left-sided prosthetic valve thrombosis.[36]

Warfarin treatment during pregnancy

The use of warfarin during pregnancy carries important risks.

1. A significant teratogenic potential during the first trimester of pregnancy.

2. An increased risk of fetal intracranial bleeding both during the pregnancy and around the time of delivery. Fetal microcephaly may develop and this is thought to be due to repeated small haemorrhages during the pregnancy.

3. An increased risk of maternal haemorrhage particularly around the time of delivery.

The risks to the fetus can be greatly reduced by using heparin rather than warfarin. Heparin in a large, highly polarised molecule which does not cross the placenta to the fetus. However, there are real concerns as to whether heparin provides adequate anticoagulation for a pregnant woman with a non-biological prosthetic valve.

Anticoagulant regimens during pregnancy

Various different anticoagulation regimens have been used during pregnancy, including:

1. Warfarin throughout the pregnancy.

2. Heparin in the first trimester, warfarin in the second trimester and heparin in the third trimester.

3. Intravenous, unfractionated heparin throughout the pregnancy.

4. Subcutaneous, low molecular weight heparin throughout the pregnancy.

In all regimens in which warfarin is used, it is replaced by heparin well in advance of anticipated delivery.

No randomised, controlled trials have been performed. All of the available data are from observational studies. Patient compliance, monitoring and the target therapeutic ranges vary within the published literature. It is, therefore, impossible to make any evidence-based recommendation on the best anticoagulation regimen for a pregnant woman with a non-biological prosthetic valve.

The European Society of Cardiology (Expert Consensus Document of the Task Force on the Management of Cardiovascular Diseases During Pregnancy)[29] presented data comparing the fetal and maternal risks of heparin during the first trimester or throughout pregnancy with those of vitamin K antagonists (predominantly warfarin) throughout. The results are presented in Table 3. It should be noted that these data were taken originally from the study by Chan, Anand and Ginsberg,[29a] who conducted a literature review of 1234 pregnancies in 976 women with mechanical heart valve prostheses. Two-thirds of the patients had prosthetic valves in the mitral position and 49.7% had (the older) 'ball and cage' type of valve (most commonly Starr-Edwards valves). The probability is that modern prosthetic valves will be less thrombogenic but similar large data sets in relation to such modern prosthetic valves do not appear to be available.

More recently, there have been an increasing number of case reports and small series describing of the use of supra-therapeutic doses of low molecular

Table 3 Adapted from the Expert Consensus Document on management of cardiovascular diseases during pregnancy (The Task Force on the Management of Cardiovascular Diseases during Pregnancy of the European Society of Cardiology), *Eur Heart J* 2003; **24**: 761–781. The data were derived from the earlier literature review of Chan et al.[29a]

Anticoagulant regimen	Embryo-pathy (%)	Spontaneous abortion (%)	Thrombo-embolic complications (%)	Maternal death (%)
Vitamin K antagonist throughout	6.4	25	3.9	1.8
Low-dose heparin throughout	0	20	60	40
Adjusted dose heparin throughout	0	25	25	6.7
Heparin in first trimester, then vitamin K antagonists	3.4	25	9.2	4.2

weight heparin throughout the pregnancy, although these have not been without maternal complications.[37–40]

It is clear that there is no risk-free option. There is not even a low-risk option. The decision whether to continue with warfarin throughout pregnancy (undoubtedly the safest course for the mother) or to use heparin (safer for the fetus) is one which should be made at the earliest opportunity (preconception, if possible) after full discussion with the patient and her partner. Women should be offered a choice between the higher rates of fetal loss or damage associated with the use of warfarin and the higher risk of maternal valve thrombosis and death with subcutaneous heparin.[5,41]

If warfarin is used, the INR has to be kept in the range recommended for the particular prosthesis, but should be as low within this range as possible. There is evidence that the risk to the fetus is lower when less than 5 mg warfarin per day is needed.[42]

In women with mechanical heart valves who elect to use subcutaneous heparin, the use of dosage based on maternal weight is totally inadequate. It is essential that the dose of low molecular weight heparin is adjusted in response to peak and trough measurements of anti-Factor Xa levels. These must be maintained at all times at therapeutic levels, guided by monitoring of anti-Factor Xa activity, at least monthly and preferably at 2-weekly intervals. The aim is to achieve peak post-dose level (usually 4 h post injection) of at least 1.0 U/ml, and a trough (pre-dose) level of at least 0.5 U/ml and preferably 0.6–0.7 U/ml.[34] Low-dose aspirin (75–150 mg) daily is a safe and possibly effective adjunct to low molecular weight heparin in women with mechanical heart valves.[5]

CARDIAC ARRHYTHMIAS DURING PREGNANCY

Pregnancy is associated with an increased frequency of arrhythmias both in those with, and in those without, underlying heart disease. The cause of the increased incidence is not known with confidence but hormonal changes, stress, autonomic changes and electrolyte shift could all play a part. Atrial and ventricular ectopic (premature) beats are by far the commonest of the rhythm disturbances. Provided no more serious rhythm disturbances are present, these arrhythmias usually have no significant impact on maternal or fetal well-being and re-assurance is then appropriate.

There is also some suggestion that paroxysmal supraventricular tachy-cardias are more common in the pregnant state. The commonest forms of supraventricular tachycardia are atrioventricular nodal re-entrant tachycardia (AVNRT) and atrioventricular re-entrant tachycardia (AVRT). AVRT presupposes the existence of an accessory pathway (the anatomical substrate of the Wolff–Parkinson–White syndrome).

In general, there are two indications for treating any arrhythmia. The first is because the arrhythmia may be prognostically significant (*e.g.* ventricular tachycardia, *torsades de pointes*, pre-excited atrial fibrillation, or any rhythm disturbance with a dangerously high or dangerously low ventricular rate) and the second is to relieve symptoms. During pregnancy, to this list may be added maternal haemodynamic deterioration, in particular hypotension (or the anticipation of such), sufficient to give rise to concerns about the adequacy of the placental circulation.

In the management of any arrhythmia (except in the context of an acute emergency), the first steps would be an overall assessment of the cardiac status with a check on the serum potassium level and on the thyroid status. A high-quality 12-lead ECG is essential for a reliable diagnosis of the arrhythmia (even with such a record, a definitive diagnosis is not always possible). A single lead monitor or strip recording will not provide nearly as much information although it may be adequate for the recognition of some of the more straight-forward arrhythmias. If time and circumstances permit, an echocardiogram is likely to be extremely useful.

In terms of the management of arrhythmias, the general principle during pregnancy is to avoid all but the (almost) absolutely safe or necessary treatments.[43] Any significant arrhythmia in a pregnant patient requires simultaneous input from the obstetrician and the cardiologist and may also require advice and attention from the anaesthetist. AVNRT and AVRT nearly always respond to intravenous adenosine. This drug has an extremely short half-life. It is cleared from the maternal circulation within seconds and appears to have no effect on the fetal heart rate.[44–46] Data relating to the use of this drug during the first trimester are limited.[47] With any sustained ectopic tachydysrhythmia during pregnancy, DC cardioversion should be considered (*vide infra*).

DC CARDIOVERSION

DC cardioversion may be necessary during pregnancy (as at other times) to deal with such arrhythmias as ventricular tachycardia, pre-excited atrial fibrillation, atrial fibrillation, atrial flutter, atrial tachycardia. It can also be used in cases of AVNRT or AVRT although in these cases intravenous adenosine is usually effective and carotid sinus massage is sometimes effective.

There is naturally some anxiety about the application of a high-energy DC shock during pregnancy but the evidence is that DC cardioversion is a safe procedure at all stages of pregnancy.[3,48,49] It is the preferred method of management of sustained atrial flutter or sustained atrial fibrillation developing during pregnancy. The Expert Consensus Document from the European Society of Cardiology recommends that cardioversion should be used during pregnancy 'for any sustained tachycardia causing haemodynamic instability and therefore threatening fetal security'.[28]

Data on the optimal approach to anticoagulant therapy in relation to DC cardioversion in pregnancy are very limited. In general (*i.e.* not in relation to pregnancy), full warfarin anticoagulation for 4 weeks prior to and for 3 months following (successful) cardioversion is recommended for patients with a atrial fibrillation and either significant valve disease or significant myocardial disease, or when the atrial fibrillation has been present for 48 h or longer. In pregnancy, the onset of atrial flutter or fibrillation will usually be recognised early on; if cardioversion is considered appropriate, it is best done at the earliest safe opportunity, within 48 h of the onset or the arrhythmia. Intravenous heparin can be given acutely to 'cover' the procedure, though there is no clear evidence base for this. The anticoagulant management requires thoughtful consideration by the responsible team (including obstetrician and cardiologist). The indications for immediate and for subsequent anticoagulation are greatly increased in the presence of significant valve disease or myocardial disease or if there is knowledge of any previous embolic event. These considerations, however, have to be set against the risks of any form of anticoagulation in pregnancy.

MANAGEMENT OF CARDIAC ARREST DURING PREGNANCY

The management of cardiac arrest needs to be modified when the subject of the arrest is a pregnant woman. All midwives, obstetricians, cardiologists, coronary care staff and accident and emergency staff should be aware of how to modify their management of a cardiac arrest for a pregnant woman.

The weight of a gravid uterus may compress the inferior vena cava producing orthostatic hypotension and reducing cardiac output. In the critically ill patient, this may be sufficient to precipitate arrest. It substantially reduces the effectiveness of cardiac massage. Pregnant women should be nursed or resuscitated using 15–30% lateral tilt.

The combination of the physiological relaxation of the gastric sphincter and the upward pressure of the gravid uterus pressing against the stomach make inhalation of gastric contents more likely in an unconscious pregnant patient. The airway needs to be protected by a cuffed endotracheal tube as early as possible during the resuscitation.

If initial attempts at resuscitation fail, a perimortem caesarean section should be performed promptly (after 5 min of resuscitation) to empty the uterus. This is done to optimise maternal resuscitation, rather than to save the baby. Emptying the uterus reduces compression of the inferior vena cava allowing the woman to be laid flat, facilitating more effective cardiac compressions. It also reduces the splinting of the diaphragm, facilitating more effective ventilation, reduces oxygen requirements and reduces the risk of aspiration of gastric contents.

Key points for clinical practice

- Heart disease is the second most common cause of maternal death and there is frequently some degree of substandard care.

- There are profound cardiovascular changes during pregnancy. Women with cardiac disease may decompensate during pregnancy.

- A proactive approach should be taken to preconceptual counselling. This is particularly important for adolescent girls as they begin their reproductive years. Advice on safe and effective contraception and information on how to access services should be included.

- Throughout pregnancy, the safety and well-being of the mother should be prioritised over that of the fetus.

- Access to tertiary care by a multidisciplinary team should be facilitated. The strength of multidisciplinary management lies in the team's being aware of the physiological and pathological interactions between pregnancy and the underlying cardiac condition. The team would also be aware of any effects proposed therapies may have on both the pregnancy and the cardiac condition.

(continued on next page)

Key points for clinical practice *(continued)*

- There is a lack of evidence on which to base recommendations for antibiotic prophylaxis around the time of delivery. Decisions must be based on the likelihood of significant bacteraemia and the susceptibility to infective endocarditis posed by the specific cardiac condition. For women with pre-existing cardiac disease deemed to be at low risk, the administration of antibiotics is unnecessary. For women at high risk, a policy of antibiotic cover is likely to reduce the small, but very important, group who suffer the catastrophic consequences of endocarditis.

- In view of the high maternal mortality, women with pulmonary hypertension should be advised against pregnancy, given clear contraceptive advice and offered termination should they become pregnant.

- Cyanosis is a risk factor for both a poor fetal and maternal outcome.

- The immediate post partum period is a time of increased, rather than reduced, risk of maternal death. Close monitoring should be maintained.

- Owing to the lack of evidence, it is impossible to make any recommendations on the best anticoagulation regimen for a pregnant woman with a non-biological prosthetic valve. The risks and benefits of the different regimens should be discussed with the woman. The potentially fatal consequences of valve thrombosis should be stressed. The importance of good compliance should be stressed. Close anticoagulant monitoring must be instituted whichever regimen is chosen.

- All clinicians should be aware of how to modify their management of a cardiac arrest for a pregnant woman.

References

1. Drife JO, Lewis G, Clutton-Brock T. (eds) *Why Mothers Die: The Sixth Report of the Confidential Enquiries into Maternal Deaths in the United Kingdom 2000–2002*. London: RCOG, 2004.
2. Royal College of Obstetricians and Gynaecologists. Why mothers die 1997–1999, the confidential enquiries into maternal deaths in the United Kingdom. London: RCOG, 2001.
3. Elkayam U, Gleicher N. Hemodynamic and cardiac function during normal pregnancy and the puerperium. In: Elkayam U, Gleicher N. (eds) *Cardiac Problems in Pregnancy*, 3rd edn. New York: Wiley-Liss, 1998; 3–20.
4. Thorne SA. Pregnancy in heart disease. *Heart* 2004; **90**: 450–456.
5. Steer PJ, Gatzoulis MA, Baker P. (eds) *Consensus views arising from the 51st Study Group: Heart Disease in Pregnancy Heart Disease and Pregnancy*. London: RCOG, 2006; 329.
6. Sui SC, Sermer M, Colman JM *et al*. Cardiac Disease in Pregnancy (CARPEG) Investigators. Prospective multicenter study of pregnancy outcomes in women with heart disease. *Circulation* 2001; **104**: 515–521.

7. Harper PS. *Practical Genetic Counselling*, 5th Edn. Oxford: Butterworth Heinemann, 1998; 242.

8. Liling J, Cross I, Burn J, Daniel CP, Tawn EJ, Parker L. Frequency and predictive value of 22q11 deletion. *J Med Genet* 1999; **36**: 794–795.

9. Pyeritz RE, McKusick VA. Basic defects in the Marfan syndrome. *N Engl J Med* 1981; **305**: 1011–1012.

10. Weiss BM, Hess OM. Pulmonary vascular disease and pregnancy: current controversies, management strategies, and perspectives. *Eur Heart J* 2000; **21**: 104–115.

11. Kingdom J, Huppertz B, Seaward G, Kaufmann P. Development of the placental villous tree and its consequences for fetal growth. *Eur J Obstet Gynecol Reprod Biol* 2000; **92**: 35–43.

12. Whittemore R, Hobbins JC, Engle MA. Pregnancy and its outcome in women with and without surgical treatment of congenital heart disease. *Am J Cardiol* 1982; **50**: 641–651.

13. Durack DT, Prevention of infective endocarditis. *N Engl J Med* 1995; **332**: 38–44.

14. ACC/AHA. ACC/AHA 2006 guidelines for the management of patients with valvular heart disease. *J Am Coll Cardiol* 2006; **48**: e1–e148.

15. Horstkotte D, Follath F, Gutschik E *et al*. Guidelines on prevention, diagnosis and treatment of infective endocarditis. The task force on infective endocarditis of the European Society of Cardiology. *Eur Heart J* 2004; **25**: 267–276.

16. Seaworth BJ, Durack DT. Infective endocarditis in obstetric and gynecologic practice. *Am J Obstet Gynecol* 1986; **154**: 180–188.

17. Elkayam U, Bitar F. Valvular heart disease and pregnancy. Part I: native valves. *J Am Coll Cardiol* 2005; **46**: 223–230.

18. Boggess KA, Watts DH, Hillier SL *et al*. Bacteremia shortly after placenta separation during cesarian delivery. *Obstet Gynecol* 1996; **87**: 779–784.

19. Petanovic M, Zagar Z. The significance of asymptomatic bacteremia for the newborn. *Acta Obstet Gynecol Scand* 2001; **80**: 813–817.

20. Furman B, Shohan-Vardi I, Bashire A *et al*. Clinical significance and outcome of preterm pre-labour rupture of membranes: population based study. *Eur J Obstet Gynecol Reprod Biol* 2000; **92**: 209–216.

21. Campuzans K, Rogue H, Bolwick A *et al*. Bacterial endocarditis complicating pregnancy: case report and systematic review of the literature. *Arch Gynecol Obstet* 2003; **268**: 251–255.

22. Sawhney H, Agarwal N, Surv V *et al*. Maternal and perinatal outcome in rheumatic heart disease. *Int J Gynaecol Obstet* 2003; **80**: 9–14.

23. Bhatla N, Lal S, Behera G *et al*. Cardiac disease in pregnancy. *Int J Gynaecol Obstet* 2003; **82**: 153–159.

24. Gould FK, Elliott TSJ, Foweraker J *et al*. Guidelines for the prevention of endocarditis: report of the Working Party of the British Society for Antimicrobial Chemotherapy. *J Antimicrob Chemother* 2006; **57**: 1035–1042.

25. Li W, Somerville J. Infective endocarditis in the grown-up congenital heart (GUCH) population. *Eur Heart J* 1998; **19**: 166–173.

26. Ashrafian H, Bogle RG. Antimicrobial prophylaxis for endocarditis: emotion or science? *Heart* 2006; **93**: 5–6.

27. Stuart G. Consensus views arising from the 51st Study Group: Heart Disease in Pregnancy. In: Steer PJ, Gatzoulis MA, Baker P. (eds) *Heart Disease and Pregnancy*. London: RCOG, 2006; 275.

28. Weiss BM, Hess OM. Pulmonary vascular disease and pregnancy: current controversies, management strategies, and perspectives. *Eur Heart J* 2000; **21**: 104–115.

29. The Task Force on the Management of Cardiovascular Diseases during Pregnancy of the European Society of Cardiology. Expert consensus document on management of cardiovascular diseases during pregnancy. *Eur Heart J* 2003; **24**: 761–781.

29a. Chan WS, Anand S, Ginsberg JS. Anticoagulation of pregnant women with mechanical heart valves. A systematic review of the literature. *Arch Int Med* 2000; **160**: 191–196

30. Weiss BM, Zemp L, Seifert B, Hess OM. Outcome of pulmonary vascular disease in pregnancy: a systematic overview from 1978 through 1996. *J Am Coll Cardiol* 1998; **31**: 1650–1657.

31. Roth A, Elkayam U. Acute myocardial infarction associated with pregnancy. *Ann Intern*

Med 1996; **9**: 751–762.

32. Pearson GD, Veille JC, Rahimtoola S *et al*. Peripartum Cardiomyopathy National Heart, Lung, and Blood Institute and Office of Rare Diseases (National Institutes of Health) Workshop Recommendations and Review. *JAMA* 2000; **283**: 1183–1188.

33. Elkayam U, Tummala PP, Rao K *et al*. Maternal and fetal outcomes of subsequent pregnancies in women with peripartum cardiomyopathy. *N Engl J Med* 2001; **344**: 1567–1571.

34. Elkayam U, Bitar F. Valvular heart disease and pregnancy. Part II: prosthetic valves. *J Am Coll Cardiol* 2005; **46**: 403–410.

35. Weiss BM, Von Segesser LK, Alon E *et al*. Outcome of cardiovascular surgery and pregnancy: a systematic review of the period 1984–1996. *Am J Obstet Gynecol* 1998; **179**: 1643–1653.

36. Lengyel M, Fuster V, Keltai M *et al*. Guidelines for management of left-sided prosthetic valve thrombosis: a role for thrombolytic therapy. Consensus Conference on Prosthetic Valve Thrombosis. *J Am Coll Cardiol* 1997; **30**: 1521–1526.

37. Montalescot G, Polle V, Collet JP *et al*. Low molecular weight heparin after mechanical heart valve replacement. *Circulation* 2000; **101**: 1083–1086.

38. Lee LH. Low molecular weight heparin for thromboprophylaxis during pregnancy in 2 patients with mechanical mitral valve replacement. *Thromb Haemost* 1996; **76**: 628–629.

39. Tenconi PM, Gatti L, Acaia B. Low molecular weight heparin in a pregnant woman with mechanical heart valve prosthesis: a case report. *Thromb Haemost* 1997; **79**: 733.

40. Lev-Ran O, Kramer A, Gurevitch J *et al*. Low-molecular weight heparin for prosthetic heart valves: treatment failure. *Ann Thorac Surg* 2000; **69**: 264–265.

41. Sbarouni E, Oakley CM. Outcome of pregnancy in women with valve prostheses. *Br Heart J* 1994; **71**: 196–201.

42. Vitale N, De Feo M, De Santo LS, Pollice A, Tedesco N, Cotrufo M. Dose-dependent fetal complications of warfarin in pregnant women with mechanical heart valves. *J Am Coll Cardiol* 1999; **33**: 1637–1641.

43. Page RL. Treatment of arrhythmias during pregnancy. *Am Heart J* 1995; **130**: 871–876.

44. Harrison JK, Greenfield RA, Wharton JM. Acute termination of supraventricular tachycardia by adenosine during pregnancy. *Am Heart J* 1992; **123**: 1386–1388.

45. Leffler S, Johnson DR. Adenosine use in pregnancy: lack of effect on fetal heart rate. *Am J Emerg Med* 1992; **10**: 548–549.

46. Afridi I, Moisw Jr KJ, Rokey R. Termination of supraventricular tachycardia with intravenous adenosine in a pregnant woman with the Wolff–Parkinson–White syndrome. *Obstet Gynecol* 1992; **80**: 481–483.

47. Elkayam U. Pregnancy and heart disease. In: Zipes DP, LibbyP, Bonow RO, Braunwald E (eds) *Braunwald's Heart Disease*, 7th edn. Amsterdam: Elsevier Saunders, 2005; Chapter 7.

48. Brown O, Davidson N, Palmer J. Cardioversion in the third trimester of pregnancy. *Aust NZ J Obstet Gynecol* 2001; **41**: 241–242.

49. Oktay C, Kesapli M, Altekin E. Wide-QRS complex tachycardia during pregnancy: treatment with cardioversion and review. *Am J Emerg Med* 2002; **20**: 492–493.

Sanjay Sharma William J. McKenna

7

Sudden cardiac death in young athletes

Participation in regular exercise is associated with an overall reduction in the risk of developing atherosclerosis,[1-4] as well as increasing stamina and psychological well-being. Many exercising individuals are capable of extraordinary physical achievements and are perceived by many as the epitome of health. However, exercise is also a recognised trigger for fatal cardiac arrhythmias and sudden cardiac death (SCD) in athletes harbouring sinister cardiac conditions.[5,6] Approximately 80% of all non-traumatic sudden deaths in athletes are attributed to a cardiac disorder.[7]

The SCD of an athlete with unsuspected cardiovascular disease tends to attract a great deal of publicity, particularly when high-profile athletes are involved, generating alarm in the lay public as well as among fellow athletes, coaches and sports physicians.[8] The steady trickle of sudden deaths in high profile athletes has become an increasing public health issue over the past two decades and has evoked the development and implementation of pre-participation screening programmes and formulation of disqualification criteria in athletic individuals harbouring potentially serious cardiac conditions in an aim to reduce the risk of sudden death.

This chapter aims to provide a comprehensive review of the causes, diagnosis and management of conditions causing SCD in young athletes and outlines the current perspective on pre-participation screening.

Sanjay Sharma BSc FRCP MD (for correspondence)
Consultant Cardiologist, Department of Cardiology, King's College Hospital, Denmark Hill, London SE3 9RS, UK
E-mail: ssharma21@hotmail.com

William J. McKenna DSc FACC FESC FRCP
Professor of Cardiac Medicine, Centre of Cardiology in the Young, The Heart Hospital, 16–18 Westmoreland Street, London WIG 8PH, UK
E-mail: wmckenna@ucl.ac.uk

DEFINITIONS

Before proceeding further, it is prudent to define some terminologies to place the article in perspective. Sudden cardiac death is defined as an event which is non-traumatic, non-violent, unexpected and resulting from sudden cardiac arrest within 6 h of previously witnessed normal health.

Although a substantial proportion of the population consider themselves to be athletes, we consider an 'elite' or 'competitive athlete' as an individual who undergoes organised training and participates in a team or an individual sport in which regular competition is a component.

The term 'young' refers to an individual who is aged < 35 years. The age cut-off is arbitrary and based on the fact that deaths in athletes aged < 35 years are usually due to inherited or congenital abnormalities of the cardiovascular system;[5,6,9] deaths in athletes aged > 35 years deaths are largely due to coronary artery disease.[10,11]

INCIDENCE

Fortunately, SCD in young athletes is rare; however, the precise incidence of SCD in young athletes is unknown. Estimates from the US suggest an incidence of 1–2 in 100,000 athletes.[12,13] These statistics probably underestimate the true incidence of SCD in athletes for three important reasons. First, the lack of a national systematic registry in the US for sudden death during sport means that compilation of statistics relies on media reports, which usually concentrate on high profile athletes and voluntary information from pathologists with an interest in conditions causing SCD in an athlete. Second, an expert pathologist with experience in conditions causing SCD is rarely responsible for conducting post mortem examination on athletes; thus, rare pathologies or atypical histopathological manifestations of otherwise well-recognised conditions causing SCD and accessory pathways may not be detected. Finally, some young athletes who die suddenly have no identifiable cause at post mortem examination but it is well established that a significant proportion of such deaths are due to the disorders affecting cardiac ion channels or abnormalities of cardiac conduction tissue.

More accurate estimates relating to the incidence of SCD in athletes are derived from Northern Italy which has a systemic registry of recording deaths in athletes, specifically epidemiological and pathological data on SCD in athletes. Between 1979 and 1980, prior to the implementation of the national screening programme for young competitive athletes, the incidence of SCD in this group was 3.6 per 100,000.[14]

DEMOGRAPHICS

Almost 90% of all SCDs in young athletes occur during, or immediately after, strenuous physical activity indicating that exercise is a trigger for fatal ventricular arrhythmias in athletes harbouring potentially lethal cardiac conditions. Indeed, the relative risk of an athlete dying from a cardiac disorder is 2.5 times more than that of a non-athlete.[15] Adrenergic surges, increased myocardial oxygen demand, hyperthermia, lactic acidosis and electrolyte derangement resulting from strenuous exertion are all potential contributing factors. Male athletes are more susceptible to sudden death than their female counterparts with a ratio of 9:1. The gender difference may be partly explained by the fact that males have a higher participation rate in sport and engage in more physically demanding sporting disciplines.

The most vulnerable group of athletes at risk of SCD are adolescent athletes and athletes in early adulthood. In an American series of 157 deaths in young competitive athletes, the mean age of sudden death was 17.1 years.[16] Approximately 40% of sudden deaths occur in athletes under 18 years and 33% in athletes under 16 years.[17] The vast majority of athletes are asymptomatic and sudden death is usually the first presentation with prodromal symptoms being present in only 18% of cases within 36 months of death.[16] Our own experience of screening athletes in the UK agrees with the observation that most young athletes harbouring potentially serious cardiac disorders are asymptomatic.

Most deaths have been reported in American football, basketball and soccer reflecting the popularity of these sporting disciplines in US and Northern Italy where most of the reports in the literature on SCD have been compiled.

CAUSES

The cause of SCD in during sport is influenced by the age of the athlete. In athletes > 35 years, more than 80% of all SCDs are due to atheromatous coronary artery disease.[10,11,18] Most deaths occur in competitive, long-distance racing, jogging and other vigorous sports such as rugby and squash. About 50% of athletes

Table 1 Causes of sudden cardiac death in young athletes

Congenital/inherited causes	
Disease of the myocardium	• Hypertrophic cardiomyopathy • Arrhythmogenic ventricular cardiomyopathy • Dilated cardiomyopathy
Coronary artery disease/anomalies	• Anomalous insertion of coronary arteries • Premature atheromatous coronary artery disease
Cardiac conduction tissue abnormalities	• Wolff–Parkinson–White syndrome • Right ventricular out-flow tachycardia
Valvular heart disease and disorders of the aorta	• Mitral valve prolapse • Congenital aortic stenosis • Marfan's syndrome
Ion-channelopathies	• Congenital long QT syndrome • Catecholeaminergic polymorphic ventricular tachycardia
Acquired heart disease • Infections (myocarditis) • Drugs (cocaine, amphetamine) • Electrolyte disturbances (hypokalaemia or hyperkalaemia) • Hypothermia • Hyperthermia • Trauma (commotio cordis)	

who die suddenly have prodromal symptoms suggestive of myocardial ischaemia and many have significant risk factors for coronary artery disease which include smoking, hypertension, diabetes mellitus, hypercholesterolaemia and a family history of myocardial infarction before the age of 55 years. Pathological findings in joggers and marathon runners dying suddenly reveal severe and extensive coronary atherosclerosis, involving two or more large coronary arteries in over 70% of cases. Myocardial scarring is evident in approximately 40% and fresh infarcts are seen in 15% of cases.[11]

Most SCDs in young athletes are due to inherited or congenital abnormalities resulting in a structural cardiac abnormality or a primary electrical abnormality. The latter is associated with a structurally normal heart. Disorders can be divided into those affecting cardiac muscle, coronary arteries, the valves, the aorta, and the conduction system and ion channels. Many athletes harbouring potentially serious cardiac abnormalities are capable of excelling in competition at national and international level. Sudden cardiac death may also occur due to acquired conditions such as myocarditis, drug abuse and trauma (Table 1). Most conditions predisposing to sudden death in athletes result in the same final common denominator (cardiac arrest) on presentation to an emergency physician. Primary ventricular tachyarrhythmias are the predominant mechanisms of SCD in these inherited conditions, except in Marfan's syndrome where death is often from rupture of aneurysmal aorta.

SUDDEN CARDIAC DEATHS DUE TO INHERITED OR CONGENITAL STRUCTURAL HEART DISEASE

Cardiomyopathies

The most common causes of SCD in young athletes are the cardiomyopathies which, together, account for almost 50% of all deaths reported in the literature. The main cardiomyopathies implicated in sudden death during sport are hypertrophic cardiomyopathy (HCM) and arrhythmogenic right ventricular cardiomyopathy (ARVC). Reports from the US indicate that the commonest cause of SCD is HCM, accounting for 36% of all deaths (Fig. 1) whereas data from Northern Italy suggest that the leading cause of sudden death is ARVC. In one Italian study of 22 SCDs in young athletes, ARVC accounted for 22% of

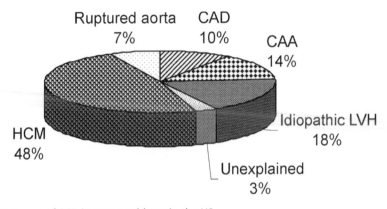

Fig. 1 Causes of SCD in young athletes in the US.

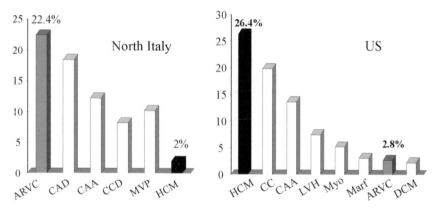

Fig. 2 The distribution of causes of SCD in young athletes in the US and Northern Italy.

all deaths whereas HCM was responsible for only 2% of deaths (Fig. 2).[19] The difference between the US and Italian series may be partly explained by the fact that individuals with HCM are identified early in the mandatory Italian pre-participation screening programme and subsequently disqualified from sport.[20] Interestingly, SCD rates from HCM in Italian athletes have been significantly lower than in American athletes even prior to the development of the Italian screening programme suggesting that the lower HCM related SCD rate is partly explained by the lower genetic cluster of HCM in the relatively homogeneous population of Northern Italy.

Hypertrophic cardiomyopathy (HCM) is the commonest recognised cause of SCD in young athletes world-wide. It is genetic disorder of sarcomeric contractile proteins characterised by unexplained left ventricular hypertrophy, non-dilated left ventricular cavity, impaired myocardial relaxation, left ventricular outflow obstruction in about 25% of cases and myocardial ischaemia. Sudden death is usually the most common mode of presentation but some athletes may present with angina, exertional dizziness or syncope.

The structural and functional changes associated with HCM preclude efficient left ventricular filling and augmentation of stroke volume required to generate a sustained increase in cardiac output for prolonged periods.[21] However, the disorder exhibits marked morphological and functional heterogeneity allowing a small proportion of affected individuals to compete at national and international level. Most deaths occur in sports associated with a 'start-stop' nature such as soccer, where excellence is dependent largely on skill rather than endurance; however, there are also reports of exceptional athletic achievements in endurance events including triathlon and marathon running. Thus, in some circumstances, the disorder defies the theoretical principles of cardiovascular physiology.[22]

Although it is well established that the prevalence of HCM in the general population is 1 in 500,[23] there are few data relating to the prevalence of HCM in the young athletic population. Calculations based on identification of HCM in the Italian screening programme indicate a prevalence of 1 in 1533 young athletes. An American study evaluating 5165 young athletes failed to detect any cases of HCM.[24] Our own 10-year experience of screening 4000 athletes in the UK, competing at regional or national level, has failed to identify any cases of HCM. The low identification rate of HCM in highly trained young athletes suggests that the structural and functional cardiac abnormalities associated with the disorder select most affected individuals out of the athlete arena.

Reports from the US indicate that deaths from HCM are more common in young athletes of Afro-Caribbean origin than in white athletes. In some cases, post mortem studies in black athletes have revealed left ventricular hypertrophy and heart weights of 400–490 g; however, subsequent histological analysis of cardiac tissue blocks has failed to reveal myocyte disarray, the histological hallmark of HCM. These cases have been attributed to idiopathic left ventricular hypertrophy rather than HCM and may represent pathological left ventricular hypertrophy due to previously diagnosed hypertension, or exaggerated left ventricular hypertrophy resulting from the stresses of exercise to the point that is becomes pathological.[16]

Arrhythmogenic right ventricular cardiomyopathy is the commonest cause of SCD in athletes in Italy and is being increasingly diagnosed as a cause of SCD in other countries as experience in the pathological identification of the condition increases.[14,15,19,20] It is a genetically determined disorder of cardiac desmosomal proteins which are responsible for the adhesive cell junction and is characterised by progressive loss of myocardium from the right ventricle, with fibro fatty replacement. The condition manifests with arrhythmias of right ventricular origin and morphological changes affecting the right ventricle. Most deaths in athletes occur during sport, particularly soccer. It is

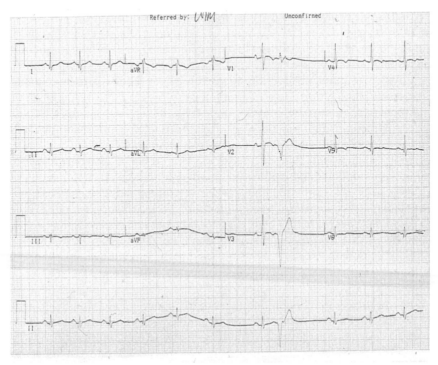

Fig. 3 T-wave inversions in V_1–V_5 and ventricular extra systoles of left bundle branch block morphology (right ventricular origin) in an individual with ARVC.

postulated that, under conditions of mechanical stress, the inherent weakness of cell junctions results in myocyte detachment and predisposes the athlete to fatal ventricular arrhythmias and sudden death. The myocardium is subsequently repaired by fibro fatty replacement which forms further substrate for ventricular arrhythmias.[25] The prevalence of genetic ARVC in the general population ranges from 0.2–1 in 1000; however, the prevalence in athletes is unknown. Most athletes are asymptomatic and SCD is usually the first presentation; however, a small number present with palpitation, dizziness and exertional syncope.

Although the right ventricle is amenable to endocardial biopsy, histological diagnosis of ARVC is rarely possible and potentially dangerous because the disease is patchy, characteristically affects the thinnest portions of the right ventricle (notably the right ventricular inflow and outflow tract) and requires transmural tissue sampling for definitive diagnosis.

The diagnosis of ARVC is difficult and generally requires a combination of electrocardiographic and imaging studies which include 12-lead ECG, surface average,[24] Holter monitoring, exercise ECG, echocardiography with contrast to improve endocardial definition and cardiac magnetic resonance.[26] Phenotypic manifestations of ARVC on the 12-lead ECG include T-wave inversions and prolonged QRS duration in right ventricular leads (V_1–V_3), epsilon waves (delayed repolarisation) and ventricular extra systoles of right ventricular origin (manifest with left bundle branch block morphology; Fig. 3). Holter monitoring and exercise testing are useful for identifying sustained or non-sustained ventricular arrhythmias with left bundle branch block morphology (Fig. 4). Echocardiography reveals thinning of the akinetic and dyskinetic

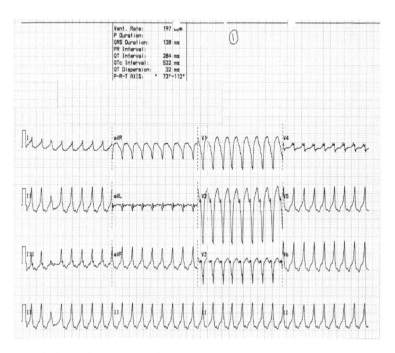

Fig. 4 Ventricular tachycardia or right ventricular origin (left bundle branch block morphology) in an athlete diagnosed with ARVC.

segments affecting the right ventricle or overt right ventricular dilatation and hypokinesia but may be normal in the early phases of the disease. The sensitivity of echocardiographic diagnosis is improved with contrast agents. Cardiac magnetic resonance imaging may be more sensitive than echocardiography for the diagnosis of ARVC provided it is performed by an experienced operator.

Disorders of coronary arteries and the aorta

Coronary artery anomalies and premature atheromatous coronary artery disease. Coronary artery anomalies (CAAs) are a relatively common form of congenital abnormality and are estimated to be present in 0.64% of the general population. They are a well-recognised cause of SCD in athletes and are second only to the cardiomyopathies.[27] Origins of the left main coronary artery or the right coronary artery from the wrong sinus are the most common anomalies associated with SCD. The resulting acute passage of the coronary arteries along the aortic wall causes their origins to become slit-like. During exercise, there is compression of the anomalous artery between the aorta and pulmonary trunk causing acute ischaemia and ventricular fibrillation. Almost all deaths in athletes occur in individuals during exercise and are mostly confined to individuals aged < 30 years. Many individuals are asymptomatic prior to death but recognised premorbid symptoms include exertional chest pain and syncope.

Premature coronary artery disease is almost always a manifestation of familial hypercholesterolaemia which has a prevalence of 1 in 500. Sudden death is almost always the first presentation in young athletes. Prodromal symptoms of myocardial ischaemia may be absent; however peripheral stigmata of hypercholesterolaemia including xanthelesma, corneal arcus, palmer and eruptive xanthomata are common and their presence should raise the suspicion of the disorder.

Marfan's syndrome is a collagen disorder caused by mutations in the gene encoding fibrillin. It is inherited as an autosomal dominant trait and has a prevalence of 1 in 5000. The condition is characterised by skeletal, cardiac and ocular abnormalities. Cystic medial necrosis in the tuna media of the aorta results in aortic dilatation and rupture or aortic dissection. Affected patients are excessively tall and, by virtue of the habitus, usually excel in basketball. Exercise-related increases in aortic pressure may expedite aortic root dilatation, dissection and rupture causing instantaneous death during sport.[28]

Valvular heart disease

Mitral valve prolapse and aortic stenosis. Mitral valve prolapse (MVP) is probably the commonest congenital valvular disorder and affects 3–5% of the general population. Most individuals are asymptomatic; in rare instances, the condition is associated with ventricular tachycardia. The exact mechanism for ventricular tachycardia is unknown. Only 60 cases of sudden death have been reported where MVP was the only abnormality identified in the literature and only three occurred during physical exertion.[29] The relatively high frequency MVP in the general population begs the question whether the identification of MVP in a victim of SCD is causal or coincidental. The current guidelines state that an athlete with MVP is at low risk of SCD unless there is a history of syncope or documented ventricular arrhythmias, family history of premature SCD, disabling and protracted chest pain during sport, or associated moderate-to-severe mitral regurgitation. Athletes with MVP as part of the spectrum of Marfan's syndrome or co-existent long QT are also precluded from participating in strenuous physical exertion.

Aortic stenosis due to a congenital bicuspid aortic valve is a rare but a recognised cause of SCD in young athletes which can be identified through basic screening efforts involving cardiovascular physical examination.

SUDDEN CARDIAC DEATHS DUE TO GENETIC OR CONGENITAL ABNORMALITIES PREDISPOSING TO PRIMARY ELECTRICAL DISORDERS OF THE HEART

About 2% of athletes who die suddenly do not have an identifiable cause at post mortem examination and, by definition, are victims of sudden adult death syndrome.[30] Experience from studies in first-degree relatives of victims of sudden adult death syndrome indicates that a proportion of these deaths are attributable to inherited ion channelopathies. Fatal tachyarrhythmias due to undiagnosed accessory pathways comprise other potential causes (Table 2).

Congenital long QT syndrome

The congenital long QT syndromes (LQTSs) are inherited as autosomal dominant or recessive traits and characterised by abnormalities in cardiac sodium or potassium ion channels. Abnormal shifts in electrical currents result in membrane instability during cardiac repolarisation and predispose to polymorphic ventricular tachycardia and ventricular fibrillation. There are currently 8 different identified loci accounting for the disorder termed LQT1–8, respectively, but LQTS1 (potassium ion channel), LQTS2 (potassium ion channel) and LQTS3 (sodium ion channel) account for approximately 95% of all known cases of the disorder. Adrenergic surges provoke ventricular arrhythmias, particularly in individuals with the LQT1 genotype.[31] Most deaths in sport occur in young females during swimming and are attributed to the adrenergic surge associated with diving suddenly into cold water. The disorder is usually diagnosed on a resting ECG which reveals a long QT interval in about 60% of cases. It is prudent to state that a

Table 2 Sudden cardiac deaths in structurally normal hearts

- Congenital long QT syndrome
- Brugada syndrome
- Catecholaminergic polymorphic tachycardia
- Short QT syndrome
- Wolff–Parkinson–White syndrome
- Right ventricular outflow tachycardia
- Coronary vasospasm
- Commotio cordis
- Electrolyte disturbances
- Hypo- or hyperthermia
- Drugs (amphetamine or cocaine)

prolonged QT interval is not part of the recognised spectrum of electro-cardiogaphic changes observed in highly trained athletes and that it warrants further investigation.

The prevalence of congenital LQTS in the general population is between 0.2–1 in 1000. However, based on the findings from screening programmes in athletes, we suspect that the prevalence of LQTS may be even higher than currently estimated. In the Italian screening programme, the prevalence of a long QT interval on the ECG of competitive athletes was 0.69%. Our own experience of screening competitive British athletes reveals a prevalence of 0.42%. The low death rate from sudden adult death syndrome in athletes in the context of a relatively high prevalence of long QT observed in this group suggests that many long QT mutations may run a relatively benign course.

Wolff–Parkinson–White syndrome

Wolff–Parkinson–White syndrome (WPW) is characterised by the presence of an accessory conduction pathway between the atria and ventricles with a predilection to re-entrant supraventricular tachyarrhythmias, which may degenerate to ventricular fibrillation. It is a rare cause of SCD in athletes. The prevalence of WPW syndrome is 1 in 750. The risk of SCD in WPW syndrome is believed to be approximately 0.4%. Most deaths occur in athletes with previous symptoms of palpitation, dizziness or syncope. The accessory pathway can be identified by the presence of delta wave and a short PR interval on the 12-lead ECG. Electrophysiological studies to assess the refractory period of the pathway are essential to gauge the risk of atrial fibrillation with high ventricular rates. Radiofrequency ablation is the definitive treatment in athletes with high-risk pathways who wish to continue to participate in competitive sport.

ACQUIRED CAUSES OF SUDDEN CARDIAC DEATH IN ATHLETES

In a few cases, SCD may be due to acquired causes, the commonest of which include viral myocarditis, illicit drug abuse and commotio cordis.

Myocarditis

Myocarditis is usually due to a viral illness and accounts for 7% of all SCDs in athletes. The inflammation and subsequent focal necrosis of the myocardium is thought to be the substrate for malignant ventricular tachyarrhythmias causing sudden death. Most affected individuals experience coryzal symptoms and a mild febrile illness but sudden death in a relatively asymptomatic athlete is the commonest presentation. Overt cardiac symptoms are rare and include chest pain, dyspnoea and palpitation. The ECG usually reveals non-specific ST and T-wave abnormalities but may be normal. Echocardiography may also be normal in mild cases. A raised serum cardiac troponin is useful in confirming the diagnosis in an athlete with a febrile illness associated with chest pain, palpitation and non-specific electrocardiographic abnormalities. Athletes with proven myocarditis should abstain from strenuous exertion and competitive sport for 6 months.

Commotio cordis

Commotio cordis refers to SCD from ventricular fibrillation resulting from blunt trauma to the chest wall. The precise frequency of the problem is unknown but it has been reported with increasing frequency in the past decade. The incidence is more common in children and adolescents due to relatively thin and compliant chest walls. Sports usually associated with commotio cordis include baseball, hockey, ice-hockey, karate and judo. The victim is often struck by an innocent appearing blow or projectile objects regarded as standard implements of the game. Sudden death is instantaneous.[32]

Animal experiments using a juvenile swine model have provided insights into the mechanism responsible ventricular fibrillation. Induction of ventricular fibrillation occurs following chest wall blows during a vulnerable window just before the peak of the T-wave. A rapid rise in left ventricular pressure follows which is thought to activate ion channels via mechano-electric coupling. The generation of an inward current via mechano-sensitive ion channels results in augmentation of repolarisation and non-uniform myocardial activation, and is the cause of premature ventricular depolarisations that trigger ventricular fibrillation in commotio cordis. Survival after commotio cordis is only 15% and only possible with prompt cardiac defibrillation. The velocity and hardness of the projectile object are recognised determinants of ventricular fibrillation. Several measures to prevent commotio cordis have been suggested, which include use of softer balls than traditional, standard, hard balls in hockey and base ball and the use of chest barriers in sports vulnerable to commotio cordis. Automatic external defibrillators in young athletic individuals vulnerable to such trauma have saved lives.

EVALUATION OF AN ATHLETE AT RISK

HISTORY AND PHYSICAL EXAMINATION

Most athletes are evaluated as part of cardiovascular programmes implemented by certain sporting organisations to exclude potentially sinister inherited or congenital cardiac disorders prior to acceptance for competition. Rarely, cardiovascular evaluation may be triggered because of symptoms of cardiovascular disease or a family history of premature cardiovascular disease or SCD in a first-degree relative. Ideally, athletes should be investigated at centres with expertise in conditions capable of causing SCD, particularly cardiomyopathy, as well as knowledge regarding the impact of cardiovascular training on the cardiac size to enable the differentiation of physiological adaptation from cardiac pathology.

Most athletes are asymptomatic but the presence of chest pain, dyspnoea disproportionate to the exercise performed, palpitation, dizziness or syncope during exercise are ominous symptoms and warrant thorough evaluation. It is prudent to ascertain any family history of premature cardiac disease or SCD in first-degree relatives as most conditions discussed above are hereditary. Ventricular arrhythmias in family members may present as syncope, epilepsy or unexplained drowning and enquiry into these circumstances may provide further important information regarding sinister familial cardiac disease. Where possible, it is important to obtain post mortem reports on first-degree relatives who have been victims of premature SCD as this may prove useful in differentiating death from a hereditary disorder such as HCM and a sporadic disorder such as CAA.

PHYSICAL EXAMINATION

General physical examination may prove useful in identifying a Marfanoid habitus and peripheral stigmata of familial hypercholesterolaemia. Cardiac auscultation may raise suspicion of aortic stenosis and approximately 25% of cases of HCM with resting left ventricular outflow obstruction.

12-LEAD ECG

The 12-lead ECG permits the diagnosis of WPW and congenital LQTS and provides vital information regarding the possibility of an underlying heart muscle disorder; the ECG is abnormal in over 90% of individuals with HCM.

The presence of deep (> 0.2 mV) T-wave inversions in leads other than III, aVr and V_1 should result in further investigation for cardiomyopathy. Contrary to previously published literature, our experience suggests that deep T-wave inversions are rare manifestation of cardiovascular adaptation in adult and adolescent athletes[33] but are common in HCM and may be present in almost any lead (Fig. 5). Additional electrocardiographic abnormalities in HCM include voltage criteria for left atrial enlargement, extreme left-ward axis, ST segment depression, pathological q waves and left bundle branch block. Although individuals with HCM commonly exhibit high voltage QRS complexes, the presence of isolated Sokolow–Lyon voltage criterion for left ventricular hypertrophy is rare in HCM and more suggestive of physiological cardiac adaptation. T-wave inversions in leads V_1–V_3 may be normal in juvenile athletes and Afro-Caribbean athletes but their persistence in Caucasian adolescent or adult athletes should prompt further investigation for ARVC. T-wave inversions may also present in dilated cardiomyopathy and LQTS.

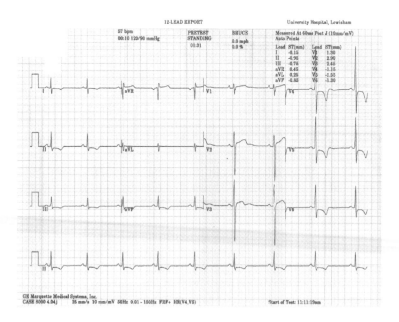

Fig. 5 ECG in individual with HCM showing deep T-wave inversions and ST segment depression.

ECHOCARDIOGRAPHY

Echocardiography is the gold standard investigation for the diagnosis of HCM and valvular heart disease and proves diagnostic in advanced cases of ARVC. The echocardiographic assessment of an athlete with chest pain or syncope should also involve identification of the origins[34] of the coronary ostia to refute the diagnosis of anomalous coronary origins as exercise testing lacks sensitivity and is invariably normal in these conditions.

FURTHER INVESTIGATIONS

Some athletes require further electrocardiographic, imaging and invasive electrophysiological investigations for the purposes of diagnostic clarification and risk stratification for SCD. Exercise testing and 24-h Holter monitoring provide prognostic information in HCM and diagnostic information in ARVC and LQTS. Cardiac magnetic resonance facilitates the diagnosis of ARVC and magnetic resonance coronary angiography is the investigation of choice for confirming the diagnosis of CAA. Electrophysiological studies provide prognostic information in WPW.

In the past 15 years, there have been major advances in the molecular genetics of HCM, ARVC and LQTS. However, marked genetic heterogeneity and incomplete knowledge of causal mutations does not currently allow timely diagnosis in the majority of affected individuals and failure to identify an abnormality when screening for known mutations for a particular disorder such as HCM cannot be regarded as exclusion as many mutations are yet to be identified. Continuing advances in molecular genetics and refinement of genetic analytical techniques holds promise and may prove invaluable in facilitating diagnoses in difficult clinical scenarios.

DIFFERENTIATING PHYSIOLOGICAL CARDIAC HYPERTROPHY FROM HCM AND ARVC

HYPERTROPHIC CARDIOMYOPATHY VERSUS PHYSIOLOGICAL LEFT VENTRICULAR HYPERTROPHY

Regular participation in regular sport is associated with modest increases in ventricular wall thickness and cavity size as well as enhanced diastolic filling. This reversible physiological cardiac remodelling enables enhanced left ventricular filling and the augmentation of a large stroke volume even at rapid heart rates for sustained increases in cardiac output.[35] A small proportion of male athletes involved in endurance sports may demonstrate extreme adaptations with left ventricular wall thickness measurements ranging from 13–15 mm.[36] Whilst most individuals with HCM have a mean left ventricular wall thickness of 18–20 mm, approximately 8% have morphologically mild hypertrophy in the same range. Therefore, a male athlete with a wall thickness of 13–15 mm represents a grey zone where the differentiation between physiological left ventricular hypertrophy is crucial since diagnostic errors have the potential for serious consequences. This distinction may prove challenging even for the most experienced sport cardiologists.

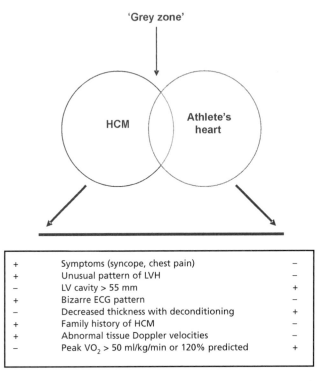

'Grey zone'

HCM

Athlete's
heart

+	Symptoms (syncope, chest pain)	−
+	Unusual pattern of LVH	−
−	LV cavity > 55 mm	+
+	Bizarre ECG pattern	−
−	Decreased thickness with deconditioning	+
+	Family history of HCM	−
+	Abnormal tissue Doppler velocities	−
−	Peak VO$_2$ > 50 ml/kg/min or 120% predicted	+

Fig. 6 Non-invasive methods for differentiating HCM from physiological left ventricular hypertrophy.

In the majority of athletes, the differentiation between athlete's heart and HCM is possible with 2-D echocardiography alone. Physiological left ventricular hypertrophy is homogeneous and associated with enlarged chamber size and normal indices of diastolic function. In contrast individuals with HCM often show bizarre patterns of left ventricular hypertrophy, small chamber size and impaired diastolic function. In equivocal cases further information regarding personal and family history, 12-lead ECG and cardiopulmonary exercise testing usually helps to resolve the clinical dilemma. The presence of a family history of HCM, bizarre ECG patterns including deep T-wave inversions and low peak oxygen consumption favour HCM. In some individuals, re-evaluation of the cardiovascular system with ECG and echocardiogram following a period (8–12 weeks) of detraining may be the only practical method of differentiating between the two entities (Fig. 6).[37]

ARRHYTHMOGENIC RIGHT VENTRICULAR CARDIOMYOPATHY VERSUS PHYSIOLOGICAL RIGHT VENTRICULAR DILATATION

The diagnosis of ARVC in athletes is challenging in the early 'concealed phase' of the disease and requires a high level of expertise. Minor electrocardiographic abnormalities in right ventricular leads, infrequent ventricular extra systoles of right ventricular origin and subtle morphological changes of the right ventricle, may be the only objective manifestations of the disorder and may

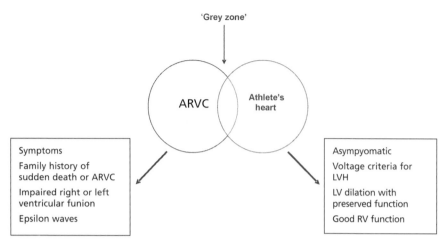

'Grey zone'

ARVC

Athlete's heart

Symptoms

Family history of
sudden death or ARVC

Impaired right or left
ventricular funion

Epsilon waves

Asympyomatic

Voltage criteria for
LVH

LV dilation with
preserved function

Good RV function

Fig. 7 Non-invasive methods of differentiating ARVC from physiological enlargement of the right ventricle.

overlap with physiological adaptation of the right ventricle to regular exercise. However, the presence of epsilon waves or late potential on the signal averaged ECG, non-sustained ventricular tachycardia of left bundle branch block morphology, regional wall motion abnormalities of the right ventricle favour the diagnosis of ARVC (Fig. 7). Unravelling the molecular genetics of ARVC and subsequent genotype–phenotype correlations have identified individuals with left ventricular involvement;[38] therefore, concomitant left ventricular dilatation associated with a depressed ejection fraction in an individual with a dilated right ventricle may also support ARVC although the diagnosis of dilated cardiomyopathy may also be possible in this situation.

MANAGEMENT OF ATHLETES HARBOURING CONDITIONS WHICH PREDISPOSE TO SCD

Definitive management of an athlete is dependent on the pathology identified. Most deaths are potentially triggered by physical exertion; therefore, the most pragmatic approach in preventing such catastrophes is to recommend abstinence from medium- and high-intensity competitive sports. Guidelines from the 26th Bethesda Conference and the European Cardiac Society recommend abstinence from strenuous physical exertion and competitive sport.[39,40] Persuading a high-profile athlete to refrain from competitive sports can be difficult and sometimes impossible. Some athletes may accept the risk of SCD and continue to be involved in competitive sports in order to be in the athletic arena.

β-Blockers are important in controlling symptoms in HCM, retarding aortic root dilatation in Marfan's syndrome and preventing syncope and SCD in congenital LQTS. The prophylactic use of implantable intracardiac defibrillators is recommended in some patients with HCM, ARVC and congenital LQTS who are considered to be at high risk of life-threatening ventricular tachyarrhythmias Pre-excitation syndromes are best managed with radiofrequency ablation of the culprit electrical pathways. Potentially fatal CAA are treated by surgical correction.

PREPARTICIPATION SCREENING

The sudden death of a young athlete is a highly visible event. The perceived well-being of the individual, potential life years lost, impact on peers and family members and the potential to prevent such tragedies by life-style modification and/or defibrillator implantation often call upon the medical and sporting community to implement preparticipation cardiovascular screening to permit identification of a potentially fatal cardiac disorders prior to competition.

The relatively low prevalence of conditions associated with SCD in young athletes means that several thousand athletes would have to be screened to identify a handful with a serious disorder and this questions the cost-effectiveness of such screening programmes. Most countries do not offer preparticipation cardiac evaluation to athletes. In the UK, preparticipation screening is confined to highly commercial sporting organisations such as the British Lawn Tennis Association and (football) Premier League.

The US has traditionally offered a long-standing, low-cost, preparticipation programme which is limited to medical history-taking and physical examination. Unfortunately, the efficacy of the programme for detecting potentially lethal cardiac disease is questionable since most athletes are asymptomatic and physical examination is rarely helpful. In the series of 157 deaths in the US, the preparticipation programme failed to identify all young athletes dying from HCM.[16]

In Italy, a unique, state-sponsored, mandatory, national, screening programme has been operating for 25 years. All competitive athletes are required to undergo physical examination as well as additional 12-lead ECG and limited exercise testing for the identification of predominantly hereditary or congenital abnormalities causing SCD. Athletes with abnormalities on the initial evaluation undergo further investigations and those diagnosed with a potentially serious cardiac disorder are disqualified from sport. The programme generates a small number of false positives creating anxiety and the need for further investigation in a healthy individual; however, it has been shown to be effective in identifying individuals with HCM,[20] the leading cause of SCD in young athletes world-wide.

Until recently, the true benefit of such a screening programme in reducing SCD in sport has been unresolved. However, a recent report on the 25-year experience of screening in Italian athletes has shown a reduction in death rate from 3.6 per 100,000 athletes to 0.4 per 100,000 athletes.[14] These figures represent a 90% reduction in SCD (predominantly due to reduced cardio-myopathy deaths) and provide the most compelling evidence available, to date, that cardiovascular screening does indeed reduce death rates in sport. The findings of the study have led to the endorsement of a cardiovascular screening programme with additional 12-lead ECG testing by the European Society of Cardiology and the International Olympic Committee.

The practicalities of adopting the systematic Italian approach *de novo* in countries such as the UK and US remains an enormous task when one takes into consideration financial constraints, lack of appropriate personnel and infrastructure. In the current era, the most pragmatic approach in the UK is to raise awareness of the familial nature of disorders causing SCD and their presenting symptoms amongst the athlete community.

Key points for clinical practice

- Sudden cardiac death in athletes is rare; the prevalence ranges from 1–4 per 100,000.

- Most sudden cardiac deaths in young athletes are due to hereditary or congenital abnormalities of the heart whereas deaths in older athletes are predominantly due to atheromatous coronary disease.

- Cardiomyopathies are the commonest cause of exercise-related sudden cardiac death in young athletes. Hypertrophic cardiomyopathy is the commonest cause world-wide.

- The vast majority of athletes harbouring potentially fatal cardiac disorders are asymptomatic.

- The mean age of sudden cardiac death in young athletes is 17.1 years and males are more vulnerable than females.

- A small proportion of athletes with potentially fatal cardiac disorders are capable of excelling in sport at national and international level.

- The evaluation of an athlete should occur in centres with expertise in the diagnosis and management of conditions causing sudden cardiac death.

- The differentiation of physiological cardiac enlargement from cardiomyopathy is possible in most cases but may prove challenging for the most able cardiologist.

- The early identification of athletes with potentially sinister cardiac disorders and subsequent disqualification from sport saves lives.

- In athletes diagnosed with serious cardiac disorders, sudden death is preventable with life-style medication and a variety of therapeutic modalities ranging from pharmacotherapy to cardiac surgery.

References

1. Paffenbarger RS, Hyde RT, Wing AL, Hsieh CC. Physical activity, all cause mortality and longevity of college alumni. *N Engl J Med* 1986; **314**: 605–613.
2. Powell KE, Thompson PD, Caspersen CJ, Kendrick JS. Physical activity and the incidence of coronary artery disease. *Annu Rev Public Health* 1987; **8**: 253–287.
3. Slattery ML, Jacobs DR, Nichmann MZ. Leisure time physical activity and coronary artery disease. The US rail-road study. *Circulation* 1989; **79**: 304–311.
4. Siskovick DS, Weiss NS, Fletcher RH. The incidence of primary cardiac arrest during vigorous exercise. *N Engl J Med* 1994; **311**: 874–877.
5. Maron BJ, Roberts WC, McAllister HA, Rosing DR, Epstein SE. Sudden death in young athletes. *Circulation* 1980; **62**: 218–229.
6. Maron BJ, Epstein SE, Roberts WC. Causes of death in competitive athletes. *J Am Coll Cardiol* 1986; **7**: 204–214.

7. Van Camp SP, Bloor CM, Mueller FO et al. Non traumatic sports death in high school and college athletes. Med Sci Sports Exer 1995; 27: 641–647.

8. Maron BJ. Sudden death in young athletes: lessons from the Hank Gathers affair. N Engl J Med 1993; 329: 55–57.

9. Maron BJ. Sudden death in young athletes. N Engl J Med 2003; 349: 1064–1075.

10. Waller BF, Roberts WC. Sudden death whilst running in conditioned runners aged 40 years or over. Am J Cardiol 1980; 45: 1292.

11. Noakes TD, Opie HL, Rose AG. Autopsy proved coronary atherosclerosis in marathon runners. N Engl J Med 1979; 310: 86–95.

12. Epstein SE, Maron BJ. Sudden death and the competitive athlete: perspectives on preparticipation screening studies. J Am Coll Cardiol 1986; 7: 220–230.

13. Maron BJ, Gohman TE, Aeppli D. Prevalence of sudden cardiac death during competitive sports activities in Minnesota high school athletes. J Am Coll Cardiol 1998; 32: 1881–1884.

14. Corrado D, Cristina B, Pavei A. Trends in sudden cardiovascular death in young competitive athletes after implementation of a preparticipation screening program. JAMA 2006; 296: 1593–1601.

15. Corrado D, Basso C, Rozzoli G, Schiavon M, Thiene G. Does sports activity enhance the risk of sudden cardiac death in adolescents and young athletes? J Am Coll Cardiol 2003; 42: 1964–1966.

16. Maron BJ, Shirani J, Poliac LC, Mathenge R, Roberts WC, Mueller FO. Sudden death in young competitive athletes: clinical, demographic, and pathological profiles. JAMA 1996; 276: 199–204.

17. Bille K, Fiquiras D, Schamasch P. Sudden cardiac death in athletes. The Lausanne recommendations. Eur J Cardiovasc Prev Rehabil 2006; 13: 859–875.

18. Thompson PD, Funk EJ, Carleton RA. Incidence of death during jogging in Rhode Island from 1975 through 1980. JAMA 1982; 247: 2535–2538.

19. Corrado D, Thiene G, Nava A et al. Sudden death in young competitive athletes: clinicopathological correlation in 22 cases. Am J Med 1990; 89: 588.

20. Corrado D, Basso C, Schiavon M. Screening for hypertrophic cardiomyopathy in young athletes. N Engl J Med 1998; 339: 364–369.

21. Sharma S, Elliott PM, Whyte G et al. Utility of cardiopulmonary exercise in the assessment of clinical determinants of functional capacity in hypertrophic cardiomyopathy. Am J Cardiol 2000; 86: 162–168.

22. Maron BJ, Klues H. Surviving competitive athletics with hypertrophic cardiomyopathy. Am J Cardiol 1994; 73: 1098–1104.

23. Maron BJ, Gardin JM, Flack JM et al. Prevalence of hypertrophic cardiomyopathy in a general population of young adults: echocardiographic analysis of 4111 subjects in the CARDIA study. Circulation 1995; 92: 785–789.

24. Fuller CM, McNulty CM, Spring DA et al. Prospective screening of 5,615 high school athletes for risk of sudden cardiac death. Sci Sports Exerc 1997; 29: 1131–1138.

25. Sen-Chowdhry S, Lowe MD, Sporton S, McKenna WJ. Arrhythmogenic right ventricular cardiomyopathy: clinical presentation, diagnosis, and management. Am J Med 2004; 117: 685–695.

26. McKenna WJ, Thiene G, Nava A et al. Diagnosis of arrhythmogenic right ventricular dysplasia/cardiomyopathy. Task force of the Working Group Myocardial and Pericardial Disease of the European Society of Cardiology and the Scientific Council on Cardiomyopathies of the International Society and Federation of Cardiology. Br Heart J 1994; 71: 215–218.

27. Taylor AJ, Rogan KM, Virmani R. Sudden cardiac death with isolated congenital coronary artery anomalies. J Am Coll Cardiol 1992; 20: 640–647.

28. Yetman AT, Bornemeier RA, McCrindle BW. Long-term outcome in patients with Marfan syndrome: is aortic dissection the only cause of sudden death? J Am Coll Cardiol 2003; 41: 329–332.

29. Jeresaty RM. Mitral valve prolapse: definition and implications in athletes. J Am Coll Cardiol 1986; 7: 231–236.

30. Behr E, Wood DA, Wright M et al., Sudden Arrhythmic Death Syndrome Steering Group. Cardiological assessment of first-degree relatives in sudden arrhythmic death syndrome.

Lancet 2003; **362**: 1457–1459.

31. Schwartz PJ, Priori SG, Spazzolini C *et al.* Genotype–phenotype correlation in the long-QT syndrome: gene-specific triggers for life-threatening arrhythmias. *Circulation* 2001; **103**: 89–95.

32. Madias C, Maron BJ, Weinstock J, Estes 3rd NA, Link MS. Commotio cordis – sudden cardiac death with chest wall impact. *J Cardiovasc Electrophysiol* 2007; **1**: 115–122.

33. Sharma S, Whyte G, Elliott PM *et al.* Electrocardiographic changes in 1000 highly trained elite athletes. *Br J Sports Med* 1999; **30**: 319–324.

34. Zipelli P, dello Russo A, Santini C *et al. In vivo* detection of coronary artery anomalies in asymptomatic athletes by echocardiographic screening. *Chest* 1998; **114**: 89–93.

35. Maron BJ. Structural features of the heart as defined by echocardiography. *J Am Coll Cardiol* 1986; **7**: 190–203.

36. Pellicia A, Maron BJ, Spataro A, Proschan MA, Spirito P. The upper limit of physiological hypertrophy in highly trained elite athletes. *N Engl J Med* 1991; **324**: 295–301.

37. Maron BJ, Pellicia A, Spirito P. Cardiac disease in young trained athletes. Insights into methods for distinguishing athletes heart from structural heart disease, with particular emphasis on hypertrophic cardiomyopathy. *Circulation* 1995; **91**: 1596–1601.

38. Norman M, Simpson M, Mogensen J *et al.* Novel mutation in desmoplakin causes arrhythmogenic left ventricular cardiomyopathy. *Circulation* 2005; **112**: 636–642.

39. Maron BJ, Isner JM, McKenna WJ. 26th Bethesda conference: recommendations for determining eligibility for competition in athletes with cardiovascular abnormalities. Task Force 3: hypertrophic cardiomyopathy, myocarditis and other myopericardial diseases and mitral valve prolapse. *J Am Coll Cardiol* 1994; **4**: 880–85.

40. Pelliccia, A, Fagard R, Bjornstad HH *et al.* Recommendations for competitive sports participation in athletes with cardiovascular disease: a consensus document from the Study Group of Sports Cardiology of the Working Group of Cardiac Rehabilitation and Exercise Physiology and the Working Group of Myocardial and Pericardial Diseases of the European Society of Cardiology. *Eur Heart J* 2005; **14**: 1422–1445.

Tony M. Heagerty

8

The current approach to the treatment of hypertension: a response to trials and guidelines

Hypertension now affects about 1 billion people world-wide and is estimated to cause 1.7 million deaths annually from cardiovascular disease.[1,2] Unless greater effort is paid to control hypertension, it will afflict 1.56 billion by 2025. The Australian Heart Foundation has reported that roughly half of all people with hypertension are completely untreated and that 8.1% of the Australian population with untreated high blood pressure already have cardiovascular disease or are at high risk of developing it.[3]

In recent years, a variety of guidelines has been published from national and international bodies addressing the issue of how to control hypertension and minimise the risks associated with it.[1-4] These have been greeted with varying acceptance rates and there is some evidence world-wide that the detection of hypertension has improved and in some acculturated societies the number of patients adequately treated is rising. However, there is still a large number of patients who have not been identified and, for those that have, treatment programmes remain unsatisfactory.

This review is designed to look at developments that have taken place since the most recent guidelines have been published. It will underline some of the recommendations that have been almost unanimous and addresses issues which have occurred or are outstanding subsequently as a result of evidence that has appeared in recent studies.

TREATMENT OF HYPERTENSION

WHAT LEVEL OF BLOOD PRESSURE SHOULD BE ACHIEVED?

In terms of a target level of blood pressure to be achieved with a management programme, the guidelines are largely in agreement. The evidence for the

Tony M. Heagerty MD FRCP FMedSci
Professor of Medicine, Division of Cardiovascular and Endocrine Sciences, University of Manchester, Core Technology Facility (3rd floor), 46 Grafton Street, Manchester M13 9NT, UK
E-mail: tony.heagerty@manchester.ac.uk

Table 1 What level of blood pressure should be achieved?

BHS (2004)[1]	< 140/85 mmHg (< 130/80 mmHg for diabetics)
ESH/ESC (2003)[2]	< 140/80 mmHg (< 130/80 mmHg for diabetics)
JNC-7 (2003)[3]	< 140/90 mmHg (< 130/80 mmHg for diabetics)
NICE (2004)[4]	< 150/90

stipulated levels comes from the Hypertension Optimum Treatment (HOT) Trial.[5] Admittedly, the levels chosen are arbitrary and the HOT study was looking at whether assiduous control of blood pressure was safe. The target levels stated in each of these guidelines are shown in Table 1. One will note also that there are separate targets for patients with diabetes and concomitant hypertension. Outcome studies of the treatment of mild-to-moderate hypertension have clearly demonstrated that: (i) the risk associated with the combination of diabetes and hypertension is far greater than hypertension alone; (ii) the protection afforded to such individuals is greater than that given to hypertensives without diabetes; and (iii) there is clear evidence that the control of hypertension in diabetic patients is much more difficult. For this reason, the targets are set at less than 140/80 mmHg and 130/80 mmHg, respectively. For all such individuals there should be counselling on life-style and these measures are clearly delineated and emphasised in all the guidelines. Most germane to reducing blood pressure is a reduction in weight as it is acknowledged that the majority of hypertensives are obese. Although a cessation of smoking will not necessarily reduce blood pressure *per se*, it will reduce the risk associated with blood pressure, which is multiplied when cigarette smoking is combined. Attention to diet will also have beneficial

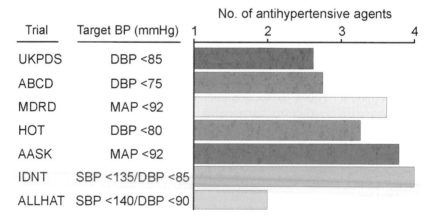

DBP, diastolic blood pressure; MAP, mean arterial pressure; SBP, systolic blood pressure.
Bakris GL *et al. Am J Kidney Dis* 2000;**36**:646–661
Lewis EJ *et al. N Engl J Med* 2001;**345**:851:860
Cushman WC *et al. J Clin Hypertens* 2002;**4**:393–404

Fig. 1 Multiple antihypertensive agents are needed to achieve target blood pressure values.

effects on blood pressure especially an increase in food stuffs rich in potassium and a decrease in salt-containing dietary constituents.

The inevitable consequence of setting strict and rigorous targets for blood pressure control across all age groups is that many patients will require more than one hypertensive drug (Fig. 1).

ARE ALL HYPERTENSIVE DRUGS THE SAME?

There has been a large amount of publicity suggesting that newer classes of drug may be superior to more established agents when it comes to protecting the circulation in the management of hypertension. Two points need to be made: (i) in repeated meta-analyses, it is the level of blood pressure control that is achieved that is paramount and not the drug involved;[6–8] and (ii) in attempting to reach the targets stipulated above, a large number of patients will receive two and maybe three classes of antihypertensive medication in addition to lipid-lowering and antiplatelet treatment. However, there is some evidence to suggest that, when it comes to protecting against the development of new diabetes mellitus, ACE inhibitors, angiotensin receptor blockers and calcium channel blockers do appear to be superior to diuretics and β-blockers. The evidence in favour of this has most recently emerged from a variety of studies including the VALUE and the ASCOT trials.[9,10] A number of mechanisms has been proposed including the possibility of these agents acting through vasodilatation and improving the blood supply to the skeletal muscle and decreasing insulin resistance in consequence. Also, there is the possibility of small changes in potassium influencing pancreatic function. It is important to point out that the evidence in favour of new classes of drug protecting against the development of diabetes comes from secondary observations in primary outcome studies. The most recent evidence provided by the DREAM trial[11] where the development of diabetes was a primary end-point was disappointingly negative when it came to the use of ACE inhibitors to protect against diabetes development. This notwithstanding, there is a body of evidence to suggest that diuretics and β-blockers are associated with an adverse metabolic profile and although they will be useful in combinations, their use as primary agents has been called into question (see below). In consequence, there is an increasing emphasis being placed on the earlier use of newer classes of hypertensive drug.

ARE β-BLOCKERS A WISE CHOICE?

There is no question that physicians should continue to use β-blockers in the area of secondary prevention such as post-myocardial infarction and also in selected patients with heart failure where there is good evidence that this class of drug is very effective. However, in the primary setting of hypertension management, the protection against stroke and heart disease has been disappointing and two meta-analyses have recently appeared strongly suggesting that β-blockers should no longer be first-choice therapy in hypertension management.[12,13] This has led to the UK Government advisory body, The National Institute for Clinical Excellence (NICE), to issue a new set of guidelines indicating that β-blockers should now be considered as fourth choice agents when it comes to the management of hypertension. This position is reinforced by further analyses contained within the recommendation[4] and supported further by an article by Kaplan and Opie[14] also suggesting that the evidence to support the use of β-blockers is weak. There are virtually no studies which have examined the use of β_1-selective β-blockers in the management of hypertension. It is possible that such agents are equivalent to newer classes of drugs in terms of circulatory protection when used to lower blood pressure; however, until further evidence is available, the view is that β-blockers should be used as add-on therapy rather than first-line treatment.

WHICH DRUGS SHOULD BE USED IN THE MANAGEMENT OF HYPERTENSION IN 2007?

Although some guidelines are currently being revised, the most recent recommendations in this area come from NICE.[4] Its conclusions were based on a systematic search of the literature performed on M-Base and Medline for randomised control trials comparing any combination of antihypertensive drug from among the commonly used five classes, namely ACE inhibitors (ACI), angiotensin receptor antagonists (ARB), β-receptor blockers, calcium channel blockers (CCB) and thiazide diuretics (TD). A total of 20 studies were found that satisfied the inclusion criteria for comparison using these agents. The Guideline Development Group that advises NICE drafted recommendations based upon clinical evidence provided by these studies. Then, a health economic analysis was conducted to balance the clinical outcomes and test the cost-effectiveness of the initial antihypertensive medications. The results of this analysis supported the preliminary conclusions and the document then provided a series of new recommendations (Fig. 2).

In hypertensive patients aged 55 years or over or black patients of any age, the first choice for initial therapy should either be a CCB or TD (Fig. 2). In hypertensive patients younger than 55 years, the initial choice should be an ACE inhibitor or, where this cannot be tolerated, an ARB. If initial therapy was

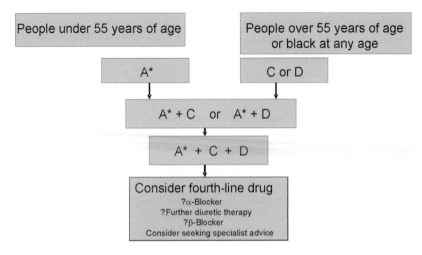

Fig. 2 Management algorithm for treatment of newly diagnosed hypertension.

with a CCB or TD and a second drug is required, then an ACI should be added. If initial therapy was with an ACI, then CCB or TD should be added. If treatment with three drugs is required the combination of ACI, CCB and TD should be used and if blood pressure remains uncontrolled, expert medical advice should be sought and a fourth drug should be considered such as a higher dose of TD, the addition of another diuretic or a β-blocker or α-adrenoreceptor antagonist such as Doxazosin. β-Blockers should be used in young patients if they have intolerance or contra-indications to ACE inhibitors or ARB or in women with child-bearing potential or patients with evidence of increased sympathetic drive. This is not to say that patients that are established on β-blockers and have their blood pressure well controlled to target should have their treatment stopped. Indeed, it is probably appropriate to continue them on their current regimen. The indications for using antiplatelet and lipid-lowering drugs are shown in Tables 2 and 3.

CAN BLOOD PRESSURE BE LOWERED TOO FAR?

Whilst there is no doubt that rapid reductions in blood pressure can bring about damage to the brain and the heart because of acute underperfusion, this is not a general consideration when oral therapy is instituted in a graded and controlled way. Also, concerns that were expressed by a J-shaped relationship between levels and vascular protection, namely that too low a blood profile would be associated with an increase in mortality and morbidity; meta-analyses have failed to confirm this. Indeed, as Table 4 demonstrates, in a series of recent outcome trials in the management of mild-to-moderate hypertension, the close-out blood pressure has incrementally fallen and there has always been a demonstrable protection in terms of risk reduction in the study participants. In consequence, the answer to this question is, unequivocally, 'no'.

Table 2 Aspirin/antiplatelet therapy

A 75-mg daily dose is recommended for hypertensive patients aged > 50 years who have:
•   No contra-indications
•   Blood pressure controlled to < 150/90 mmHg
•   CVS complications
•   Target organ damage
•   CV risk > 2%

Table 3 Statin recommendations

•   All patients up to 80 years with active CHD, PVD, CVD, diabetes if cholesterol > 3.5
•   Patients with 10-year CVD risk > 20% if cholesterol > 3.5
Aim to reduce by 30%
GMS: reduce total to < 5 mmol/l

Table 4 Blood pressure levels in other clinical trials

Trial	Publication	Final blood pressure (mmHg)
HOT	*Lancet* (1998)	142/83
CAPPP	*Lancet* (1999)	150/90
STOP-2	*Lancet* (1999)	159/81
ALLHAT	*JAMA* (2000)	136/76
NORDIL	*Lancet* (2000)	151/88
INSIGHT	*Lancet* (2000)	138/82
LIFE	*Lancet* (2002)	145/81
VALUE	*Lancet* (2004)	138/79
ASCOT	*Lancet* (2005)	136/79

SHOULD THE MANAGEMENT OF HYPERTENSION IN DIABETES BE DIFFERENT FROM HYPERTENSION WITHOUT CONCOMITANT CONDITIONS?

Most recent guidelines have all pointed to stricter blood pressure control in patients with type 2 diabetes. This is because there is clear evidence that the lower the blood pressure, the more protection is afforded to this high-risk group of individuals. Inevitably there will be the need for more than one antihypertensive drug. There is a compelling argument for the use of agents that interfere with the renin–angiotensin system such as ACE inhibitors or angiotensin receptor blockers especially at an early stage, not least because of trial evidence in favour of nephro-protection. However, in order to achieve the level stipulated in guidelines, a variety of drugs will be necessary and it is important to achieve these levels and minimise the side affects experienced by any patient. In other words, the most important maxim to adopt in such individuals is to optimise blood pressure control with the minimum of side affects using a series of antihypertensive agents, which are tolerated best by individual patients. The CARDS trial provided irrefutable evidence the majority of diabetic patients should be on lipid-lowering therapy.[15] Such patients also should be seriously considered for antiplatelet therapy in addition.

Key points for clinical practice

- It is the level of achieved blood pressure that largely determines outcome.
- Hypertension in diabetics needs even more aggressive control.
- Antiplatelet and lipid-lowering drugs need to be used in at-risk patients.
- β-Blocking drugs are no longer regarded as first-line treatment in uncomplicated hypertension.
- Evidence for a J-curve in mortality if blood pressure is lowered too far is limited..

References

1. Guidelines Committee: European Society of Hypertension – European Society of Cardiology. Guidelines for the management of arterial hypertension. *J Hypertens* 2003; **21**: 1011–1053.
2. British Hypertension Society. Guidelines for management of hypertension: report of the Fourth Working Party of the British Hypertension Society, 2004 – BHS IV. *J Hum Hypertens* 2004; **18**: 139–185.
3. Seventh Report of the Joint National Committee on Prevention, Detection, Evaluation and Treatment of High Blood Pressure. National High Blood Pressure Education Programme, August 2004.
4. National Institute for Clinical Excellence. Essential hypertension: managing adult patients in primary care. North of England Hypertension Guideline Development Group. London: NICE, 2004.
5. Zanchetti A, Hansson L, Ménard J *et al*. Risk assessment and treatment benefit in intensively treated hypertensive patients of the Hypertension Optimal Treatment (HOT) Study for the HOT Study Group. *J Hypertens* 2001; **19**: 819–825.
6. Blood Pressure Lowering Treatment Trialists' Collaboration. Effects of ACE inhibitors, calcium antagonists, and other blood-pressure-lowering drugs: results of prospectively designed overviews of randomised trials. *Lancet* 2000; **356**: 1955–1964.
7. Staessen JA, Wang JG, Thijs L. Cardiovascular protection and blood pressure reduction: a meta-analysis. *Lancet* 2001; **358**: 1305–1315. Erratum in: *Lancet* 2002; **359**: 360.
8. Turnbull F. Blood Pressure Lowering Treatment Trialists' Collaboration. Effects of different blood-pressure-lowering regimens on major cardiovascular events: results of prospectively-designed overviews of randomised trials. *Lancet* 2003; **362**: 1527–1535.
9. Julius S, Kjeldsen SE, Weber M *et al*. Cardiac events, stroke and mortality in high-risk hypertensives treated with valsartan or amlodipine: main outcomes of the VALUE Trial. *Lancet* 2004; **363**: 2022–2031.
10. Dahlof B, Sever PS, Poulter NR *et al*., ASCOT Investigators. Prevention of cardiovascular events with an antihypertensive regimen of amlodipine adding perindopril as required versus atenolol adding bendroflumethiazide as required, in the Anglo-Scandinavian Cardiac Outcomes Trial-Blood Pressure Lowering Arm (ASCOT-BPLA): a multicentre randomised controlled trial. *Lancet* 2005; **366**: 895–906.
11. DREAM Trial Investigators. Effect of ramipril on the incidence of diabetes. *N Engl J Med* 2006; **355**: 1551–1562.
12. Carlberg B, Samuelsson O, Lindholm LH. Atenolol in hypertension: is it a wise choice? *Lancet* 2004; **364**: 1684–1689.
13. Lindholm LH, Carlberg B, Samuelsson O. Should beta blockers remain first choice in the treatment of primary hypertension? A meta-analysis. *Lancet* 2005; **366**: 1545–1553.
14. Kaplan NM, Opie LH. Controversies in hypertension. *Lancet* 2006; **367**: 168–176.
15. Colhoun HM, Betteridge DJ, Durrington PN *et al*., on behalf of the CARDS Investigators. Primary prevention of cardiovascular disease with atorvastatin in type 2 diabetes in the Collaborative Atorvastatin Diabetes Study (CARDS): a multicentre randomised placebo-controlled trial. *Lancet* 2004; **364**: 685–696.

Mimi R. Bhattacharyya Andrew Steptoe

9

Triggering of acute coronary syndromes

The idea that an acute coronary syndrome (ACS) can be triggered by stimuli such as vigorous exertion or emotional stress has been studied extensively over the past 20 years.[1–3] Our purpose in this chapter is to: (i) review the evidence for triggering; (ii) outline the biological mechanisms that may be involved; and (iii) describe the clinical implications of this work. Although most research has focused on acute myocardial infarction, triggers may be relevant to the broader spectrum of ACS including ST segment elevation myocardial infarction, non-ST segment elevation myocardial infarction, and unstable angina, with related processes being involved in sudden cardiac death.

A trigger can be defined as a stimulus or an activity that produces acute physiological or pathophysiological changes leading directly to onset of acute cardiovascular disease.[1,3] There is no general agreement about how long before symptom onset the stimulus must occur to be regarded as an acute trigger, rather than a more general aetiological factor. Most research has focused on a 1–2-h period before the onset of symptoms, but there are possible triggers such as infection that have a longer time course. Triggering typically takes place against a background of long-term coronary artery disease (CAD), although Tofler and Muller[3] have argued that there is an inverse association between plaque vulnerability and trigger intensity, implying that intense triggers might precipitate acute syndromes in patients without vulnerable coronary lesions. Apical ballooning syndrome or takostubo cardiomyopathy may be an instance

Mimi R. Bhattacharyya BSc MBBS MRCP
Clinical Research Fellow, Psychobiology Group, Department of Epidemiology and Public Health, University College London, 1–19 Torrington Place, London WC1E 6BT, UK

Andrew Steptoe MA DPhil DSc (for correspondence)
British Heart Foundation Professor of Psychology, Psychobiology Group, Department of Epidemiology and Public Health, University College London, 1–19 Torrington Place, London WC1E 6BT, UK
E-mail: a.steptoe@ucl.ac.uk

of this phenomenon.[4] This syndrome is characterised by left ventricular dysfunction without clinically significant CAD, even though many patients have clinical symptoms including chest pain and elevated troponin levels. The syndrome may be driven by elevated catecholamines and sympathoadrenal activation following sudden extreme emotional distress.[5]

METHODOLOGICAL CHALLENGES

The scientific study of acute triggers presents particular methodological challenges. Since triggers are unpredictable, they are difficult to study prospectively. Most of the evidence is, therefore, collected retrospectively from survivors of ACS. Information of this type is susceptible to memory loss, biases concerning the social acceptability of the activities preceding onset (such as drug use or sexual activity), and to the influence of patients' private beliefs about the causes of heart disease. Clinical studies of the triggering of fatal cardiac events are difficult, unless the circumstances are witnessed by others. An additional problem is that of comparison groups or control periods. Vigorous exertion, smoking or emotional distress may occur frequently in patients' lives, so their association with ACS onset may be coincidental. Case-control methods can be used, but there are difficulties in identifying appropriate control groups.[1]

A special method of data analysis has been developed to minimise the limitations of interview-based studies. The case-crossover method involves questioning patients about possible triggers during the hazard period, and then in control periods, and comparing the two on a within-subject basis.[6] For example, ACS patients might be questioned about activities and emotions in the 2 h preceding symptom onset, and also about the corresponding 2 h that occurred 24 h earlier (pair-matched interval approach), or another time period such as the previous 12 months (usual frequency method). If a patient is habitually physically active or emotionally stressed, then he or she will report exertion or stress for both time periods. By comparing hazard and control periods, the relative risk that a trigger episode is followed by an ACS can be computed. This method has several advantages in the analysis of transient events, since self-matching removes selection and individual reporting biases. Any differences in chronic cardiovascular risk profile between cases and controls are also eliminated, reducing the risk of residual confounding.

TRIGGERS OF ACUTE CORONARY SYNDROMES

PHYSICAL EXERTION

Physical exertion has a paradoxical association with ACS: people who are regularly physically active or fit are at reduced risk, but vigorous exertion has been found transiently to increase the likelihood of both myocardial infarction and sudden cardiac death. The proportion of patients who reported moderate or vigorous physical activity in the hours before acute myocardial infarction onset was 23% in the Multicenter Investigation of Limitation of Infarct Size (MILIS) study, 18.7% in the Thrombolysis in Myocardial Infarction Phase II (TIMI-II) study, but rather lower in the Determinants of Myocardial Infarction

Onset (Onset) and Triggers and Mechanisms of Myocardial Infarction (TRIMM) study.[1,7,8] Using case-crossover methods, the relative risk of having engaged in vigorous activity in the hour prior to cardiac events was estimated at 5.9 (95% CI 4.6–7.7) and 2.1 (95% CI 1.6–3.1) in different samples. The paradox is to some extent resolved by the observation of a strong protective effect of regular exercise on acute triggering.[3] For instance, in the TRIMM study, the relative risk was 6.9 among those who exercised fewer than four times a week, compared with 1.3 for those who were more active.[7]

Vigorous activity is a trigger for sudden cardiac death as well as non-fatal events. A case-crossover analysis of deaths in the Physician's Health Study compared activity over the 30 min preceding symptom onset with habitual exercise levels measured by questionnaire.[9] The relative risk was 10.9 (95% CI 4.5–26.2) in patients who exercised regularly, increasing to 74.1 (95% CI 22.0–249) in sedentary individuals. More recently, Whang et al.[10] analysed sudden cardiac deaths in the Nurses' Health Study. Although the absolute risk during exercise was very low (estimated at less than 1 in 35 million hours of exertion), there was evidence of a transient increase in risk when participants were active. This was only significant among women who did less than 2 h of exercise per week.

These studies, therefore, show a consistent pattern, despite the variation in relative risks. Heavy exertion is an acute trigger for ACS, particularly in otherwise sedentary people, but the absolute risks are low and should not discourage regular physical activity. Several mechanisms implicated in ACS may be stimulated by physical exertion. Plaque rupture is associated with the majority of exertion-related deaths. An autopsy study of 141 men with advanced CAD who died suddenly following exertion showed plaque rupture in 68%, compared with 23% in those dying at rest, and haemorrhage into the plaque was also frequent.[11] Myocardial ischaemia during exercise testing is, of course, a common phenomenon, and physical activity also provokes ischaemia during everyday life in CAD patients. Epicardial coronary artery vaso-constriction has been reported during exercise in stenosed vessels. Physical exertion elicits an acute increase in sympathetic activity and release of catecholamines. The imbalance of autonomic activity in favour of sympathetic over parasympathetic tone can lead to cardiac electrical instability and risk of ventricular fibrillation. The haemodynamic changes associated with exertion may cause rupture of previously non-significant plaques. The catecholamine response to exercise stimulates surface expression of adhesion molecules, and there is a pronounced rise in the concentration of circulating interleukin 6 (IL-6). Physical exertion stimulates both coagulation and fibrinolytic pathways, and there is some evidence that more intensive activity tips the balance towards procoagulatory responses.[12]

INFECTIOUS ILLNESS

Upper respiratory and other infectious illnesses induce inflammatory responses and vascular endothelial dysfunction, so might be expected to increase risk of acute coronary events in vulnerable individuals. A study of a large UK database showed that there was a substantial increase in risk of acute myocardial infarction (RR 4.95; 95% CI 4.43–5.53) and stroke over the 3 days following physician diagnosis of a respiratory tract infection.[13]

SEXUAL ACTIVITY

The role of recent sexual activity as a trigger of acute myocardial infarction has been studied in both the Onset and Stockholm Heart Epidemiology Program (SHEEP) with similar results.[1] Sexual activity was reported within 2 h of myocardial infarction by 1–3% of survivors, with relative risks of 2.5 (95% CI 1.7–3.7) and 2.1 (95% CI 0.7–6.5). The absolute risk is very low, estimated at about one in a million, and is greater in sedentary patients, suggesting that the mechanisms may be similar to those operating with physical exertion. Sexual activity is often carried out as part of a loving intimate relationship. Since social support and good marital relationships are strongly protective for cardiovascular and other health end-points,[14] the benefits of sexual activity may offset the costs.

TOBACCO SMOKING

Smoking increases risk of coronary heart disease (CHD), and smokers have more procoagulant haemostatic profiles, impaired endothelial function and higher plasma IL-6 and C-reactive protein concentrations than non-smokers. Acutely, smoking increases catecholamine and cortisol levels, stimulates an elevation in heart rate and blood pressure, and impairs endothelial function.[15] Despite these effects, there is little evidence of direct triggering of ACS by tobacco smoking. This is because of the habitual nature of cigarette smoking; a heavy smoker is likely to have smoked tobacco within 1–2 h of symptom onset, but this may be no different from other times when an ACS did not occur. There is more evidence for triggering of ACS by substances such as cocaine in a small proportion of patients.[16]

ALCOHOL CONSUMPTION

There is a J-shaped relationship between alcohol consumption and CHD mortality in the general population, with the lowest levels in moderate drinkers. Moderate consumption is also protective in patients with diagnosed coronary artery disease.[17] It is possible that heavy drinking is a trigger for ACS, but definite proof is lacking. One study reported a protective effect of drinking up to 8 drinks in men and 4 drinks in women over the previous 24 h, in comparison with not drinking.[18] However, the drinkers who abstained from consumption in the previous 24 h may have been experiencing prodromal symptoms or cardiac problems, so may not be an appropriate comparison group. In a case control study of patients admitted for acute brain infarction, the relative risk for those who had consumed a large amount of alcohol in the previous 24 h was 4.19, while light drinking was not associated with increased risk.[19] Survivors of ACS who binge drink have a doubled mortality rate over the next 2–3 years.[20]

There can be difficulties in estimating the effect of factors such as tobacco smoking, drug use and alcohol consumption, since patients may not accurately report activities that they might consider socially unacceptable. It should also be remembered that many risk behaviours of this type can increase in frequency or intensity at times of emotional stress.

EMOTIONAL STRESS

Two broad strategies have been used to investigate emotional triggers of ACS. The first is to study the effects of stressful events that affect large numbers of people such as natural disasters or terrorist attacks. The advantages of this strategy are that the stimulus is objective, a population-based sampling frame can be used, and fatal as well as non-fatal cardiac events can be evaluated. Very often, however, the circumstances surrounding natural disasters or conflict are not well suited to systematic data collection, and most cardiac events take place in individuals who are not exposed to major traumatic events. The second method is to collect data from patients after they have suffered an ACS, asking them about their experiences in the period before symptom onset. This information is particularly susceptible to patients' beliefs or cognitive representations about the causes of heart disease.

Earthquakes

Rates of cardiac events following earthquakes have been studied in the US, Japan, Australia and Europe.[2] The most thorough analyses were carried out following the Northridge earthquake that took place in January 1994 in the Los Angeles area. Admissions for acute myocardial infarction in the local area increased from 149 in the week before to 201 in the week after the earthquake, and sudden deaths from cardiac causes increased from an average of 4.6 per day in the preceding week to 24 on the day of the earthquake. Only three cases were associated with unusual physical exertion. Studies of the Hanshin-Awaji earthquake in 1995 in the Kobe region of Japan showed similar effects, with a large increase in the number of patients admitted with acute myocardial infarction on the day of the event. Somewhat smaller increases in rates were recorded following earthquakes in Greece and Australia. By contrast, the 1989 Loma Prieta earthquake in the San Francisco Bay area was not associated with increased ACS admissions. A possible explanation may lie in the timing of these events. The Northridge earthquake occurred at 4:31 am on a Monday morning in winter, and the Hanshin-Awaji earthquake early on a Tuesday morning in winter. By contrast, the Loma Prieta earthquake struck at 17:04 pm on a Tuesday in October. There is a greater susceptibility to acute myocardial infarction in winter months, and a Monday morning in the winter may be a particularly vulnerable moment.

There have been few direct studies of the pathophysiological mechanisms that might underlie triggering by earthquakes. But a major earthquake happened by chance to take place in Taiwan as a group of patients with suspected CAD were undergoing Holter monitoring.[21] Spectral analysis showed a marked increase in the low to high frequency ratio for about 40 min after the earthquake, indicative of vagal withdrawal and heightened sympathetic cardiac drive.

War and terrorist acts

Studies of the impact of war and terrorist acts have produced mixed findings. Research in Israel showed that there was a 58% increase in total mortality on the day of the first missile strikes during the 1991 Gulf War that was largely attributable to acute myocardial infarction and sudden cardiac death.[22] It might be anticipated that terrorist incidents would have similar effects. A study of 200 patients with implantable cardioverter defibrillators (ICDs) in New York City showed an increase in serious arrhythmias following the attacks on 11 September, 2001;[23] however, there was no increase in cardiac death and admissions to acute coronary care in New York City in the period surrounding 11 September.[24]

Festivals, public holidays and sporting events

A controversial literature has emerged relating anniversaries and culturally significant dates with heightened cardiac mortality. It has been argued that mortality and vascular event rates are raised around Christmas and New Year, on birthdays, following Passover among Jewish Americans, and other significant dates.[2,25] The reliability of these effects has been doubted, and it has been suggested that they may depend on the comparison periods used. There is also evidence that sports fans are at risk of acute cardiac events when their teams lose dramatically. A good example is the study of the quarter-final of the 1996 European football championships between the French and Dutch teams. This match resulted in a draw at the end of extra time, and so went to a penalty shoot-out (sudden death) which the French won. An analysis of mortality in the complete population of Dutch men and women aged 45 years or more showed a relative risk of death from acute myocardial infarction or stroke of 1.51 (95% CI 1.08–2.09) for men on the day of the match, compared with the 5 days on either side, with no effect on women.[26] A question that arises with these studies is whether effects are driven by emotional responses or other factors that might coincide with these situations such as binge drinking, overeating, difficulties in obtaining medical assistance, and hospital staffing issues during holiday periods.[2]

ANGER AS AN ACUTE TRIGGER

Studies of triggers based on interviews allow patients' emotional experiences to be defined in some detail. These analyses have identified anger as a possible trigger of ACS. The Onset study interviewed 1623 patients, 39 of whom reported being very angry or furious in the 2 h prior to acute myocardial infarction (an incidence of 2.4%).[27] The odds of ACS onset following acute anger relative to no anger in the pair-matched analysis were 4.0 (95% CI 1.9–9.4). This effect was independent of age, sex, cardiovascular risk factors, and the use of β-blockers, although aspirin had a protective effect. Interestingly, the risk of anger triggering was inversely related to socio-economic status, so was more common in patients with little formal education.

Our group tested the role of anger as a trigger not only of acute myocardial infarction but of other forms of ACS in a cohort of 295 patients selected for their ability to recall the onset of symptoms, and excluding individuals with co-morbid conditions that might have affected mood and emotion.[28] Episodes of anger, including arguments with neighbours, anger during commuting, and family conflict, were reported by 17.4%. The odds ratio for onset of ACS after anger compared with no anger in the pair-matched analysis was 2.06 (95% CI 1.12–3.92). Anger triggering was again more common in socio-economically deprived patients, echoing the findings from the Onset study. Anger triggering was not related to cardiovascular risk factors, having a previous myocardial infarction, or to the presence of premonitory symptoms, but was more common in patients admitted with ST elevation myocardial infarction compared with non-ST elevation myocardial infarction or unstable angina.

ACUTE STRESS

The role of work stressors as acute triggers has been studied in a Swedish patient cohort.[29] It was found that work stressors such as having high pressure deadlines in the previous 24 h were associated with substantial increases in risk (OR 6.0; 95% CI 1.8–20.4), in comparison with the period 24–48 h before the myocardial infarction. This finding is significant in view of the evidence that high job demands, either alone or in conjunction with low control, predict future CHD.[14]

Other researchers have assessed general emotional distress. For instance, emotional upset was reported by 4.4% of patients in the 24 h prior to onset in the TRIMM study, with a relative risk in a case-control analysis of 2.7 (95% CI 1.1–6.6).[30] Stress resulting from exposure to heavy traffic has been evaluated in Augsburg, Germany.[31] The odds of myocardial infarction following exposure to traffic in the hour before onset of symptoms were 2.92 (95% CI 2.22–3.83).

ACUTE DEPRESSION

Depression has not been widely studied as an acute triggering of ACS, although it is relevant both to the long-term development of CHD and to prognosis following cardiac events.[32] In our recent study, we enquired about the occurrence of episodes of acute depressed mood prior to ACS symptom onset.[33] Discrete episodes of depression or sadness were reported by 18.2% of patients in the 2 h before symptom onset. The odds of ACS following depressed mood were 2.50 (95% CI 1.05–6.56) in the case-crossover analysis. When we limited analyses to severe depression only, the odds were greater (5.08; 95% CI 1.07–47.0). As with anger triggering, depressed mood in the hazard period was more common in lower socio-economic patients. It was unrelated to the clinical severity of the ACS, extent of coronary artery stenosis, or to a history of depression.

METHODOLOGICAL ISSUES

The use of case-crossover designs has greatly increased the confidence with which we can draw conclusions about triggers. These methods overcome many of the biases present in studying acute causes, but a cautious attitude to the evidence is still needed.[1] Neither case-crossover nor case-control designs can completely eliminate reporting biases. Even though the same individuals provide information for hazard and control periods in the case-crossover design, patients may emphasise triggers in the period just before symptom onset, as it is likely to be especially vivid. The control periods are more distant in time, and may lack the salience of the hours preceding symptom onset.

PATHOPHYSIOLOGICAL PROCESSES UNDERLYING TRIGGERING

The key pathological events underlying ACS are the disruption of coronary plaque and the subsequent development of a thrombus.[3] Plaque rupture is the commonest type of disruption, accounting for some 70% of fatal acute myocardial infarction and sudden cardiac deaths. Rupture occurs when the fibrous cap of the plaque is mechanically disturbed, or degraded by the action of matrix metalloproteinases released by macrophages. In other cases, injury is due to plaque erosion, as thrombus is superimposed on a plaque which is intact except for the loss of the endothelial cell layer. Vulnerable plaques are characterised by active inflammation, macrophage accumulation and activated T-cells, a thin fibrous cap with a large lipid core, and endothelial denudation with platelet aggregation. Episodes of high haemodynamic shear stress may stimulate plaque disruption, so acute increases in heart rate, blood pressure, myocardial oxygen demand, and coronary vasoconstriction are potentially important.

Atherosclerotic plaques are dynamic structures in which the constituents of the lipid-rich core and the fibrous cap regularly change. The most angiographically severe lesions are not necessarily at highest risk of rupture. It is evident from histological and intravascular ultrasound imaging studies that episodic rupture is a frequent event that only occasionally results in an ACS.[34] Two other factors, therefore, need to be taken into account. The first is the presence of a procoagulatory milieu. After plaque disruption, the local balance between circulating prothrombotic and thrombolytic factors will determine whether vessel occlusion takes place. The second is the presence of a

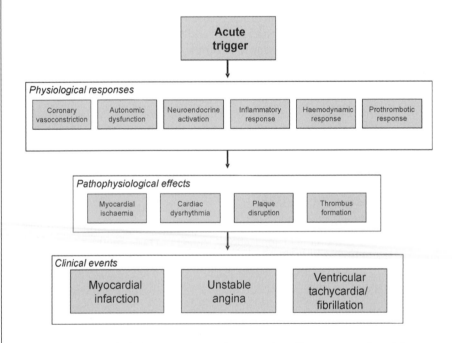

Fig. 1 Hypothesised links between acute triggers and cardiac events mediated through physiological responses and pathophysiological effects.

myocardium that is susceptible to ischaemia. Autonomic processes strongly influence outcome after plaque disruption, with sympathetic hyperactivity provoking potentially life-threatening ventricular tachyarrhythmias, while vagal activity is protective. When sudden cardiac death occurs in the absence of thrombosis, coronary spasm may be particularly relevant, whilst ventricular tachycardia and ventricular fibrillation are the most common causes of out of hospital cardiac arrest.

Figure 1 outlines some of the pathways through which triggers might contribute to the onset of acute cardiac events. Both sudden physical exertion and emotional stress stimulate sympathetic nervous system activation, vagal withdrawal, pressor responses, catecholamine release, increases in circulating IL-6 and other inflammatory markers, together with platelet activation and prothrombotic responses.[35] Emotional stress also induces coronary artery vasoconstriction in patients with CAD, particularly in regions of stenosis. Acute mental stress administered under controlled laboratory conditions induces transient myocardial ischaemia as defined by decreased ejection fraction, wall motion abnormalities or ST segment changes in around 30–50% of patients with CAD.[36] Stress-induced haemodynamic responses, particularly increases in systemic vascular resistance, coronary artery vasoconstriction, and microvascular changes may all contribute to transient myocardial ischaemia. CAD patients who are prone to emotional triggering of ACS show larger haemodynamic responses and platelet activation following acute stress compared with patients whose ACS was unrelated to emotional stress.[37]

CLINICAL IMPLICATIONS OF RESEARCH ON TRIGGERING

The identification of acute stimuli as triggers of ACS may have important implications for primary and secondary prevention. Tofler and Muller[3] have argued that a clinical strategy directed against risk of triggering should complement long-term risk management, and advocate a triggered acute risk prevention (TARP) approach. Triggering might be prevented by building resources that will ameliorate the impact of specific stimuli, while an understanding of the circumstances in which triggering is particularly likely may alert clinical staff to the increased risk experienced by vulnerable patients.

Table 1 summarises some of the potential approaches to managing ACS triggering. They are divided into two types: (i) interventions that could reduce the risk of cardiac events when patients are exposed to potential triggers; and (ii) precautions that could be implemented in high-risk situations. A good example of the first type is exercise training for reducing the risk of triggering by exertion. As noted earlier, the onset of ACS during vigorous exercise is greatly lessened in people who are physically fit and exercise regularly, so exercise training programmes should reduce the likelihood of exertion-related triggering. In the same vein, triggering by infectious illness could be reduced by increasing the uptake of influenza vaccination in people at elevated cardiovascular risk, while triggering by binge drinking and cocaine use may be lessened by targeted, tailored, health education and individual treatment.

The prevention of emotional triggering is more difficult. Informing patients about the possible dangers of emotional triggers must be handled delicately, since it is important not to give the impression that all excitement

Table 1 A comprehensive approach to the prevention of ACS triggering

ACS trigger	Tailored management
Reducing exposure to triggers	
Physical exertion	Exercise training programme
Alcohol, cocaine use	Public health education awareness programmes, individual treatment
Infectious illness	Influenza vaccination, antibiotic treatment, public health education awareness programme
Anger	Anger management programme
Stress and heightened emotion	Stress management, cognitive behaviour therapy, medication
Precautions in high-risk situations	
Festivals/public holidays/sporting events	Improved access to defibrillators, increased medical cover, public health awareness programmes
Natural disasters/industrial and transport accidents/terrorist acts	Programmes to increase public and clinical awareness of triggering, appropriate emergency care
Anniversaries, significant dates	Social support
Time-of-day effects	Appropriate medication schedules

and intense emotion should be avoided, and that the patient should withdraw into a restricted style of living.[38] Patients should be reassured that the absolute risk levels are low even though relative risk may be high. Nevertheless, there are cognitive behavioural therapies that can assist people with the inappropriate or excessive expression of emotions such as anger and distress. For example, anger management programmes can help people appraise situations differently, escape from the cycle of irritation and suspicion that spirals into outbursts of anger, and replace it with more measured methods of coping with difficult social interactions. Similarly, stress management training can help people cope with apparently overwhelming or mutually exclusive demands by more effective time management, prioritising, and re-appraisal of the importance of different pressures. Pharmacological methods may also be appropriate, including β-blockers and selective serotonin re-uptake inhibitors (SSRIs). There is some evidence that emotional triggering is less common in patients taking β-blockers, but this is not a universal finding.[27,28] Anger has been implicated in provoking vascular spasm,[39] and medications such as calcium channel blockers could be helpful in this regard.

Table 1 also details some of the precautions that might be adopted in situations in which triggering is more common. Both the public and medical profession need to be informed that festivals, major sporting events, and public holidays are associated with increased risk. Greater provision of defibrillators in public places and increased public education in their correct use could help reduce the number of triggered fatal ventricular arrhythmias and sudden cardiac deaths in these settings. Similarly, greater understanding of the impact of natural and human disasters on the heart could lead to more rapid and effective management of acute cardiac symptoms, thereby reducing morbidity.[23] Anniversaries of significant events such as bereavements or birthdays may be moments of increased risk for susceptible individuals, and steps could to be taken to ensure that they are not alone but have adequate social support on such occasions. Onset of ACS is especially common in the early hours of the day,[2] and is related to morning surges in blood pressure, neuro-endocrine responses and inflammatory cytokines. Appropriate scheduling of cardiovascular medication will help ensure adequate pharmacological coverage in the early morning hours, and some long-acting β-blockers and calcium channel blockers can reduce the frequency of early morning ischaemic episodes.[40,41] Low-dose aspirin has also been shown markedly to reduce morning peak of onset of myocardial infarction.[42]

The management methods outlined in Table 1 have not yet been systematically implemented to help prevent triggering, so their effectiveness in clinical practice remains to be demonstrated empirically. The prevention of triggering is challenging because the absolute rates are low. So, even in high risk cases, the chances of a trigger stimulus actually inducing an ACS on any particular occasion are small. It should also be emphasised that these special management techniques are supplementary, rather than alternatives, to sound risk factor control.

CONCLUSIONS

Studies involving a range of different methodologies provide convergent evidence on the role of diverse stimuli in the acute triggering of ACS. The pathophysiological processes underlying triggering remain to be fully elucidated, but include processes that may promote plaque rupture, together with a prothrombotic vascular environment that encourages thrombosis formation, and neuro-endocrine and autonomic processes stimulating rhythm disturbances. There has been little utilisation of this knowledge in clinical management to date, and the development of a systematic approach to risk stratification and prevention is a priority. The study of triggers promises important insight into the timing of acute cardiac events, and opens up possibilities for new methods of clinical management.

Key points for clinical practice

- Triggers are stimuli or activities that provoke acute pathophysiological changes leading to the onset of acute coronary syndromes (ACS).
- Most triggers operate over a period of 1–2 h before symptom onset.

Key points for clinical practice *(continued)*

- ACS triggering takes place against a backdrop of advanced coronary artery disease.

- Vigorous exertion leads to a transient increase in risk of ACS and sudden cardiac death, with larger effects in sedentary individuals.

- Binge drinking, cocaine use and acute severe respiratory infection may also act as triggers in susceptible individuals.

- Emotional triggers include acute anger and stress.

- Triggers provoke autonomic, inflammatory, neuro-endocrine and haemostatic responses that promote plaque disruption, myocardial ischaemia, thrombus formation and cardiac dysrhythmia.

- Although the relative risk of ACS onset is increased by triggers, absolute risks are low.

- Clinical management strategies include techniques that reduce exposure to triggers, and precautions that heighten alertness to high-risk situations so as to ameliorate the impact of triggers on cardiac health.

- Risk stratification of high-risk patients could be a precursor to individually tailored pharmacological and non-pharmacological management programmes that address both biological factors and the concurrent socio-economic and emotional environment.

ACKNOWLEDGEMENT

The authors' work was supported by the British Heart Foundation.

References

1. Strike PC, Steptoe A. Behavioral and emotional triggers of acute coronary syndromes: a systematic review and critique. *Psychosom Med* 2005; **67**: 179–186.
2. Kloner RA. Natural and unnatural triggers of myocardial infarction. *Prog Cardiovasc Dis* 2006; **48**: 285–300.
3. Tofler GH, Muller JE. Triggering of acute cardiovascular disease and potential preventive strategies. *Circulation* 2006; **114**: 1863–1872.
4. Gianni M, Dentali F, Grandi AM *et al*. Apical ballooning syndrome or takostubo cardiomyopathy: a systematic review. *Eur Heart J* 2006; **27**: 1523–1529.
5. Wittstein IS, Thiemann DR, Lima JA *et al*. Neurohumoral features of myocardial stunning due to sudden emotional stress. *N Engl J Med* 2005; **352**: 539–548.
6. Maclure M, Mittleman MA. Should we use a case-crossover design? *Annu Rev Public Health* 2000; **21**: 193–221.
7. Willich SN, Lewis M, Lowel H *et al*. Physical exertion as a trigger of acute myocardial infarction. *N Engl J Med* 1993; **329**: 1684–1690.
8. Mittleman MA, Maclure M, Tofler GH *et al*. Triggering of acute myocardial infarction by heavy physical exertion. Protection against triggering by regular exertion. *N Engl J Med* 1993; **329**: 1677–1683.
9. Albert CM, Mittleman MA, Chae CU *et al*. Triggering of sudden death from cardiac causes by vigorous exertion. *N Engl J Med* 2000; **343**: 1355–1361.

10. Whang W, Manson JE, Hu FB *et al*. Physical exertion, exercise, and sudden cardiac death in women. *JAMA* 2006; **295**: 1399–1403.

11. Burke AP, Farb A, Malcom GT *et al*. Plaque rupture and sudden death related to exertion in men with coronary artery disease. *JAMA* 1999; **281**: 921–926.

12. El-Sayed MS, El-Sayed Ali Z, Ahmadizad S. Exercise and training effects on blood haemostasis in health and disease: an update. *Sports Med* 2004; **34**: 181–200.

13. Smeeth L, Thomas SL, Hall AJ *et al*. Risk of myocardial infarction and stroke after acute infection or vaccination. *N Engl J Med* 2004; **351**: 2611–2618.

14. Kuper H, Marmot M, Hemingway H. Systematic review of prospective cohort studies of psychosocial factors in the aetiology and prognosis of coronary heart disease. In: Elliott P, Marmot M. (eds) *Coronary Heart Disease Epidemiology*, 2nd edn. Oxford: Oxford University Press, 2005: 363–413.

15. Ambrose JA, Barua RS. The pathophysiology of cigarette smoking and cardiovascular disease: an update. *J Am Coll Cardiol* 2004; **43**: 1731–1737.

16. Mittleman MA, Mintzer D, Maclure M *et al*. Triggering of myocardial infarction by cocaine. *Circulation* 1999; **99**: 2737–2741.

17. Mukamal KJ, Maclure M, Muller JE, Sherwood JB, Mittleman MA. Prior alcohol consumption and mortality following acute myocardial infarction. *JAMA* 2001; **285**: 1965–1970.

18. McElduff P, Dobson AJ. How much alcohol and how often? Population based case-control study of alcohol consumption and risk of a major coronary event. *BMJ* 1997; **314**: 1159–1164.

19. Hillbom M, Numminen H, Juvela S. Recent heavy drinking of alcohol and embolic stroke. *Stroke* 1999; **30**: 2307–2312.

20. Mukamal KJ, Maclure M, Muller JE, Mittleman MA. Binge drinking and mortality after acute myocardial infarction. *Circulation* 2005; **112**: 3839–3845.

21. Lin LY, Wu CC, Liu YB *et al*. Derangement of heart rate variability during a catastrophic earthquake: a possible mechanism for increased heart attacks. *Pacing Clin Electrophysiol* 2001; **24**: 1596–1601.

22. Kark JD, Goldman S, Epstein L. Iraqi missile attacks on Israel. The association of mortality with a life-threatening stressor. *JAMA* 1995; **273**: 1208–1210.

23. Steinberg JS, Arshad A, Kowalski M *et al*. Increased incidence of life-threatening ventricular arrhythmias in implantable defibrillator patients after the World Trade Center attack. *J Am Coll Cardiol* 2004; **44**: 1261–1264.

24. Chi JS, Poole WK, Kandefer SC, Kloner RA. Cardiovascular mortality in New York City after September 11, 2001. *Am J Cardiol* 2003; **92**: 857–861.

25. Saposnik G, Baibergenova A, Dang J, Hachinski V. Does a birthday predispose to vascular events? *Neurology* 2006; **67**: 300–304.

26. Witte DR, Bots ML, Hoes AW, Grobbee DE. Cardiovascular mortality in Dutch men during 1996 European football championship: longitudinal population study. *BMJ* 2000; **321**: 1552–1554.

27. Mittleman MA, Maclure M, Sherwood JB *et al*. Triggering of acute myocardial infarction onset by episodes of anger. *Circulation* 1995; **92**: 1720–1725.

28. Strike PC, Perkins-Porras L, Whitehead DL, McEwan J, Steptoe A. Triggering of acute coronary syndromes by physical exertion and anger: clinical and sociodemographic characteristics. *Heart* 2006; **92**: 1035–1040.

29. Moller J, Theorell T, de Faire U, Ahlbom A, Hallqvist J. Work related stressful life events and the risk of myocardial infarction. Case-control and case-crossover analyses within the Stockholm heart epidemiology programme (SHEEP). *J Epidemiol Community Health* 2005; **59**: 23–30.

30. Willich SN, Maclure M, Mittleman M, Arntz HR, Muller JE. Sudden cardiac death. Support for a role of triggering in causation. *Circulation* 1993; **87**: 1442–1450.

31. Peters A, von Klot S, Heier M *et al*. Exposure to traffic and the onset of myocardial infarction. *N Engl J Med* 2004; **351**: 1721–1730.

32. Nicholson A, Kuper H, Hemingway H. Depression as an aetiologic and prognostic factor in coronary heart disease: a meta-analysis of 6362 events among 146 538 participants in 54 observational studies. *Eur Heart J* 2006; **27**: 2763–2774.

33. Steptoe A, Strike PC, Perkins-Porras L, McEwan JR, Whitehead DL. Acute depressed mood as a trigger of acute coronary syndromes. *Biol Psychiatry* 2006; **60**: 837–842.

34. Naghavi M, Libby P, Falk E *et al*. From vulnerable plaque to vulnerable patient: a call for new definitions and risk assessment strategies: Part I. *Circulation* 2003; **108**: 1664–1672.

35. Steptoe A, Brydon L. Psychosocial factors and coronary heart disease: the role of psychoneuroimmunological processes. In: Ader R. (ed) *Psychoneuroimmunology*, 4th edn. San Diego, CA: Elsevier, 2007: 945–974.

36. Strike PC, Steptoe A. Systematic review of mental stress-induced myocardial ischaemia. *Eur Heart J* 2003; **24**: 690–703.

37. Strike PC, Magid K, Whitehead DL *et al*. Pathophysiological processes underlying emotional triggering of acute cardiac events. *Proc Natl Acad Sci USA* 2006; **103**: 4322–4327.

38. Thompson DR, Lewin RJ. Coronary disease. Management of the post-myocardial infarction patient: rehabilitation and cardiac neurosis. *Heart* 2000; **84**: 101–105.

39. Boltwood MD, Taylor CB, Burke MB, Grogin H, Giacomini J. Anger report predicts coronary artery vasomotor response to mental stress in atherosclerotic segments. *Am J Cardiol* 1993; **72**: 1361–1365.

40. Deanfield JE, Detry JM, Lichtlen PR *et al*. Amlodipine reduces transient myocardial ischemia in patients with coronary artery disease: double-blind Circadian Anti-Ischemia Program in Europe (CAPE Trial). *J Am Coll Cardiol* 1994; **24**: 1460–1467.

41. Deedwania PC, Pool PE, Thadani U, Eff J. Effect of morning versus evening dosing of diltiazem on myocardial ischemia detected by ambulatory electrocardiographic monitoring in chronic stable angina pectoris. *Am J Cardiol* 1997; **80**: 421–425.

42. Ridker PM, Manson JE, Buring JE, Muller JE, Hennekens CH. Circadian variation of acute myocardial infarction and the effect of low-dose aspirin in a randomized trial of physicians. *Circulation* 1990; **82**: 897–902.

Ghada W. Mikhail

10

Coronary heart disease in women: under-diagnosed and under-treated

Cardiovascular disease remains the leading cause of death in men and women world-wide exceeding the number of deaths from all cancers combined. In the UK, cardiovascular disease was responsible for over 216,000 deaths in 2004.[1] Cardiovascular disease, including stroke, is responsible for 36% of deaths in women compared to 4% of deaths caused by breast cancer with coronary heart disease (CHD) killing almost 4 times more women than breast cancer.[1] In Europe, cardiovascular disease kills a higher percentage of women (55%) than men (43%).[2]

It is well established that the prevalence and incidence of cardiovascular disease in both men and women increases with age.[3] The prevalence of CHD is lower in younger women compared to men, but with increasing age there is a significant rise in CHD seen in women with a clear narrowing in gender differences. Yet CHD is still considered a disease of men and there is little recognition of its importance in women. Many women, themselves, lack the basic awareness that CHD is their main killer, with their biggest fear being breast cancer. Of greater concern, however, is the fact that there appears to be a disturbing lack of a general understanding and awareness of cardiovascular disease in women amongst healthcare professionals.

RISK FACTORS

Age is an important risk factor for both men and women. At the time of presentation, women tend to be 10 years older than men and, at the time of their first myocardial infarction, they are usually 20 years older.[4,5] This is largely due to the protective effects of oestrogen up until the menopause. In

Ghada W. Mikhail BSc MD MRCP
Consultant Cardiologist and Honorary Senior Lecturer, Imperial College London, St Mary's Hospital
NHS Trust, Praed Street, London W2 1NY, UK
E-mail: g.mikhail@btopenworld.com

addition, risk factors for coronary disease tend to predominate and have a higher prevalence in older women. As CHD is a disease of the 'older woman', many women believe that reducing risk factors can be postponed. Furthermore, the misconception and lack of awareness amongst women of the importance of cardiovascular disease is a major cause of morbidity and mortality and hinders their active reduction of risk factors.

Although risk factors are common to both genders, diabetic women have a higher risk of CHD mortality than men. Diabetes increases the risk of CHD 2.5-fold in men compared to over 4-fold in women. When mortality is adjusted for other cardiovascular risk factors, however, there is no difference in outcomes according to gender.[6] Systemic hypertension is associated with a 2–3-fold increased risk of coronary events in women with isolated systolic hypertension being the main form of hypertension seen in menopausal women.[4] In addition, more women than men develop hypertension in their later years (above 45 years).[7] In women, total cholesterol levels tend to peak approximately 10 years later than in men. Although elevated cholesterol levels are associated with increased cardiovascular events in both genders, low levels of high-density lipoprotein (HDL) appear to be a better predictor of coronary risk in women, especially in older women, compared to high low-density lipoprotein (LDL) levels.[4] Furthermore, high triglyceride levels are associated with a greater risk for women compared to men.[4] There is clear evidence that lipid lowering therapy, especially with statins, reduces the risk of cardiovascular events in both genders. Women, however, appear to be less effectively treated and do not reach the required cholesterol levels specified by guidelines.[8]

Although smoking poses significant cardiovascular risk in both genders, women who smoke have almost twice the risk of coronary events with a relative risk of 2.24 for women compared with a 1.43 for men.[9] There is also a higher risk in young women who smoke and who use oral contraceptives. Although the prevalence of tobacco use is slighter higher in men than in women, the decrease in smoking rates appears to be less in women than in men. Obesity and physical inactivity are also associated with significant cardiovascular risk in both genders and metabolic syndrome has a higher prevalence in women than in men.[8]

PRESENTATION AND INVESTIGATIONS

Coronary heart disease in women continues to pose a challenge to the physician. There are features of heart disease which are unique to women, including the presenting symptoms, investigations, treatment and overall prognosis. Compared to men, women tend to present with more atypical symptoms such as breathless, upper back pain, burning in the chest, abdominal discomfort, nausea or fatigue making the diagnosis more difficult. Women are also less likely to seek medical help and their presentation tends to be late in their disease process. They are also less likely to undergo appropriate investigations such as coronary angiography.[10] This, together with their late presentation to hospital, may well result in delays in receiving effective treatment.

As women with CHD continue to go unrecognised and under-treated, it is imperative that timely and accurate diagnosis is made in order to institute early preventative and therapeutic measures. In all age groups, women are less likely than men to have obstructive coronary artery disease including triple vessel and left main coronary artery disease. This decreased prevalence in women, therefore, increases the rates of false positive results and decreases the diagnostic accuracy of non-invasive tests. The exercise electrocardiogram only moderately predicts CHD in females. Exercise testing has a sensitivity and specificity of 61% and 71%, respectively, compared to 68% and 77%, respectively, in men.[4] In addition, the exercise test may not be as useful in women because of the large number of women who tend to have a lower exercise capacity and who are unable to exercise to an appropriate intensity. The American College of Cardiology/American Heart Association (ACC/AHA) Task Force on Exercise Testing has also stated the lower sensitivity of the exercise ECG in women compared to men[11] and proposed that non-invasive imaging may be a better first choice for women. Non-invasive imaging such as myocardial perfusion scans, although more sensitive and specific in women compared to exercise testing, continue to pose a challenge. The reasons are: (i) CHD is less prevalent before the menopause; (ii) women have smaller sized coronary vessels and less obstructive CHD compared to their male counterparts; and (iii) the presence of breast tissue as well as the increased body fat seen in women can lead to artefacts and attenuation during non-invasive imaging.

The ACC/AHA guidelines recommend that symptomatic women with an intermediate probability of CHD should be investigated with an exercise test as the initial test of choice.[12] Stress echocardiography and stress myocardial gated perfusion SPECT imaging are both recommended for symptomatic women with an intermediate-to-high pretest probability of CHD and who have an abnormal resting 12-lead ECG as well as for symptomatic women with established coronary artery disease.[12]

DIAGNOSIS AND TREATMENT

PERCUTANEOUS CORONARY INTERVENTION

Gender differences in coronary revascularisation exist with the majority of trials and registries showing a worse clinical outcome in women.[13–19] The recent Euro Heart Survey in the management and clinical outcomes of stable angina investigated 3779 patients of which 42% were women.[10] Women were less likely to be referred for coronary angiography (OR 0.59; 95% CI 0.48–0.72) compared to men.[10] Furthermore, women with confirmed coronary artery disease were less likely to undergo revascularisation compared to men and were twice as likely to suffer a non-fatal myocardial infarction or death during the first year (HR 2.09; 95% CI 1.13–3.85).[10] This worse outcome is mostly explained by the higher risk profile seen in women.[20] At the time a woman presents with coronary artery disease, she is older and has more co-morbid factors such as diabetes mellitus, hypertension, hypercholesterolaemia, heart failure and peripheral vascular disease. Women also have smaller coronary arteries making them more difficult to revascularise both percutaneously and surgically.[21] In clinical trials and registries, however, adjustment for these co-morbid factors demonstrates that the female gender *per se* is not responsible for the worse clinical outcome.[22–24] Furthermore, a number of studies have demonstrated no gender differences in long-term mortality (longer than 1 year) following percutaneous coronary intervention (PCI).[18,23,25–27]

In recent years, with improvement in interventional techniques and devices, there has been a general trend towards improved outcomes in women undergoing coronary revascularisation.[22,23,28,29] Registries from the late 1980s and early 1990s, which compared gender-related differences following plain balloon angioplasty have shown a lower procedural rate, a higher complication rate (death, dissection, abrupt vessel closure, vasospasm and ventricular fibrillation) in women.[30] Later studies, however, have shown a general improvement in outcome in women undergoing PCI. Data from the NHLBI Dynamic Percutaneous Coronary Intervention Registry, reported in 2002, also showed a general improvement in the overall success rate in women undergoing PCI, despite women having more co-morbid factors at the time of angioplasty.[28] In the Northern New England Cardiovascular Disease Study Group, gender differences in outcome following PCI were studied in 33,666 patients from 1994 to 1999.[29] In this study, there was a greater use of stents (> 75% in 1999). Although women had more co-morbid factors, there was a reduction over time in procedure related myocardial infarction (by 29.7%, P_{trend} = 0.378) and need for emergency coronary artery bypass graft (CABG) surgery (in 1999: 0.06%, P_{trend} = 0.001) with no significant differences in mortality between genders (mean 1.21% in women, 1.06% in men; P = 0.096). Data from the National Cardiovascular Network (NTN) from 1994–1998 in almost 110,000 patients was published in 2001 by Peterson *et al*.[22] In this study, 33% were women and stents were used in 37% of them. Despite procedural success being about 90% in both genders, women continued to have a higher mortality after stent implantation compared to men (1.8% versus 1.0%; P < 0.001). Women were twice as likely to have a stroke (0.4% versus 0.2%; P < 0.001), vascular complications (5.4% versus 2.7%; P < 0.001) or myocardial infarction (odds ratio [OR] 1.28; 95% CI 1.1–1.5). Following adjustment for base-line risk factors especially body surface area, there were no gender differences in mortality risks.[22] A pooled analysis of 7 prospective investigational device exemption (IDE) stent trials was performed in 7171 patients (2179 women) who underwent elective stenting with a tubular slotted stent design.[31] In this study, women were older (66 years versus 61 year; P = 0.001), had more diabetes (27% versus 18%; P = 0.001), hypertension (67% versus 53%; P = 0.001) and smaller vessel size (3.03 ± 0.54 mm versus 2.90 ± 0.49 mm; P = 0.001) compared to men. Although women had a higher frequency of co-morbid factors, women had a similar unadjusted in-hospital mortality compared to their male counterparts (0.28% versus 0.14%; P = NS). In addition, there was no difference in periprocedural myocardial infarction or need for CABG. At 1 year, the mortality risk was higher in women compared to men (2.25% versus 1.44%; P = 0.15). After adjusting for gender differences in co-morbid factors, this difference was no longer apparent between men and women (OR = 1.2, P = 0.383).[31]

Despite women having smaller vessel size and more co-morbid factors such as diabetes mellitus at the time of presentation with coronary artery disease, various studies have reported either similar or lower target vessel revascularisation in women compared to men.[27,30,32,33] In a meta-analysis of 31 studies, gender did not appear to have an influence on the rate of restenosis.[32] In contrast, a more recent study in 4374 consecutive patients (1025 women and

3349 men) demonstrated that women had significantly lower restenosis compared to men.[33] Clinical restenosis was present in 14.8% of women compared to 17.5% of men (P = 0.048).[12] The incidence of angiographic restenosis was also significantly lower in women compared to men (28.9% versus 33.9%; P = 0.01).[33] This is an unexpected finding considering the fact that women have smaller coronary arteries and a higher incidence of diabetes mellitus. A possible explanation for gender differences in restenosis rates is the lower rate of follow-up revascularisation in women. This may either reflect a referral bias amongst women who are less likely to be admitted for subsequent revascularisation or a true reduction in the need for repeat revascularisation. A further possible explanation could be that the protective effect of oestrogen may attenuate the response of the vessel wall to balloon injury. Furthermore, oestrogen may prevent restenosis by accelerating endothelial cell growth resulting in the increased production of nitric oxide.[33] It must also be noted that the above studies were performed using bare metal stents. A recent study investigated gender-based outcomes using the Paclitaxel eluting TAXUS stent.[24] In this study, 187 women received the TAXUS stent. Compared to men, women were older, had more hypertension, diabetes mellitus, renal impairment, unstable angina and heart failure. Although women had a higher unadjusted 1-year rates of target lesion revascularisation compared to men (7.6% versus 3.2%; P = 0.03), female gender *per se* was not an independent predictor of target lesion or target vessel revascularisation after TAXUS stent implantation. Multivariate analysis demonstrated that the increase in absolute revascularisation rates seen in women compared to men was mainly because of the increased incidence of co-morbid factors in women, including diabetes mellitus, body surface area and small reference vessel diameter. Furthermore, the TAXUS stent resulted in an almost identical 70% reduction in angiographic restenosis in both sexes. In women, randomisation to the TAXUS stent was the only independent predictor of a reduction in restenosis.[24] This study, therefore, concluded that the benefits of TAXUS stents in reducing clinical and angiographic restenosis were applicable to both genders.[24] Similarly, the SIRIUS trial using the Sirolimus eluting stent in patients with *de novo* coronary artery lesions demonstrated that restenosis rates, reductions in target vessel revascularisation and major cardiac events at 1 year were similar in both genders.[34]

Studies from the 1990s have shown that women, because of their smaller vessel size, had had more frequent peripheral vascular complications compared to men. With the advancement of interventional techniques, smaller sheath sizes as well as weight-adjusted heparin are now current practice and have helped to reduce vascular complications in women. The benefits of adjunctive medical therapy in women appear to be beneficial, although their use may be complicated by a higher prevalence of bleeding complications. The pooled analysis from the EPIC (Evaluation of 7E3 for the Prevention of Ischemic Complications), EPILOG (Evaluation in Percutaneous Transluminal Coronary Angioplasty to Improve Long-Term Outcome with Abciximab GP IIb/IIIa Blockade) and EPISTENT (Evaluation of Platelet IIb/IIIa Inhibitor for Stenting) trials have shown that abciximab reduced the 30-day major adverse cardiac events (MACE) in women from 12.5% to 6.5% (P < 0.0001).[35] Although women had a higher rate of major and minor bleeding complications with abciximab compared to men, in women major bleeding was similar with and without abciximab (3.0% versus 2.9%; P = 0.96) with a small significant increased risk of minor bleeding (6.7% versus 4.7%; $P = 0.01$) with abciximab versus placebo, respectively.[35] The gender sub-analysis of the CADILLAC (Controlled Abciximab and Device Investigation to Lower Late Angioplasty Complications) investigated 2082 patients with acute myocardial infarction who were treated with primary angioplasty with or without the use of abciximab.[23] Of the total study population, 27% were female. The unadjusted MACE rate at 1 year was higher in women than men (23.9% versus 15.3%; $P < 0.001$), respectively. Female gender was an independent predictor of bleeding complications and MACE. However, the presence of co-morbid factors and body surface area, but not gender, predicted 1-year death. Also, the addition of abciximab to primary stenting reduced the 30-day target vessel revascularisation without increasing bleeding risk in females.[23]

Although heparin has been conventionally used during PCI, the benefit of the direct thrombin inhibitor, bivalirudin, in women has been shown in REPLACE 2 (Randomization Evaluation in PCI Linking Angiomax to Reduced Clinical Events).[36] This study demonstrated that bivalirudin with provisional glycoprotein IIb/IIIa inhibition was not inferior to heparin plus planned glycoprotein IIb/IIIa blockade in the prevention of acute ischaemic end-points.[36] In all patient subgroups, there was a non-significant trend towards lower 1-year mortality with bivalirudin which was of greatest magnitude in the high-risk patients such as women.[36] In addition, the use of bivalirudin was also associated with significantly less bleeding at 30 days after PCI (2.4% versus 4.1%; $P < 0.001$).

ACUTE CORONARY SYNDROMES

Women with acute coronary syndromes (ACSs) tend to be older and are more likely to have diabetes mellitus and hypertension.[4] An elevated troponin level, however, equally predicted the risk for men and women for mortality. In the Euro Heart Survey of ACS, women under 65 years were more likely to present with unstable angina and were less likely to have ST elevation myocardial infarction compared to men.[37] Women older than 65 years, however, had a similar distribution of presentation and diagnosis compared to men.[37] The Fragmin and fast Revascularization during InStability in Coronary artery disease (FRISC II) study, compared an early invasive therapy with revascularisation within 7 days to a conservative strategy.[38] At 12 months, there was no difference in death, myocardial infarction rate for women in the invasive versus non-invasive groups (12.4% versus 10.5%; $P = NS$), respectively. This is in contrast to the favourable effect seen in the invasive group in men (9.6% versus 15.8%; $P < 0.001$). When comparing both genders, however, there was a significant difference ($P = 0.008$) with a worse outcome seen in women undergoing early invasive therapy with a suggestion of possible harm in females.[38] The notably higher mortality in patients undergoing CABG in this study (9.9% in women versus 1.2% in men; $P < 0.001$) may have accounted for the worse outcome seen in women in the revascularisation group.[38] Furthermore, the delay in the timing of the intervention may also have contributed to the worse outcome seen in women. Similar findings were demonstrated in the Randomized Intervention Trial of unstable Angina-3 (RITA-3),[39] where an early invasive therapy had no benefit for women and was associated with a worse outcome. At 1 year, death or myocardial infarction occurred in 5.1% versus 8.6% of women and 10.1% versus 7.0% of men in the conservative and invasive groups, respectively. In contrast, in the Thrombolysis In Myocardial Infarction 18 (TACTICS-TIMI 18) trial, an early invasive strategy (within 48 h of presentation) was equally beneficial in both genders with an improved benefit in women at high risk (dynamic ST segment changes, elevated troponin level; OR 0.47, 95% CI 0.26–0.83).[40] From the above trials, the best strategy in terms of invasive versus non-invasive therapy in the setting of ACS in women remains controversial with the suggestion that only women at high risk benefit from an early invasive therapy. As well as the delay in the timing of intervention, and the high risk of women treated with CABG in the FRISC II trial, other possible explanations that may account for the differences between TACTICS-TIMI 18, FRISC-II and RITA III include the apparent low rate of events for women in the conservative arm in the latter two studies. The above trials, however, were conducted before the era of drug eluting stents. With the current practice which includes an increasing use of drug eluting stents and glycoprotein IIb/IIIa inhibitors as well as a shorter delay in the timing of coronary intervention, more studies are needed to evaluate further gender differences in the use of early invasive therapy in the setting of ACS.

ACUTE MYOCARDIAL INFARCTION

At the time of presentation with acute myocardial infarction (AMI), women tend to be 20 years older and have more co-morbid factors compared to their male counterparts. Women with AMI also tend to present with more atypical symptoms than men. This, together with their late presentation to hospital is likely to result in delays in receiving treatment including thrombolysis and angioplasty. Women younger than 50 years have been shown to have almost twice the in-hospital mortality compared to men.[41] Most studies in women with AMI have reported a higher rate of complications such as cardiogenic shock, congestive cardiac failure, bleeding, stroke and re-infarction. Most strokes have been shown to occur in women who have received thrombolysis. In the PAMI trial,[42] 5.3% of women who received thrombolysis had cerebral bleeding compared to 0.7% of men. In the GUSTO study, women had a 2-fold risk of stroke compared to men.

There is a clear benefit for women with AMI receiving treatment with primary PCI compared to thrombolysis. The PAMI-1 trial was one of the first multicentre trials to compare primary PCI with thrombolysis and which specifically analysed gender differences.[42] In women, the in-hospital mortality was 3.3 times higher compared to men mainly because of a higher mortality rate in women 65 years or older who were treated with thrombolysis.[42,43] In contrast, there were no gender differences in outcome in the primary PCI group in all ages. Furthermore, the mortality rate was 22% in women aged 65 years who received thrombolysis compared to 6% treated with primary angioplasty.[42,43] From this study, it appeared that primary PCI was more effective than thrombolysis in women because of the associated reduced risk of haemorrhagic stroke. There appears, therefore, to be a similar relative risk reduction in both genders treated with primary PCI. Women, however, derive a larger absolute benefit because of their higher risk profile. The GUSTO II-B trial has shown that, in women treated with primary PCI, 56 deaths could be prevented for every 1000 women compared with 42 deaths per 1000 males.[44] Also, there is an important reduction in the risk of haemorrhagic stroke in women treated with primary PCI compared to thrombolysis.

Two large studies compared the treatment of AMI with primary stenting versus primary balloon angioplasty. The stent PAMI (Primary Angioplasty for Myocardial Infarction) trial investigated 900 patients (27% women)[45] and showed that there was a significant increase in mortality in females with primary stenting using the heparin coated Palmaz-Schatz stent compared to primary balloon angioplasty.[45] The gender sub-analysis of the CADILLAC (Controlled Abciximab and Device Investigation to Lower Late Angioplasty Complications) trial, which compared the use of bare metal stents in primary PCI compared with primary balloon angioplasty with or without the use of abciximab showed that primary stenting reduced 1-year MACE from 28.1% to 19.1% ($P = 0.01$) ischaemic target vessel revascularisation from 20.4% to 10.8% ($P = 0.002$) compared to primary balloon angioplasty.[23]

CORONARY ARTERY BYPASS GRAFT SURGERY

In the majority of studies, women undergoing coronary artery bypass graft (CABG) surgery have greater operative mortality compared to men with the relative risk for women ranging from 1.4 to 4.4.[46–49] In terms of intra- and peri-operative complications, several studies have demonstrated a higher incidence of stroke, postoperative haemorrhage,[46,49] prolonged mechanical ventilation[47] and heart failure.[27,46,49] As well as having more co-morbid factors compared to men, women at the time of presentation also have a smaller body surface area, smaller coronary arteries, are older, have a higher prevalence of urgent or emergency surgery and, in some studies, have been shown to receive fewer internal mammary grafts. Similar to the finding seen with clinical outcomes following PCI, the majority of studies on CABG surgery in women have demonstrated that gender *per se* was not an independent risk factor for operative mortality following adjustment for body surface area, age, coronary artery size and risk factors. Despite the operative mortality for women being higher than men, there appears to be no difference in long-term survival between men and women.[50] Women, however, remain more symptomatic compared to men,[50] they have a greater rate of graft occlusion,[50] and at follow-up require more revascularisation which could be explained by the fact that women receive fewer internal mammary artery conduits compared to men and receive fewer grafts in general because of their smaller coronary vessel calibre. Postoperatively, women also have a worse functional status and mental health compared to men.[51]

Similar to PCI outcomes, more recent studies have demonstrated that in-hospital mortality in women undergoing CABG surgery is decreasing.[52] Nevertheless, women remain at higher risk compared to their male counterparts.[52] Vaccarino et al.[53] showed that women less than 50 years of age who undergo CABG surgery were 3 times more likely to die than men (3.4% versus 1.1%) and women 50–59 years of age were 2.4 times more likely to die than men (2.6% versus 1.1%).[53] Of the excess mortality in women. 97% was due to diabetes or urgent or emergency presentation.[53]

The BARI trial studied 1829 (27% women) patients with multivessel disease who were randomised to either CABG surgery or PCI.[27] Following CABG, in contrast to previous studies, the in-hospital mortality was similar for men and women (1.3% versus 1.4%), whereas congestive cardiac failure was more common among women (9.8% versus 1.8%; $P < 0.001$). In women, the in-hospital mortality was the same irrespective of treatment strategy. At 5-year follow-up, the unadjusted survival was similar for both genders (87% for women versus 88% for men). After adjustment for co-morbid factors, the study concluded that female gender was a predictor of a higher survival at 5 years (OR 0.60; 95% CI 0.43–0.84; $P = 0.003$). This finding, however, needs to be interpreted with caution as it does not imply that women do not have an increased procedural risk but rather that gender is not responsible for this increased risk. It is rather the adverse base-line risk profile which imparts the higher risk in women. In addition, women who had CABG surgery had an excess of Q-wave myocardial infarction, heart failure and pulmonary oedema compared to those randomised to PCI.[27]

A more recent study included 68,774 patients (15,043 women) with a follow-up of about 11 years and specifically studied long-term non-fatal outcomes in women.[54] This study showed that women were older and were more likely to present urgently or as an emergency and were less likely to receive arterial grafts compared to their male counterparts.[54] Women also had a higher rate of hospital re-admission in the first year following CABG surgery. This was mainly due to unstable angina (HR 1.3; 95% CI 1.24–1.38) and congestive cardiac failure (HR 1.1; 95% CI 1.06–1.21). Women who were propensity-matched with males, however, had similar rates of repeat revascularisation and survival.[54]

Although the use of off-pump CABG surgery, in terms of graft patency, remains controversial, the potential benefit of this form of surgery has been recently investigated in women. A study in 16,871 consecutive women comparing off-pump and on-pump CABG surgery has demonstrated that women undergoing off-pump surgery had better clinical outcome with reduced mortality, respiratory complications and length of hospital stay.[55] A more recent study investigated a total of 7376 women undergoing CABG surgery.[56] Compared to a propensity-matched sample of females who underwent conventional CABG surgery, women who underwent off-pump CABG surgery had a 32.6% lower mortality rate, a 35.1% lower complication rate due to bleeding, a 118.6% lower rate of neurological complications and a 49.3% lower rate of respiratory complications.[56]

HORMONE REPLACEMENT THERAPY

Epidemiological studies have suggested a beneficial effect of hormone therapy in terms of the risk of CHD and its development.[57] In contrast, randomised clinical trials have failed to demonstrate a significant reduction in coronary events with the use of hormone therapy.[57] The HERS trial studied 2763 postmenopausal women with established CHD who were randomised to conjugated equine oestrogens (0.625 mg) and medroxyprogesterone acetate (2.5 mg) versus placebo.[58] After a follow-up period of 4 years, there was no significant difference between the two groups in terms of cardiovascular events.[58] The Women's Health Initiative (WHI) studies were performed to assess the role of hormone replacement therapy for the primary prevention of CHD in postmenopausal women.[59,60] Similar to the findings of the HERS trial, there was evidence of early harm (possibly related to the adverse effects on vascular remodelling and thrombogenesis) followed by later benefit (possibly related to the beneficial effects on arterial function and metabolic risk factors).[57] In addition, the dosage, route of administration, type and duration of hormone therapy for maximum cardiovascular benefit remains undefined. At the present time, there is no clear evidence that hormone replacement therapy should be used for the prevention and treatment of CHD in postmenopausal women.

CONCLUSIONS

There is no doubt that CHD in women poses significant health and economic problems. Better awareness and education, earlier and more aggressive control of risk factors and appropriate access to diagnosis and treatment are needed to tackle this potentially fatal disease.

Although the mortality for women undergoing percutaneous or surgical revascularisation appears to be improving, it still remains higher than those for their male counterparts. The role of improved procedural techniques such as off-pump and minimally invasive coronary surgery as well as the wider use of drug-eluting stents and the increasing use of adjunctive medical therapy such glycoprotein IIb/IIIa inhibitors needs further evaluation.

Women continue to be under-represented in research studies with the majority of reports including no more than 30% females. Women are, therefore, being treated on evidence extrapolated from studies mainly based on men. As gender differences continue to exist in the management of cardiovascular disease, it is imperative that gender be considered in the design and the analysis of research studies and trials. Both single gender studies and the adequate representation of women in trials are needed in order to provide reliable evidence for the management of cardiovascular disease in women.

Key points for clinical practice

- Cardiovascular disease is the leading cause of death in women.
- Coronary heart disease kills almost 4 times more women than breast cancer.
- Gender differences exist in terms of presentation, diagnosis, treatment and outcome of cardiovascular disease.
- Women with cardiovascular disease continue to be under-diagnosed and under-treated.
- Women are under-represented in research studies and trials.
- Better awareness and education amongst both healthcare professionals and the general public are needed.

References

1. British Heart Foundation 2006 Coronary Heart Disease Statistics <www.heartstats.org>.
2. World Health Organization Statistical Information System 2004 <www.who.int/whosis>.
3. Bello N, Mosca L. Epidemiology of coronary heart disease in women. *Prog Cardiovasc Dis* 2004; **46**: 287–295.
4. Wenger NK. Coronary heart disease: the female heart is vulnerable. *Prog Cardiovasc Dis* 2003; **46**: 199–229.
5. Von der Lohe E. *Coronary Heart Disease in Women*. Berlin: Springer, 2003.
6. Kanaya AM, Grady D, Barrett-Connor E. Explaining the sex difference in coronary heart disease mortality among patients with type 2 diabetes mellitus. *Arch Intern Med* 2002; **162**: 1737–1745.
7. Mosca L, Appel LJ, Benjamin EJ *et al.* American Heart Association. Evidence-based guidelines for cardiovascular disease prevention in women. *Circulation* 2004; **109**: 672–693.
8. Grundy SM, Cleeman JI, Merz CN *et al.* National Heart, Lung, and Blood Institute; American College of Cardiology Foundation; American Heart Association. Implications of recent clinical trials for the National Cholesterol Education Program Adult Treatment Panel III guidelines. *Circulation* 2004; **110**: 227–239.
9. Prescott E, Hippe M, Schnohr P *et al.* Smoking and risk of myocardial infarction in women and men: longitudinal population study. *BMJ* 1998; **316**: 1043–1047.
10. Daly C, Clemens F, Lopez Sendon JL *et al.*, on behalf of the Euro Heart Survey Investigators. Gender differences in the management and clinical outcome of stable angina. *Circulation* 2006; **113**: 490–498.
11. Gibbons RJ, Balady GJ, Beasley JW *et al.* ACC/AHA Guidelines for Exercise Testing: a report of the American College of Cardiology/American Heart Association Task Force on Practice Guidelines (Committee on Exercise Testing). *J Am Coll Cardiol* 1997; **30**: 260–315.
12. Mieres JH, Shaw LJ, Arai A *et al.* Role of noninvasive testing in the clinical evaluation of women with suspected coronary artery disease. Consensus Statement from the Cardiac Imaging Committee, Council on Clinical Cardiology, and the Cardiovascular Imaging and Intervention Committee, Council on Cardiovascular Radiology and Intervention, American Heart Association. *Circulation* 2005; **111**: 682–696.
13. Lansky AJ, Mehran R, Dangas G *et al.* New-device angioplasty in women: clinical outcome and predictors in a 7,372-patient registry. *Epidemiology* 2002; **13**: S46–S51.
14. Alfonso F, Hernandez R, Banuelos C *et al.* Initial results and long-term clinical and angiographic outcome of coronary stenting in women. *Am J Cardiol* 2000; **86**: 1380–1383.
15. Watanabe CT, Maynard C, Ritchie JL. Comparison of short-term outcomes following coronary artery stenting in men versus women. *Am J Cardiol* 2001; **88**: 848–852.
16. Abramson JL, Veledar E, Weintraub WS, Vaccarino V. Association between gender and in-hospital mortality after percutaneous coronary intervention according to age. *Am J Cardiol* 2003; **91**: 968–971.
17. Kelsey SF, Millner DP, Holubkov R *et al.* Results of percutaneous transluminal coronary angioplasty in patients greater than or equal to 65 years of age (from the 1985 to 1986 National Heart, Lung and Blood Institute's Coronary Angioplasty Registry). *Am J Cardiol* 1990; **66**: 1033–1038.
18. Mehilli J, Kastrati A, Dirschinger J, Bollwein H, Neumann FJ, Schomig A. Differences in prognostic factors and outcomes between women and men undergoing coronary artery stenting. *JAMA* 2000; **284**: 1799–1805.
19. Malenka DJ, O'Connor GT, Quinton H *et al.* Differences in outcomes between women and men associated with percutaneous transluminal coronary angioplasty. A regional prospective study of 13,061 procedures. Northern England Cardiovascular Disease Study Group. *Circulation* 1996; **94**: II99–II104.
20. Jacobs AK. Coronary revascularization in women in 2003. Sex revisited. *Circulation* 2003; **107**: 375–377.
21. Mikhail GW. Coronary revascularisation in women. *Heart* 2006; **92**: 19–23.
22. Peterson ED, Lansky AJ, Kramer J *et al.* Effect of gender on the outcomes of contemporary percutaneous coronary intervention. *Am J Cardiol* 2001; **88**: 359–364.
23. Lansky AL, Pietras C, Costa RA *et al.* Gender differences in outcomes after primary angioplasty versus primary stenting with and without abciximab for acute myocardial

infarction. Results of the Controlled Abciximab and Device Investigation to Lower Late Angioplasty Complications (CADILLAC) Trial. *Circulation* 2005; **111**: 1611–1618.

24. Lansky AJ, Costa RA, Mooney M *et al*. Gender-based outcomes after Paclitaxel-eluting stent implantation in patients with coronary artery disease. *J Am Coll Cardiol* 2005; **45**: 1180–1185.

25. Antonioucci D, Valenti R, Moschi G *et al*. Sex-based differences in clinical and angiographic outcomes after primary angioplasty or stenting for acute myocardial infarction. *Am J Cardiol* 2001; **87**: 289–293.

26. Mehilli J, Kastrati A, Dirschinger J *et al*. Sex-based analysis of outcome in patients with acute myocardial infarction treated predominantly with percutaneous coronary intervention. *JAMA* 2002; **287**: 210–215.

27. Jacobs AK, Kelsey S, Brooks MM *et al*. Better outcome for women compared with men undergoing coronary revascularization: a report from the Bypass Angioplasty Revascularization Investigation (BARI). *Circulation* 1998; **98**: 1279–1285.

28. Jacobs AK, Johnston JM, Haviland A *et al*. Improved outcomes for women undergoing contemporary percutaneous coronary intervention: a report from the national Heart, Lung, and Blood Institute Dynamic Registry. *J Am Coll Cardiol* 2002; **39**: 1608–1614.

29. Malenka DJ, Wennberg DE, Quinton HA *et al*., for the Northern New England Cardiovascular Disease Study Group. Gender-related changes in the practice and outcomes of percutaneous coronary interventions in Northern New England from 1994–1999. *J Am Coll Cardiol* 2002; **40**: 2092–2101.

30. Kelsey SF, James M, Holubkov AL *et al*. Results of percutaneous transluminal coronary angioplasty in women: 1985–1986 NHLBI coronary angioplasty registry. *Circulation* 1993; **87**: 720–727.

31. Lansky AJ, Popma JJ, Mehran R *et al*. Tubular slotted stents: a 'breakthrough therapy' for women undergoing coronary interventions. Pooled results from the STARS, ACSENT, SMART and NIRVANA randomized clinical trials. *J Am Coll Cardiol* 1999; **33**: 58A.

32. Bobbio M, Detrano R, Colombo A *et al*. Restenosis rate after percutaneous transluminal coronary angioplasty: a literature overview. *J Invas Cardiol* 1991; **3**: 214–224.

33. Mehilli J, Kastrati A, Bollwein H *et al*. Gender and restenosis after coronary artery stenting. *Eur Heart J* 2003; **24**: 1523–1530.

34. Moses JW, Leon MB, Popma JJ *et al*. SIRIUS Investigators. Sirolimus-eluting stents versus standard stents in patients with stenosis in a native coronary artery. *N Engl J Med* 2003; **349**: 1315–1323.

35. Cho L, Topol EJ, Balog C *et al*. Clinical benefit of glycoprotein IIb/IIIa blockade with abciximab is independent of gender. Pooled analysis from EPIC, EPILOG and EPISTENT Trials. *J Am Coll Cardiol* 2000; **36**: 381–386.

36. Lincoff AM, Kleiman NS, Kereiakes DJ *et al*. Long-term efficacy of bivalirudin and provisional glycoprotein IIb/IIIa blockade vs heparin and planned glycoprotein IIb/IIIa blockade during percutaneous coronary revascularization. REPLACE-2 randomized trial. *JAMA* 2004; **292**: 696–703.

37. Rosengre A, Wallentin L, Gitt AK *et al*. Sex, age, and clinical presentation of acute coronary syndromes. *Eur Heart J* 2004; **25**: 663–670.

38. Lagerqvist B, Safstrom K, Stahle E *et al*. and the FRISC II Study Group Investigators. Is early invasive treatment of unstable coronary artery disease equally effective for both women and men? *J Am Coll Cardiol* 2001; **38**: 41–48.

39. Fox KAA, Poole-Wilson PA, Henderson RA *et al*., for the Randomized Intervention Trial of unstable Angina (RITA) Investigators. Interventional versus conservative treatment for patients with unstable angina or non-ST-elevation myocardial infarction: The British Heart Foundation RITA 3 randomised trial. *Lancet* 2002; **360**: 743–751.

40. Glaser R, Hermann HC, Murphy SA *et al*. Benefit of an early invasive management strategy in women with acute coronary syndromes. *JAMA* 2002; **288**: 3124–3129.

41. Vaccarino V, Parsons L, Every NR *et al*., for the National Registry of Myocardial Infarction 2 Participants. Sex-based differences in early mortality after myocardial infarction. *N Engl J Med* 1999; **341**: 217–225.

42. Grines CL, Browne KF, Marco J *et al*. A comparison of immediate angioplasty with thrombolytic therapy for acute myocardial infarction. The Primary Angioplasty in Myocardial Study Group. *N Engl J Med* 1993; **328**: 673–679.

43. Stone GW, Grines CL, Browne KF *et al*. Comparison of in-hospital outcome in men versus women treated by either thrombolytic therapy of primary angioplasty for acute myocardial infarction. *Am J Cardiol* 1995; **75**: 987–992.

44. Tamis-Holland JE, Palazzo A, Stebbins AL *et al*. GUSTO II-B Angioplasty Substudy Investigators. Benefits of direct angioplasty for women and men with acute myocardial infarction: result of the Global Use of Strategies to Open Occluded Arteries in Acute Coronary Syndromes Angioplasty (GUSTO II-B) Angioplasty Substudy. *Am Heart J* 2004; **147**: 133–139.

45. Grines CL, Cox DA, Stone GW. Coronary angioplasty with or without stent implantation for acute myocardial infarction. Stent Primary Angioplasty in Myocardial Infarction Study Group. *N Engl J Med* 1999; **341**: 1949–1956.

46. O'Conner GT, Morton JR, Diehl MJ *et al*. for the Northern New England Cardiovascular Disease Study Group. Differences between men and women in hospital mortality associated with coronary artery bypass graft surgery. *Circulation* 1993; **88**: 2104–2110.

47. Edwards FH, Carey JS, Grover FL *et al*. Impact of gender on coronary bypass operative mortality. *Ann Thorac Surg* 1998; **66**: 125–131.

48. Aldea GS, Gaudiani JM, Shapira OM *et al*. Effect of gender on postoperative outcomes and hospital stays after coronary artery bypass grafting. *Ann Thorac Surg* 1999; **67**: 1097–1103.

49. Weintraub WS, Wenger NK, Jones EL *et al*. Changing clinical characteristics of coronary surgery patients: differences between men and women. *Circulation* 1998; **88**: 79–86.

50. Rahimtoola SH, Bennett AJ, Grunkemeier GL *et al*. Survival at 15 to 18 years after coronary bypass surgery for angina in women. *Circulation* 1993; **88**: 71–78.

51. Vaccarino V, Lin ZQ, Kasl SV *et al*. Gender differences in recovery after coronary artery bypass surgery. *J Am Coll Cardiol* 2003; **41**: 307–314.

52. O'Rourke DJ, Malenka DJ, Olmstead EM *et al*., for the Northern New England Cardiovascular Disease Study Group. Improved in-hospital mortality in women undergoing coronary artery bypass grafting. *Ann Thorac Surg* 2001; **71**: 507–511.

53. Vaccarino V, Abramson JL, Veledar E, Weintraub WS. Sex differences in hospital mortality after coronary artery bypass surgery. Evidence for a higher mortality in younger women. *Circulation* 2002; **105**: 1176–1181.

54. Guru V, Fremes SE, Austin PC, Blackstone EH, Tu JV. Gender differences in outcomes after hospital discharge from coronary artery bypass grafting. *Circulation* 2006; **113**: 507–516.

55. Brown PP, Mack MJ, Simon AW *et al*. Outcomes experience with off-pump coronary artery bypass surgery in women. *Ann Thorac Surg* 2002; **74**: 2113–2120.

56. Mack MJ, Brown P, Houser F *et al*. On-pump versus off-pump coronary artery bypass surgery in a matched sample of women. A comparison of outcomes. *Circulation* 2004; **110 (Suppl II)**: II-1–II-6.

57. Collins P. Risk factors for cardiovascular disease and hormone therapy in women. *Heart* 2006; **92**: 24–28.

58. Hulley S, Grady D, Bush T *et al*. Randomized trial of oestrogen plus progestin for secondary prevention of coronary heart disease in postmenopausal women. *JAMA* 1998; **280**: 605–612.

59. Rossouw JE, Anderson GL, Prentice RL *et al*. Risks and benefits of estrogen plus progestin in healthy postmenopausal women: principal results from the women's health initiative randomized controlled trial. *JAMA* 2002; **288**: 321–333.

60. Anderson GL, Limacher M, Assauf AR *et al*. Effects of conjugated equine estrogen in postmenopausal women with hysterectomy: the women's health initiative randomized controlled trial. *JAMA* 2004; **291**: 1701–1712.

Melanie Greaves   Derek J. Rowlands

Coronary angiography by CT: is it now feasible? Achievements, limitations, future possibilities

Coronary artery disease is the most common cause of death in the UK with approximately one in five men and one in six women dying from the disease. According to the 2006 British Heart Foundation statistics database, it was responsible for just over 105,000 deaths in the UK in 2004 (www.bhf.org.uk/professionals).

Conventional, catheter-based angiography is currently the gold standard for the diagnosis of coronary artery disease. It offers the ability to image the entire coronary tree with high spatial and temporal resolution. Haemodynamic data can be collected and there is the option to perform therapeutic intervention. It is, however, a relatively costly and invasive procedure with a small, but definite, risk of serious complications. Death related to cardiac catheterisation occurs in 0.08–0.75% of patients, depending on the population studied,[1] and about 25% of individuals investigated this way are found to have normal coronary arteries. A reliable, non-invasive imaging test to evaluate the coronary arteries is, therefore, highly desirable, particularly if it could also be used for the assessment of the early stages of coronary artery disease (CAD). Recent dramatic improvements in the technical capabilities of multi-detector-row computed tomography (MDCT) have generated considerable interest in its potential to provide non-invasive coronary angiography.

Melanie Greaves MB BS MRCP FRCR (for correspondence)
Consultant Radiologist, University Hospital of South Manchester NHS Foundation Trust, Manchester M23 9LT, UK
E-mail: mgreaves@smuht.nwest.nhs.uk

Derek J. Rowlands BSc MD FRCP FACC FESC
Consultant Cardiologist, Alexandra Hospital, The Beeches Consulting Centre, Mill Lane, Cheadle, Cheshire SK8 2PY, UK.
E-mail: djr@djr12ecg.demon.co.uk

TECHNICAL PRINCIPLES OF CARDIAC MDCT

Cardiac MDCT is an extension of the role of stationary vessel CT angiography as frequently employed to diagnose pulmonary thrombo-embolic and peripheral vascular disease. Imaging of the heart has, however, always been more challenging owing to its continuous motion, the small diameter of the coronary vessels and their complex anatomy.

INTRODUCTION TO MDCT

Helical CT requires the patient to lie on the scanning table surrounded by a ring (the gantry). On one side of the gantry is an array of detectors, on the opposite side is an X-ray source. The gantry rotates around the patient as the table moves at a constant speed, resulting in a helically acquired volume data set of attenuation information that can subsequently be manipulated for analysis. Current MDCT systems have 4, 16 or 64 rows of detectors. With increasing numbers of detectors, the speed of scanning is increased and 64-slice scanners can now acquire a full cardiac data set in about 7 s reducing the required breath-holding time.

The table can move at different speeds. If it moves by one width of the detector array for every rotation this is called a 'pitch' of one. If the table moves more rapidly, there will be gaps in the imaging data set, more slowly and there will be overlaps. Cardiac CT angiography uses a low pitch of 0.2–0.3, which results in a highly overlapped data set.

PROSPECTIVE ECG TRIGGERING AND RETROSPECTIVE GATING

In order to suppress motion artefacts, cardiac CT images are obtained either by scanning, or by retrospectively reconstructing, raw data obtained in that part of the cardiac cycle when the heart is relatively immobile. This is achieved either by prospective ECG triggering or by retrospective ECG gating. The former has been extensively used in electron-beam CT. A trigger signal is derived from the patient's ECG and the scan is started at a defined time point after an R-wave, typically during late diastole. When applied to MDCT (typically for calcium scoring), several slices are obtained simultaneously. Given that all the data obtained in the scan are used in image reconstruction, it is the most dose-efficient method for ECG-synchronised scanning. However, the technique requires a regular heart rate being very prone to misregistration (and, therefore, to degraded image quality) in the presence of rate or rhythm irregularity. Additionally, the images are acquired and reconstructed as relatively thick slices rather than as a volume data set and, therefore, are much less suitable for 3-D reconstruction of small objects such as the coronary arteries.

Retrospective ECG gating overcomes the problems of ECG triggering, but at the cost of significantly greater radiation exposure.[2] A very low table speed is needed to produce a highly overlapped data set with simultaneous recording of the ECG trace. Scan data can then be linked retrospectively to any specific phase of the cardiac cycle and image stacks can be reconstructed. This enables contiguous, phase-consistent coverage of the entire heart and adjacent anatomy. It is much more flexible than ECG triggering since the point of image reconstruction can be moved anywhere within the cardiac cycle to limit motion artefacts.

MDCT SPATIAL AND TEMPORAL RESOLUTION

High spatial resolution (the ability to distinguish between adjacent structures) is essential for diagnostic coronary MDCT, given that coronary arteries have a diameter of 2–4 mm in the proximal segments and decrease in size towards the periphery. Recent MDCT scanners achieve a spatial resolution of approximately $0.4 \times 0.4 \times 0.4$ mm^3 in comparison to conventional catheter angiograms, which have a spatial resolution of approximately 0.25×0.25 mm^2.

The coronary arteries are moving rapidly and are, therefore, subject to motion artefact if the temporal resolution (the 'shutter speed' or the time taken to acquire one image) is inadequate. Conventional catheter-based angiography has a temporal resolution of about 6 ms and motion-free imaging during every cardiac cycle requires a temporal resolution of 50 ms. Scanner gantries typically rotate in 0.3–0.5 s and image reconstruction is performed from 180° of data resulting in a temporal resolution of half of the gantry rotation time. This results in a temporal resolution of approximately 165 ms, clearly inferior to conventional coronary angiography and insufficient to obtain diagnostic image quality in every patient. Increasing the speed of gantry rotation would improve temporal resolution but current equipment design is close to engineering limits, owing to the great weight of the scanner gantries. One approach, given that the scan data are heavily overlapped, is to combine data from two or more heart beats to reconstruct an image in a particular phase. This technique is, however, very sensitive to variations in heart rate or rhythm, and may increase scan time or decrease spatial resolution. A second approach is that of the recently introduced dual source scanner (which has two sources of X-rays instead of one). These can currently provide a temporal resolution of 83 ms. Until these machines are more widely available, we primarily aim to evaluate the coronary arteries from reconstructions obtained in diastole when cardiac motion is minimal.

DIFFERENTIAL MOTION OF CORONARY ARTERIES

The coronary arteries have individual motion patterns, with the greatest degree of movement typically exhibited by the right coronary artery (RCA) and the least by the anterior descending branch of the left coronary artery (LAD). Their anatomical locations result in their having different susceptibility to movement during different phases of the cardiac cycle. It is, therefore, usual to have to reconstruct several different image series at different phases to optimise visualisation of individual vessels. The right coronary artery is best seen in early diastole, the left circumflex in mid diastole, and the anterior descending artery in late diastole.[3]

PRACTICAL ASPECTS OF CARDIAC MDCT

PATIENT PREPARATION

As discussed above, motion artefacts are a significant cause of image quality degradation. An irregular heart rhythm precludes satisfactory MDCT coronary angiography although motion artefacts caused by minor rate variations, such as the occasional ectopic beat, may be diminished by manual repositioning of the reconstruction windows. The higher the heart rate, the less is the diastolic time per minute and heart rates greater than 65 beats/min are associated with increased motion artefacts. The 64-slice scanners can achieve diagnostic image quality over a wider range of heart rates than 4- and 16-slice machines but rate variability is still reported to have a strong negative effect on image quality for all coronary segments.[4] Premedication with β-adrenergic blockers is, therefore, recommended to reduce high heart rates and heart rate variability before CT angiography.[5] Patients should also be told to avoid caffeine on the day of the examination. Sublingual nitroglycerin immediately prior to imaging is used in some centres, to induce vasodilatation of the coronary arteries.

The patient needs to be able to lie flat and to follow instructions. Adequate breath holding is required for optimal thoracic imaging and is particularly important for cardiac CT. For CT coronary angiography there should be no history of reaction to iodinated contrast. Imaging the very obese is problematic because of a reduction in the signal-to-noise ratio resulting from increased scattered radiation. In a recent study by Raff and colleagues,[6] a body mass index of ≥ 30 kg/m^2 reduced sensitivity, specificity, positive predictive value and negative predictive value of 64-slice CT angiography.

INTRAVENOUS CONTRAST DELIVERY

Intravenous contrast is not required for coronary calcium scoring but is essential in CT coronary angiography to differentiate the vessel lumen from surrounding soft tissue. Optimal contrast enhancement is necessary for detection of atherosclerotic plaque and coronary artery stenosis. An ideal contrast protocol should produce uniform, prolonged arterial contrast enhancement that is synchronised to the duration of the scan. Precise synchronisation is difficult given the short 5–7 s scan times of the 64-slice scanners and a bolus timing technique is generally used. Two types of protocol are currently available for cardiac CT – delay estimation from a test bolus injection and automatic bolus triggering. For clinically useful coronary imaging, the aim is to achieve peak attenuation values in the left ventricular outflow tract at the time of scanning. High contrast density in the superior vena cava (SVC) and right atrium have the potential to cause streak artefacts and should be avoided.

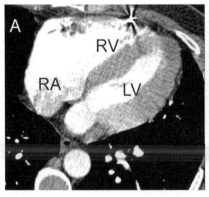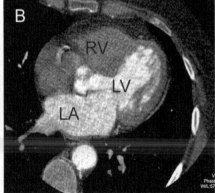

Fig. 1 Axial, contrast enhanced, 64-detector CT images, obtained through the ventricles (A) without and (B) with a saline flush. There is dense homogeneous enhancement of the cardiac chambers in (A). In (B), the saline flush has washed contrast from the right atrium and right ventricle reducing the likelihood of streak artefacts.

Currently, there are no uniform recommendations for the best cardiac CT injection protocols. A typical protocol for a 64-slice scanner is a bolus of 80–100 ml of iodinated contrast with a concentration of at least 320 mg/ml injected at a flow rate of 5 ml/s, followed by a 50-ml saline chaser bolus. Authors have also recommended the use of biphasic injection protocols with a high initial flow rate that is subsequently reduced. There is a general consensus that a saline chaser bolus of 30–50 ml should be employed.[7] A saline chaser will 'tighten' the contrast bolus and decrease the total amount required by flushing previously redundant arm vein contrast into the heart. This increases the peak concentration of contrast in the left ventricle and coronary arteries. Contrast in the SVC and right ventricle are typically reduced by the time of image acquisition reducing streak artefacts and improving the visualisation of the adjacent coronary arteries (Fig. 1).

RADIATION DOSE

The estimated average annual background radiation dose in the US is 3–3.6 mSv.[8] Calcium scoring protocols using ECG triggering typically result in an effective dose of 1 mSv[8] and conventional catheter coronary angiography 5.6 mSv.[6] The radiation dose is, however, significantly higher for coronary CT angiography. Retrospective ECG gating requires continuous data acquisition throughout the cardiac cycle, despite the fact that much of the acquired information will not be used. Radiation exposure is further increased by the requirement for very thin, highly overlapped slices. Coronary angiography using a 4-slice CT scanner results in an effective radiation dose of 9.3–11.3 mSv, a 16-slice scanner 14.7 mSv, and a 64-slice scanner up to 18 mSv.[6,8,9] Although these doses are large compared with conventional catheter angiography, it should be remembered that nuclear cardiology typically results in an effective radiation dose of 8–12 mSv per study, with thallium scans as much as 35 mSv.[10]

To maintain good image quality while reducing radiation dose, varying tube currents may be used (dose modulation). The maximal tube output is only applied during diastole, from which period the images are most likely to be reconstructed, and is decreased to about 20% of this during systole. Depending on the heart rate, an overall exposure reduction of 30–50% can be achieved.[11] The systolic images, whilst somewhat degraded, are still of sufficient quality for functional evaluation. The dose modulation technique is most suitable for patients with a slow, regular heart rate.

IMAGE RECONSTRUCTION AND DISPLAY

Reviewing data sets from multislice CT scanners (consisting of multiple stacks of several hundred individual axial images) is time consuming and not yet standardised. It remains necessary, however, for adequate visualisation of small structures. The volume data set is available for additional processing and analysis and the most frequently used reconstruction tools for MDCT coronary angiography are as follows:

2-D maximum intensity projections

These are widely used to visualise the coronary tree as they condense the diagnostic information into a smaller, more manageable format for review (Fig. 2).

2-D multiplanar reformations

These can re-slice the data along any chosen plane with image quality comparable to that of the original axial slices (Fig. 3).

3-D volume rendering

This is a means of displaying information to give an overview of what is often very complex anatomy. It is particularly helpful when reviewing coronary artery bypass grafts and anomalous coronary arteries (Fig. 4).

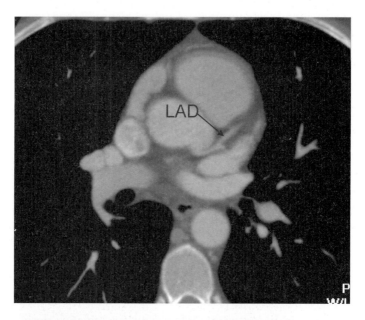

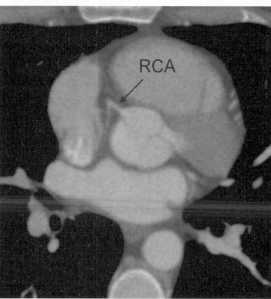

Fig. 2 Axial maximum intensity projections of the left and right coronary arteries.

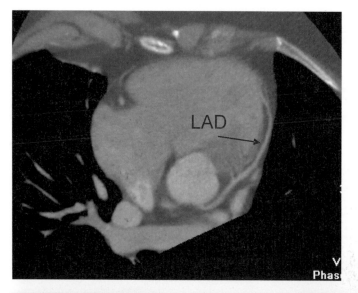

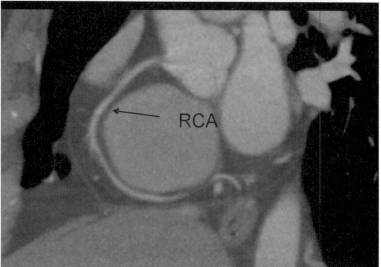

Fig. 3 Curved multiplanar reformations of the left and right coronary arteries.

Many vendors now additionally supply advanced semi-automated post processing tools to segment and extract the coronary arterial tree from the data set automatically and to visualise individual coronary arteries along their length with advanced curved multiplanar reconstructions (Fig. 4).

CLINICAL APPLICATIONS OF CARDIAC MDCT

CORONARY CALCIUM SCORING

Arterial calcification is intimately related to vessel injury and atherosclerotic plaque; the presence of calcium in the coronary arteries is evidence of

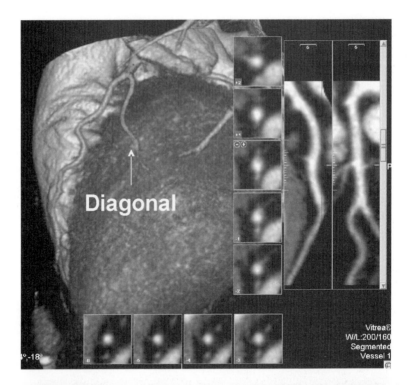

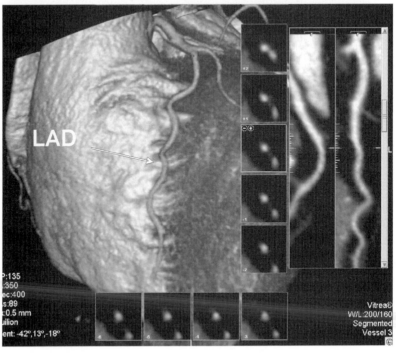

Fig. 4 Volume rendered images of normal LAD and diagonal coronary arteries with an additional advanced visualisation tool to demonstrate a curved multiplanar reformation along an automatically generated centre-line of the vessel.

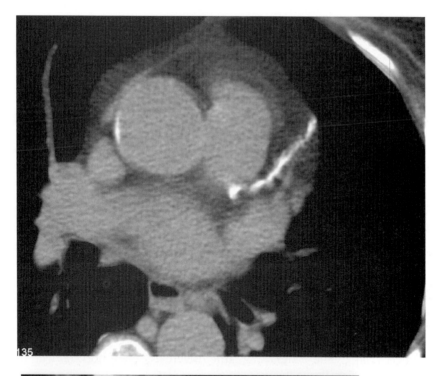

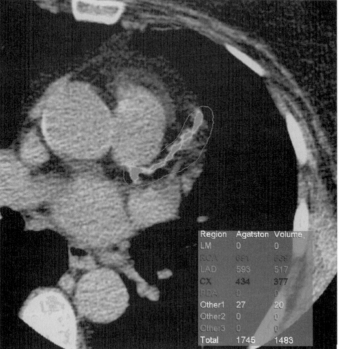

Region	Agatston	Volume
LM	0	0
RCA	691	568
LAD	593	517
CX	434	377
RDA	0	0
Other1	27	20
Other2	0	0
Other3	0	0
Total	1745	1483

Fig. 5 Detection of coronary calcification using multislice CT. Lesions exceeding a threshold of 130 HU are identified with 3-D-based picking tools and are assigned to the main coronary arteries. Our current 64-slice scanner gives measurements of Agatston score and calcium volume.

atherosclerosis. Coronary artery calcification occurs in small amounts in the early lesions of atherosclerosis but is found more frequently in advanced lesions and in older age. Calcium does not, however, concentrate exclusively at sites with severe coronary artery stenosis.

Coronary calcium assessment for the diagnosis of atherosclerosis and for risk stratification has been extensively investigated and validated. Coronary calcium is easily detected, assessed and quantified using either electron beam or MDCT and the results appear reproducible across multiple centres and scanners.[12] The procedure requires no intravenous contrast and can be performed quickly and easily using prospective ECG triggering. The amount of coronary artery calcified plaque (CACP) can be measured to provide an estimate of total coronary atheroma, although the true atherosclerotic burden will be underestimated. This is typically expressed as the 'Agatston score'. Other measures of coronary calcium such as mass and volume may also be provided (Fig. 5). The continued use of the older Agatston score (which, strictly should only be used when the slice thickness is 3 mm) is predicated upon the existence of established databases for the significance of these scores. Whatever scoring method is used, the greater the amount of calcium the greater the likelihood of occlusive coronary artery disease (CAD). It should be remembered, however, that CACP is present in the intima of both obstructive and non-obstructive lesions so a positive scan, while diagnosing atherosclerosis, does not confirm the presence of a significant stenosis.

The presence of CACP is a risk factor for future cardiac events both independent of and incremental to traditional risk factors. Coronary risk is typically stratified using conventional risk factors as they were used in the Framingham heart study.[13] Based on this estimation, patients may be classified as being at low-, intermediate- or high-risk for a cardiac event. Greenland and colleagues[14] demonstrated that patients with an intermediate Framingham risk score (FRS) and a coronary calcium score > 300 had an annual hard event rate of 2.8% and would, therefore, be reclassified as high risk. In selected intermediate risk patients, therefore, it may be reasonable to measure CACP to improve clinical risk prediction and to select patients for intensive lipid-lowering therapies.[10] A recent ACCF/AHA expert consensus document on coronary artery calcium scoring reinforced this view. It did not recommend CACP measurement in patients with either low or high coronary heart disease risk.[15]

In contrast, the absence of detectable calcium has a high negative predictive value for the presence of obstructive coronary artery disease). A negative predictive value (in respect of coronary pain or myocardial infarction) of 98% has been reported for this finding in patients with acute symptoms and equivocal ECG findings.[16] The absence of coronary calcium is most often associated with a normal nuclear scan and with the absence of obstructive disease on catheter-based angiography. A negative calcium score (total calcium = 0) implies, with a high level of confidence, that an individual does not have obstructive angiographic CAD and is consistent with a low risk (0.1% per year) of a cardiovascular event in the next 2–5 years.[10] It would, therefore, seem reasonable to perform coronary calcium scoring in low-risk, symptomatic patients with equivocal treadmill or functional testing and in those with acute

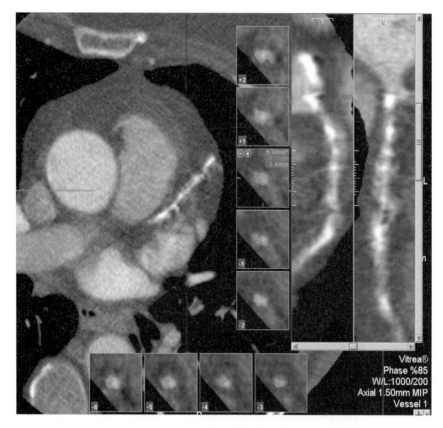

Fig. 6 Axial multiplanar reformation from a 64-slice scanner with a curved MPR view. This demonstrates the difficulty in evaluating coronary arteries in the presence of large amounts of calcified plaque. The lumen is in places completely obscured by the calcium and blooming artefact.

chest pain but equivocal or normal ECGs and normal cardiac enzyme studies.[10,15]

Severe coronary calcification obscures the coronary lumen and can lead to overestimation of lesion severity (because of blooming artefacts) resulting in a lower specificity in patients with high calcium scores. It is generally accepted that MDCT coronary angiography is unlikely to be of diagnostic quality in the presence of severe calcifications, for example, an Agatston score > 400–600 (Fig. 6). A non-enhanced coronary calcium score before contrast-enhanced coronary angiography is, therefore, usually undertaken.

MDCT CORONARY ANGIOGRAPHY

Since the first published studies on MDCT coronary angiography in 1999, there have been enormous technical advances in scanner capability. The technique has been shown to be reliable for the evaluation of coronary artery anomalies and for determining patency or occlusion of bypass grafts. Currently, it is undergoing extensive evaluation for the non-invasive identification, characterisation and quantification of atherosclerotic disease.

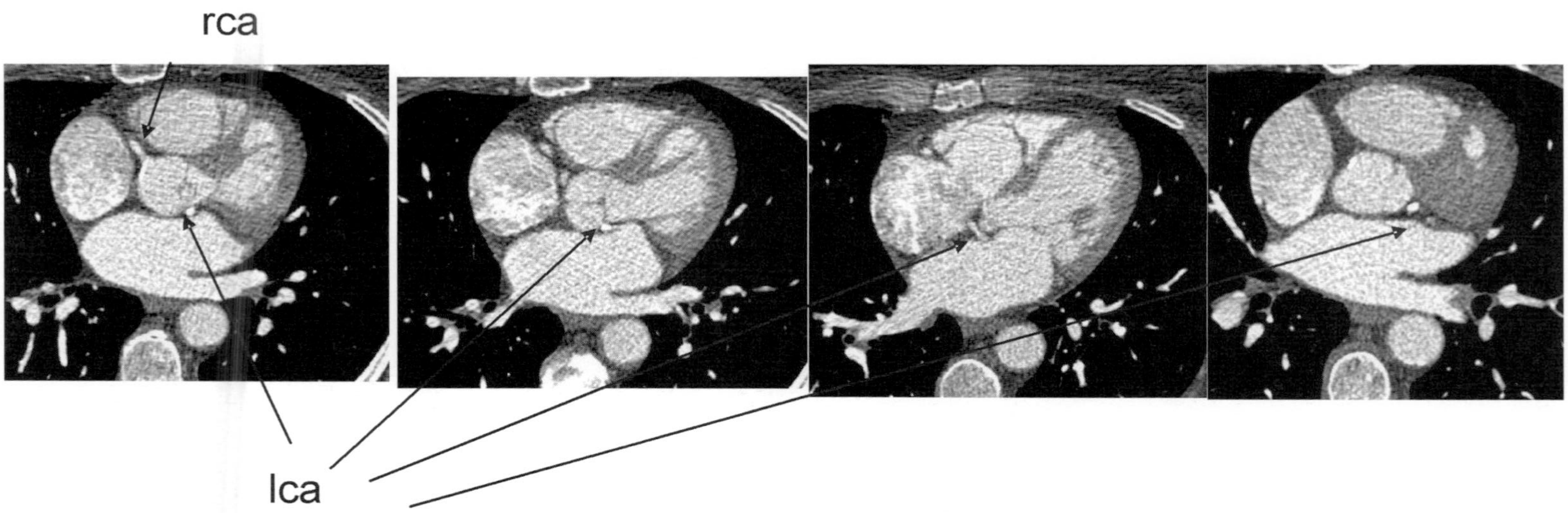

Fig. 7 Axial images from a 16-slice scanner demonstrating a single coronary artery arising from the right coronary sinus. The left coronary artery arises from the right and passes behind the aorta (a non-malignant course). The left coronary artery is heavily calcified.

CORONARY ARTERY ANOMALIES

Coronary artery anomalies are diagnosed in about 1% of coronary angiograms and 0.3% of autopsies.[17] Anomalies of the origin and course of the coronary arteries are typically classified as malignant or non-malignant dependent on

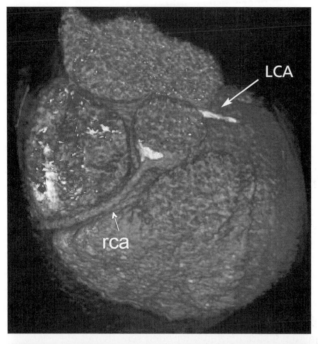

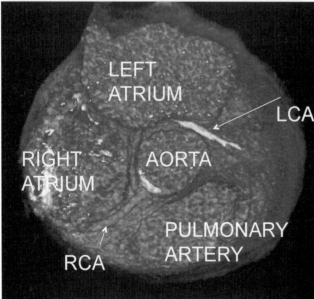

Fig. 8 Volume rendered images demonstrate the anomalous anatomy to greater effect. Note again the retro-aortic course of the LCA as opposed to a 'malignant' course between the aorta and the pulmonary artery.

their association with an increased risk of myocardial ischaemia and sudden death particularly in young adults.[18] They have been reported to be the cause of 19% of sudden deaths in athletes.[19] Anomalies most frequently associated with symptoms such as chest pain, syncope and sudden death involve origin of a coronary artery from the 'wrong' coronary sinus and a subsequent course between the pulmonary artery and the ascending aorta. The detailed assessment of anomalous coronary arteries can be difficult with conventional catheter-based coronary angiography. Numerous case reports have shown the utility of both MDCT and magnetic resonance imaging (MRI) for the evaluation of anomalous vessels, fistulas and aneurysms.[20,21] The abnormal vessel, its origin and its course can be clearly visualised. MDCT volumetric reconstructions are useful for displaying the relationship of the anomalous vessel to the adjacent mediastinal and cardiac structures and can be helpful in surgical planning (Figs 7 and 8). MRI provides an accurate assessment of the course of the anomalous vessel but is time consuming, its spatial resolution is inferior to that of current MDCT scanners, and it cannot be performed in patients with pacemakers or defibrillators.

SUSPECTED CORONARY ARTERY DISEASE

The reliable assessment of the coronary arteries for stenotic coronary artery disease has remained one of the greatest challenges for non-invasive imaging (Fig. 9). The vessels are small in calibre, have complex anatomy and are continuously moving. For MSCT to be useful clinically, complete visualisation of all clinically relevant segments of coronary arteries and a reliable quantification of coronary artery stenoses within these segments must be possible. Most published series utilising electron beam and 4-slice machines reported sensitivities of 80–90%.[22] Calculated sensitivity and specificity were often high, however, because they were based on analysable coronary segments rather than on all examined segments. Kaiser et al.[23] found that only 77% of all angiographically visible segments were evaluable by MDCT using a 16-slice scanner. Motion artefacts and coronary calcium degrade image quality and distal coronary artery segments and those of the lateral wall, particularly the left circumflex are frequently difficult to evaluate.[23] Literature published using 64-slice scanners demonstrates an increase in the number of evaluable coronary arterial segments and shows a significant improvement in stenosis detection over previous scanner generations. Leschka et al.[24] presented the first study utilising 64-slice technology. They evaluated all coronary segments and reported a high sensitivity and specificity for detecting significant lesions. Mollet and colleagues[25] demonstrated a sensitivity of 99% and a specificity of 95% compared with conventional coronary angiography. Ghostine et al.[26] compared the diagnostic accuracy of 64-slice computed tomography with subsequently undertaken coronary angiography in patients with complete left bundle branch block. Significant coronary lesions were defined at angiography as > 50% diameter narrowing. MDCT correctly excluded CAD in 35 of 37 patients. When analysed on a per artery basis, MDCT had a specificity of 99–100%, with sensitivities of 100% for the left main stem, 88% for the anterior descending, 59% for the circumflex and 52% for the right coronary artery. Improving the accuracy of CT coronary angiography is being intensively pursued and dual source CT (DSCT) with its improved temporal resolution of 83 ms shows great promise. A recent study using the DSCT demonstrated that visualisation of coronary arteries was successful in all 14 patients and that 98% of coronary artery segments were free of motion artefacts.[27]

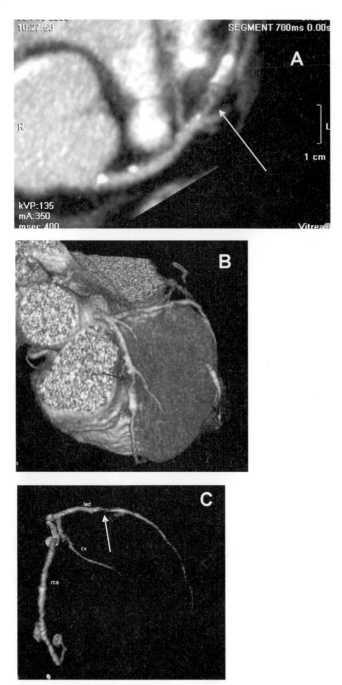

Fig. 9 (A) Curved multiplanar reformation in an oblique axial orientation; (B) volume rendered image; and (C) segmented extracted image demonstrating calcified and non-calcified plaque in the LAD. There is a significant stenosis caused by non-calcified plaque just distal to the origin of a diagonal branch (arrows).

The positive predictive value of coronary MDCT is less than the negative predictive value since limited spatial resolution results in an overestimation of coronary stenosis. All studies have, however, convincingly demonstrated a very high negative predictive value of approximately 98%.[28] A normal CT

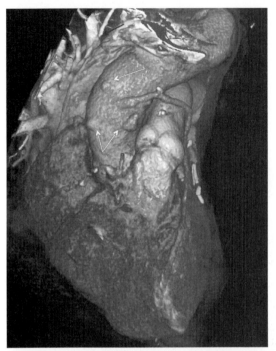

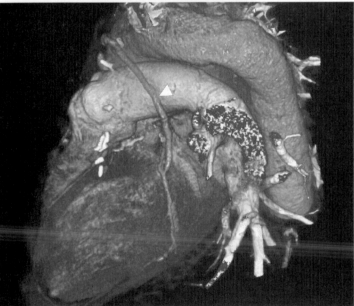

Fig. 10 Volume rendered images from a 16-slice CT demonstrating numerous occluded saphenous vein grafts (arrows). A solitary patent graft to an obtuse marginal artery is clearly visualised (arrowhead).

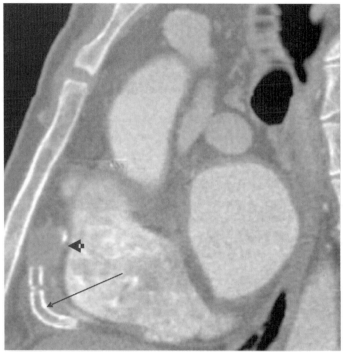

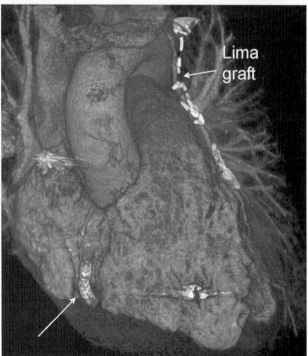

Fig. 11 (A) Coronal multiplanar reformation and (B) volume rendered image from a 16-slice scanner demonstrating a blocked stent within an occluded right coronary artery vein graft (arrows). The sagittal image also shows a thrombosed graft aneurysm immediately proximal to the (stent arrowhead). A patent LIMA graft can be seen on the volume rendered image partially obscured by surgical clips.

coronary angiogram thus allows the clinician to rule out the presence of haemodynamically relevant coronary artery stenosis with a high degree of reliability. Used clinically, it may obviate the need for invasive coronary angiography in those patients presenting with equivocal symptoms or stress test results in whom there is a low to intermediate prior probability of significant CAD.

This may be particularly applicable to patients presenting through the accident and emergency department with acute chest pain but with a non-diagnostic ECG and initially negative cardiac biomarkers. The ability of MDCT to exclude a cardiac cause of the chest pain and to diagnose non-cardiac causes such as pulmonary embolism, pneumonia, pericardial disease and thoracic aortic dissection has great appeal. Conceivably, this could reduce healthcare costs by decreasing conventional diagnostic coronary angiograms and hospital stay.

Hoffman et al.[29] evaluated 40 patients with chest pain, non-diagnostic ECG and initially negative serum markers with 16-slice CT. Significant coronary stenosis was excluded in 26 patients potentially saving unnecessary hospital admissions.

BYPASS GRAFTS

The value of CT for determining patency or occlusion of bypass grafts has been recognised for many years and bypass graft evaluation has become one of the first widely accepted indications for contrast enhanced CT angiography (Fig. 10). The sensitivity and specificity of 16-slice MDT for the detection of graft occlusion using data from multiple studies are 99% and 97%, respectively.[30] The detection of significant graft stenosis without occlusion has been more problematic as not all graft segments may be evaluable. Arterial grafts, in particular, are smaller and are frequently partially obscured by multiple metallic clips (and also by sternal wires if they course close to the anterior chest wall). MDCT is also valuable in diagnosing and localising graft aneurysms and pseudo-aneurysms (Fig. 11).

Recurrence of angina after coronary artery bypass grafting may also be related to progressive atherosclerosis in native vessels but assessment of the native vessels is often very difficult in this situation because of dense coronary artery calcification and the small calibre of distal vessels.

A recent study of 64-slice CT in the assessment of 32 patients with 96 bypass grafts has been published by Pache and colleagues.[31] Even though patients with high and irregular heart rates were included and non-evaluable segments were not excluded, sensitivity and specificity were still higher than or comparable to results from 16-slice CT. Overall sensitivity for detecting significant stenoses in both venous and arterial grafts was 97.8%, specificity was 89.3%, positive predictive value was 90% and negative predictive value was 97.7%. The negative predictive value for a separate analysis of venous grafts was 100%. On a patient-based analysis, all patients with at least one stenosis > 50% on catheter-based angiography were correctly identified by MSCT.

IMAGING THE CARDIAC SURGERY PATIENT

Re-operation following previous coronary artery bypass surgery is associated with increased morbidity and mortality, often resulting from injury to patent grafts, the right ventricle and the aorta. Furthermore, adhesions frequently distort the mediastinal anatomy, making sternal re-entry and surgical dissection potentially hazardous. Accurate pre-operative assessment with MDCT of pre-existing grafts and mediastinal anatomy may modify the surgical approach and has been shown to reduce operative morbidity.[32]

STENTS

Several studies have assessed the value of MDCT to detect restenosis following stent placement.[33-37] Metallic struts in stents result in a CT artefact known as blooming. This is caused by beam hardening and results in the struts appearing larger than they actually are. Visualisation of the lumen within the stent may be severely impaired by this artefact, which is inversely related to stent diameter and when present significantly limits the reliable detection of in-stent stenosis. Stent variables such as material, design, diameter, and strut thickness play an important role in their assessability by MDCT. If the stent diameter is less than 3.5 mm, it is unlikely to be evaluable. Increase in strut thickness can also have a detrimental role. In studies performed with 16- and 40-slice MDCT, up to 77% of stents were considered unevaluable. Additionally, if the stents were considered evaluable, sensitivities and specificities for the detection of in-stent stenosis were low. Rixe et al.[35] found that, even using 64-slice CT, 42% of stents could not be adequately assessed. They concluded that the high frequency of cases in which the stents could not be adequately visualised precluded the recommendation of MDCT for coronary angiography in unselected patients with coronary stents.[35] This view has been echoed by the American Heart Association in its scientific statement on MDCT coronary angiography.[10] Rixe et al.[35] also demonstrated, however, that if the stent was evaluable then the sensitivity for in-stent stenosis was 86%, (positive predictive value 86%, negative predictive value 98%). This implies that in selected patients, dependent on stent type and diameter, MDCT may have a clinically useful role.[36]

Supporting this is a recent study by Van Mieghem and colleagues[37] comparing MDCT with coronary angiography and intravascular ultrasound in detecting restenosis in 74 patients after left main stem drug eluting stent placement. MDCT correctly identified all patients with in-stent restenosis. The authors did, however, comment that the evaluation of relatively large, left main (LM) and proximal LAD stents provided the best case scenario for MDCT evaluation particularly as the LM and LAD run in the axial plane and are to some extent protected from motion artefact.[37]

ASSESSMENT OF NON-CALCIFIED PLAQUE

Conventional coronary angiography, which displays only the vessel lumen, consistently underestimates the atherosclerotic burden. Early manifestations of CAD are often hidden from the interventional cardiologist by coronary remodelling and angiographically normal coronary arteries may contain significant amounts of plaque. This 'hidden plaque', not associated with stenosis, may still rupture causing myocardial infarction. MDCT angiography can identify calcified and non-calcified atherosclerotic plaque within the vessel

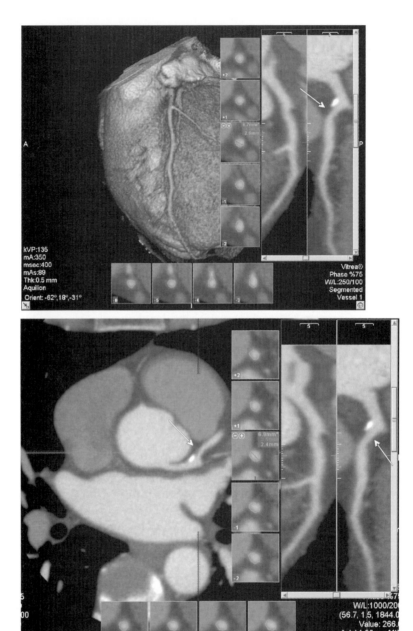

Fig. 12 Clear visualisation of a non-calcified plaque just distal to a calcified nodule at the origin of the LAD.

wall (Fig. 12). Studies with 4- and 16-slice MDCT have shown the ability of this technology to detect and classify coronary plaques and to determine remodelling.[38] Leber and colleagues[39] attempted to classify and quantify plaque volumes with 64-slice MDCT using intravascular ultrasound as the reference standard . Their results were encouraging, enabling correct detection of 83% of non-calcified plaque, 94% of mixed plaque and 95% of calcified plaque.[39]

Plaques that are frequently associated with rupture have high lipid content or demonstrate spotty calcifications. Atherosclerotic plaques can be differentiated with some success by MDCT, although sub-classification of plaque is made difficult by inadequate resolution.[39,40] Non-invasive determination of atherosclerotic plaque morphology and plaque burden may be valuable in improving risk stratification and in monitoring the course of disease. Unfortunately, the ability to determine plaque burden is currently poor, with studies demonstrating high interobserver variability.[39]

LEFT VENTRICULAR FUNCTION AND MYOCARDIAL PERFUSION

MDCT has been validated for the quantification of right and left ventricular function[41] and can also be used to obtain information about myocardial perfusion.[42] As with catheter based studies, it is usual to assess left ventricular function when MDCT coronary angiography is undertaken.

NON-CARDIAC FINDINGS

A significant proportion of the thorax is scanned during evaluation of the coronary arteries and almost the entire thorax is imaged during the evaluation of bypass grafts. Typically, images are reconstructed with small fields of view so as to demonstrate the heart and coronary arteries optimally, although the full data set is available and can be reconstructed and evaluated without additional radiation to the patient. Given that many patients with coronary artery disease are current or former smokers at risk of lung carcinoma, it would seem appropriate to review fully all the information obtained by the scan to exclude malignancy. Non-cardiac causes of the presenting symptoms may also be diagnosed. Supporting this is a study by Onuma and colleagues[43] aiming to establish the frequency of non-cardiac abnormalities on MDCT coronary angiograms. A total of 503 consecutive patients with suspected CAD were examined using either 16- or 64-slice MDCT scanners. Patients were scanned from the level of the pulmonary arteries to the base of the heart for assessment of native coronaries; more extensive coverage of the entire thorax was performed if CABG assessment was being performed. Data sets were generated with a small field of view to evaluate specifically the heart and coronary arteries and with a larger field of view to encompass the entire width of the chest. Both the lung and soft tissue windows from this latter data set were reviewed. Of these patients, 58.1% had non-cardiac MDCT abnormalities with 22.7% having significant non-cardiac pathology requiring follow-up. In 32 patients without coronary disease, non-cardiac abnormalities detected were considered sufficient to explain their symptomatology. Pathology included pulmonary nodules, pulmonary parenchymal disease, pleural effusions and aortic aneurysms. Four (0.8%) had malignancy (2 breast, 2 lung). Whilst the number of malignancies detected was relatively small, failure to diagnose cancer on readily available images is clinically unacceptable. It is, therefore, recommended that all anatomy irradiated is subsequently reviewed to avoid missing significant non-cardiac disease.

SUMMARY

MDCT is a rapidly evolving tool that shows great promise for the future. Currently, measuring calcium scores in asymptomatic patients with intermediate CHD risk may aid guide management, and may also be helpful in evaluating those patients with a low risk of coronary disease and atypical symptoms. MDCT coronary angiography, although still limited technically, is a proven non-invasive method of diagnosing coronary artery anomalies and evaluating graft patency. It may also have a role in excluding the presence of significant coronary stenoses in selected subsets of symptomatic patients.

Key points for clinical practice

- Multi-detector-row computed tomography (MDCT) coronary calcium scoring has been validated against electron-beam computed tomography (EBCT) and can document the presence of coronary atherosclerosis. It can identify patients at increased risk for myocardial infarction and can add significant predictive ability to the Framingham score.

- The absence of detectable coronary artery calcium (score = 0) makes the presence of atherosclerotic plaque and significant luminal obstructive disease highly unlikely. It is consistent with a low risk of a cardiovascular event in the next 2–5 years.

- MDCT coronary angiography is reliable, non-invasive technique for evaluating coronary artery anomalies and for determining patency or occlusion of bypass grafts.

- In selected subsets of symptomatic patients, MDCT coronary angiography may now be used to exclude the presence of significant obstructive disease.

- MDCT coronary angiography results in an effective radiation dose of up to three times that of conventional coronary angiography and radiation exposure is, therefore, a significant limitation of this technique. MDCT dose modulation techniques may significantly reduce this exposure dependent upon the patient's heart rate and should be used where possible..

References

1. Davidson CJ, Bonow RO. In: Zipes DP, Libby P, Bonow RO, Braunwald E (eds) *Braunwald's Heart Disease*, 7th edn. Amsterdam: Elsevier Saunders, 2005; Chapter 17.
2. Ohneserge B, Flohr T, Becker C *et al*. Cardiac imaging by means of ECG gated multisection spiral CT: initial experience. *Radiology* 2000; **217**: 564–571.
3. Kopp AF, Schroeder S, Kuettner A *et al*. Coronary arteries: retrospectively ECG gated multidetector row CT angiography with selective optimisation of the image reconstruction window. *Radiology* 2001; **221**: 683–688.
4. Hoffmann MH, Shi H, Manzke R *et al*. Non-invasive coronary angiography with 16-detector row CT: effect of heart rate. *Radiology* 2005; **234**: 86–97.

5. Leschka S, Wildermuth S, Boehm T *et al*. Non-invasive coronary angiography with 64-section CT: effect of average heart rate and heart rate variability on image quality. *Radiology* 2006; **241**: 378–385.
6. Raff GL, Gallagher MJ, O'Neill WW, Goldstein JA. Diagnostic accuracy of non-invasive coronary angiography using 64-slice spiral computed tomography. *J Am Coll Cardiol* 2005; **46**: 552–557.
7. Cademartiri F, Mollet N, Van der Lugt M *et al*. Non-invasive 16-row multislice CT angiography: usefulness of saline chaser. *Eur Radiol* 2004; **14**: 178–183.
8. Morin RL, Gerber TC, McCollough CH. Radiation dose in computed tomography of the heart. *Circulation* 2003; **107**: 917–922.
9. Coles DR, Smail MA, Wilde P *et al*. Comparison of radiation doses from multislice computed tomography coronary angiography and conventional diagnostic angiography. *J Am Coll Cardiol* 2006; **47**: 1840–1845.
10. Budoff MJ, Achenbach S, Blumenthal RS *et al*. Assessment of coronary artery disease by cardiac computed tomography. A scientific statement from the American Heart Association Committee on Cardiovascular Imaging and Intervention, Council on Cardiovascular Radiology and Intervention and Committee on Cardiac Imaging, Council on Clinical Cardiology. *Circulation* 2006; **114**: 1761–1791.
11. Jakobs TF, Becker CR, Ohnesorge B *et al*. Multislice helical CT of the heart with retrospective ECG gating: reduction of radiation exposure by ECG controlled tube current modulation. *Eur Radiol* 2002; **12**: 1081–1086.
12. Detrano RC, Anderson M, Nelson J *et al*. Coronary calcium measurements: effect of CT scanner type and calcium measure on rescan reproducibility – MESA study. *Radiology* 2005; **236**: 477–484.
13. Grundy SM, Balady GJ, Criqui MH *et al*. Primary prevention of coronary heart disease; guidance from Framingham. A statement for healthcare professionals from the AHA Task Force on Risk Reduction. *Circulation* 1998; **12**: 1876–1887.
14. Greenland P, LaBree L, Azen SP *et al*. Coronary artery calcium score combined with Framingham score for risk prediction in asymptomatic individuals. *JAMA* 2004; **291**: 210–215.
15. Greenland P, Bonow RO, Brundage BH *et al*. ACCF/AHA 2007 Clinical Expert Consensus Document on Coronary Artery Calcium Scoring By Computed Tomography in Global Cardiovascular Risk Assessment and in Evaluation of Patients With Chest Pain: A Report of the American College of Cardiology Foundation Clinical Expert Consensus Task Force (ACCF/AHA Writing Committee to Update the 2000 Expert Consensus Document on Electron Beam Computed Tomography) Developed in Collaboration With the Society of Atherosclerosis Imaging and Prevention and the Society of Cardiovascular Computed Tomography. *J Am Coll Cardiol* 2007; **49**: 378–402.
16. McLaughlin VV, Balogh T, Rich S. Utility of electron beam computed tomography to stratify patients presenting to the emergency room with chest pain. *Am J Cardiol* 1999; **84**: 327–328.
17. Baltaxe HA, Wixson D. The incidence of congenital abnormalities of the coronary arteries in the adult population. *Radiology* 1997; **122**: 47–52.
18. Basso C, Maron BJ, Corrado D, Thiene G. Clinical profile of congenital coronary artery anomalies with origin from the wrong aortic sinus leading to sudden death in young competitive athletes. *J Am Coll Cardiol* 2000; **35**: 1493–1501.
19. Maron BJ, Thompson PD, Puffer JC *et al*. Cardiovascular preparticipation screening of competitive athletes; a statement for health professionals from the Sudden Death Committee (clinical cardiology) and Congenital Cardiac Defects Committee (cardiovascular disease in the young), American Heart Association. *Circulation* 1996; **94**: 850–856.
20. Datta J, White C, Gilkeson RC *et al*. Anomalous coronary arteries in adults: depiction at multi-detector row CT angiography. *Radiology* 2005; **235**: 812–818.
21. Bunce NH, Lorenz CH, Keegan J *et al*. Coronary artery anomalies: assessment with free-breathing three-dimensional coronary MR angiography. *Radiology* 2003; **227**: 201–208.
22. Schoepf UJ. CT angiography of the coronary arteries. *Radiology* 2004; **232**: 18–37.
23. Kaiser C, Bremerich J, Haller S *et al*. Limited diagnostic yield of non-invasive coronary angiography by 16-slice multi-detector spiral computed tomography in routine patients referred for evaluation of coronary artery disease. *Eur Heart J* 2005; **26**: 1987–1992.
24. Leschka S, Alkadhi H, Plass A *et al*. Accuracy of MSCT angiography with 64-slice

technology: first experience. *Eur Heart J* 2005; **26**: 1482–1487.

25. Mollet NR, Cademartiri F, van Mieghem M *et al*. High-resolution spiral computed tomography coronary angiography in patients referred for diagnostic conventional coronary angiography. *Circulation* 2005; **112**: 2318–2323.

26. Ghostine S, Caussin C, Daoud B. Non-invasive detection of coronary artery disease in patients with left bundle branch block using 64-slice computed tomography. *J Am Coll Cardiol* 2006; **48**: 1929–1934.

27. Achenbach S, Ropers D, Kuettner A *et al*. Contrast-enhanced coronary artery visualisation by dual-source computed tomography-initial experience. *Eur J Radiol* 2006; **57**: 331–335.

28. Mahnken AH, Muhlenbruch G, Gunther RW, Wildberger JE. Cardiac CT: coronary arteries and beyond. *Eur Radiol* 2007; **17**: 994–1008.

29. Hoffmann U, Pena AJ, Moselewski F *et al*. MDCT in early triage of patients with acute chest pain. *AJR Am J Roentgenol* 2006; **187**: 1240–1247.

30. Stein PD, Beemath A, Skaf E *et al*. Usefulness of 4-, 8- and 16-slice computed tomography for detection of graft occlusion or patency after coronary artery bypass grafting. *Am J Cardiol* 2005; **96**: 1669–1673.

31. Pache G, Saueressig U, Frydrychowicz A *et al*. Initial experience with 64-slice cardiac CT: non invasive visualization of coronary artery bypass grafts. *Eur Heart J* 2006; **27**: 976–980.

32. Gasparovic H, Rybicki FJ, Millstine J *et al*. Three dimensional computed tomographic imaging in planning the surgical approach for redo cardiac surgery after coronary revascularization. *Eur J Cardiothoracic Surg* 2005; **28**; 244–249.

33. Kitagawa T, Fujii T, Tomohiro Y *et al*. Non-invasive assessment of coronary stents in patients by 16-slice computed tomography. *Int J Cardiol* 2006; **109**: 188–194.

34. Schuijf JD, Bax JJ, Jukema JW *et al*. Feasibility of assessment of coronary stent patency using 16-slice CT tomography. *Am J Cardiol* 2004; **94**: 427–430.

35. Pugliese F, Cademartini F, Mieghem C *et al*. Multidetector CT for visualisation of coronary stents. *Radiographics* 2006; **26**: 887–904.

36. Rixe J, Achenbach S, Ropers D *et al*. Assessment of coronary stent restenosis by 64-slice multidetector computed tomography. *Eur Heart J* 2006; **27**: 2567–2572.

37. Van Mieghem CA, Cademartiri F, Mollet NR *et al*. Multislice spiral computed tomography for the evaluation of stent patency after left main coronary artery stenting: a comparison with conventional coronary angiography and ultrasound. *Circulation* 2006; **114**: 645–653

38. Achenbach S, Moselewski F, Ropers D *et al*. Detection of calcified and noncalcified atherosclerotic plaque by contrast enhanced submillimeter multidetector spiral computed tomography: a segment based comparison with intravascular ultrasound. *Circulation* 2004; **109**: 14–17.

39. Leber AW, Becker A, Knez A *et al*. Accuracy of 64-slice computed tomography to classify and quantify plaque volumes in the proximal coronary system. *J Am Coll Cardiol* 2006; **47**: 672–677.

40. Cordeiro MAS, Lima JAC. Atherosclerotic plaque characterization by multidetector row computed tomography angiography. *J Am Coll Cardiol* 2006; **47 (Suppl)**: C40–C47.

41. Raman SV, Shah M, McCarthy B, Garcia A, Ferketich AK. Multidetector row cardiac computed tomography accurately quantifies right and left ventricular function compared with cardiac magnetic resonance. *Am Heart J* 2006; **151**: 736–744.

42. Baks T, Cademartiri C, Moelker A *et al*. Multislice computed tomography and magnetic resonance imaging for the assessment of reperfused acute myocardial infaction. *J Am Coll Cardiol* 2006; **48**: 144–152.

43. Onuma Y, Tanabe K, Nakazawa G *et al*. Noncardiac findings in cardiac imaging with multidetector computed tomography. *J Am Coll Cardiol* 2006; **48**: 402–406.

Derek J. Rowlands Philip R. Moore

12

The limb leads and the frontal plane vectors: a poorly understood and undervalued resource

The 12-lead ECG is the most extensively used cardiac investigation.[1] Well over 100 years since its first use, it remains an essential part of any cardiovascular assessment, whether in relation to health issues, to insurance or to the assessment of risk. It is still the most reliable non-invasive way of diagnosing ectopic arrhythmias and conduction disturbances, and is an essential part of the investigation of acute chest pain.

The conventional 12-lead recording consists of three bipolar limb leads (I, II and III), three unipolar limb leads (aVR, aVL and aVF) and six unipolar precordial leads (V_1–V_6). An electrocardiographic lead is defined[2] as: 'a pair of terminals with designated polarity, each connected either directly or via a passive/active network to recording electrodes'. The term 'lead' is also commonly used to refer to the wire connections to the recorder; in this text, it will refer, as implied in the definition above, exclusively to the conceptual, effective recording position and its orientation with respect to the heart.

Most of the clinically useful and prognostically significant information in the 12-lead ECG is derived from the precordial leads, but the limb leads contain an appreciable amount of clinically important information, which is often overlooked. Furthermore, there is often uncertainty about the significance of some findings, such as the presence of q-waves in III or aVL, and about when, in the limb leads, T-wave flattening or inversion is 'positional' rather than abnormal. These uncertainties arise from an incomplete understanding of the nature of these leads. **The single, most important misunderstanding is the failure to recognise the**

Derek J. Rowlands BSc MD FRCP FACC FESC (for correspondence)
Consultant Cardiologist, Alexandra Hospital, The Beeches Consulting Centre, Mill Lane, Cheadle, Cheshire SK8 2PY, UK
E-mail: djr@djr12ecg.demon.co.uk

Philip R. Moore MRCP PhD
SpR in Cardiology, Harefield Hospital, Royal Brompton & Harefield NHS Trust, Hillend Rd, Harefield, Middlesex UB9 6JH, UK
E-mail: prmoore@ukonline.co.uk

inter-relationship between these leads and the fact that the sum total of the information contained in all six leads is completely provided by any two of them.

LINEAR AND VOLUME CONDUCTORS

It is important to recognise the difference between a linear conductor and a volume conductor. The most obvious example of a linear conductor is a wire. Its fundamental property is its ability to conduct in a single direction (along the length of the wire) and to do so with minimal voltage loss (because of its low resistance) so that voltage measurements at all points along the wire (against some arbitrary reference level) are approximately equal. An example of a volume conductor would be a container full of a sodium chloride solution. In contrast to a linear conductor, a homogeneous volume conductor is capable of conducting equally well in all directions.

The torso is a volume conductor (not homogeneous) and, therefore, the nature of deflections obtained from recordings taken from the surface (*e.g.* leads V_1–V_6) is intimately dependent upon the location of the recording electrode and on its orientation with respect to the change in potential giving rise to the deflection. Furthermore, the amplitude of any recording obtained is related to the distance from the source (by the inverse square law). It follows that strictly accurate positioning (in accordance with the universally agreed positioning convention) of the precordial electrodes is essential for reliable interpretation of ECGs using available criteria datasets. The limbs, however, behave very much like linear conductors (no doubt because of their linear shape); for this reason, the precise positioning of the recording electrodes on the limbs is less critical. (It is, of course, inevitable that variations in the position [on the limbs] of the recording electrodes will have some effect, because the limbs do not behave like true wires. However, any differences are minor and the Committee on Electrocardiography of the American Heart Association, in 1975, in respect of the positioning of the limb lead electrodes, recommended only that they be placed on the arms and legs distal to the shoulders and hips).[3]

Effectively, therefore, when the right arm electrode is attached to the wrist, the right arm behaves as an extension of the wire connection to the recorder and the right arm lead is effectively 'looking' at the heart from the point where the right arm (acting as a linear conductor) attaches to the torso (at which point the properties of a volume conductor come into play). The right arm lead, therefore, 'sees' the heart from the perspective of the right shoulder, the left arm lead from the left shoulder and the foot lead from the left groin.

HISTORICAL BACKGROUND

THE BIPOLAR LIMB LEADS

The original electrocardiographic recording leads, as designed and designated by Einthoven,[4] were the limb leads, I, II and III. These were (and are) bipolar leads reflecting changes (with time) in the potential difference (measured as 'voltage') between the two recording electrodes.

By Einthoven's convention, lead I is obtained by connecting the left arm to the positive end of the recording device (originally a galvanometer, now an amplifier) and the right arm to the negative end. Thus, at any instant in time, the difference in electrical potential (E) across the electrodes of lead I (V_I volts) can be expressed as:

$$V_I = E_L - E_R \qquad \text{Eq. 1}$$

where E_L and E_R are the potentials at the left arm and right arm connections, respectively.

Lead II is obtained by connecting the foot to the positive end of the recording device and the right arm to the negative end. Thus:

$$V_{II} = E_F - E_R \qquad \text{Eq. 2}$$

where V_{II} is the voltage across the electrodes of lead II and E_F is the potential at the (left) foot connection.

Lead III is obtained by connecting the foot to the positive end of the recording device and the left arm to the negative end. Thus:

$$V_{III} = E_F - E_L \qquad \text{Eq. 3}$$

where V_{III} is the voltage across the electrodes of lead III.

It follows that

$$V_I + V_{III} = V_{II} \qquad \text{Eq. 4}$$

This is known as Einthoven's Law, which basically is a statement of Kirchoff's voltage law for a closed circuit.

The Einthoven triangle hypothesis is based on four assumptions, each one of which is only approximately true. These assumptions are:

1. The torso of the body is a homogeneous volume conductor.

2. The electrical forces generated during the cardiac cycle can be considered as originating from a dipole situated centrally in the heart.

3. The limb lead connections detect voltage changes only in the frontal plane.

4. The points of attachment of the limbs to the torso form the apices of an equilateral triangle with reference to the dipole located at its centre.

None of these assumptions is strictly true and detailed mathematical analysis[5-7] suggests that the Burger triangle (which is not necessarily confined to the frontal plane) is a closer representation of the true situation. However, the validity of Einthoven's Law does not depend upon the Einthoven triangle hypothesis. A similar relationship holds true of any three values linked in a similar way. Thus, for example, if x, y and z are the heights of three points above sea level and if 'i' is defined as the difference between y and x (as I is the difference between L and R) and 'ii' is defined as the difference between z and x (as II is the difference between F and R) and 'iii' is defined as the difference between z and y (as III is the difference between F and L) then:

$$\text{'i'} = y - x$$
$$\text{'ii'} = z - x, \text{ and}$$
$$\text{'iii'} = z - y, \text{ so}$$
$$\text{'i'} + \text{'iii'} = \text{'ii'}$$

THE UNIPOLAR LIMB LEADS

The 'indifferent' central terminal of Wilson

In 1934, Frank Wilson defined an 'indifferent electrode',[8] subsequently called the 'Wilson central terminal'. This was achieved by connecting together (via equal resistors) the right arm, left arm and (left) foot connections. If the electrical potential at the right arm is E_R, at the left arm E_L and at the foot E_F, then the potential at the central terminal (E_{CT}) will be the average of the three potentials:

$$E_{CT} = (E_R + E_L + E_F)/3 \qquad \text{Eq. 5}$$

The potential at the Wilson central terminal does not change appreciably during the cardiac cycle. (This can be understood intuitively, [and is easily proved]. If the central terminal actually consisted of an infinite number of recording positions in the form of a circle with the cardiac dipole at its centre, the two points at the ends of each and every diameter would have equal and opposite values, and would, therefore, cancel out, no matter what deflection occurred. If a finite number of recording positions were summed to give the central terminal, the same effect would be produced provided the sampling points were uniformly distributed around the cardiac dipole. Other than in relation to diameters, the minimum number of such points, geometrically, is three, and these would have to be arranged uniformly at 120° apart, *i.e.* as the apices of an equilateral triangle).

The development of the central terminal made possible the concept of a 'unipolar' recording, *i.e.* one in which the variation in potential difference (voltage) between the two electrodes is effectively the result of variation in potential at the 'exploring' electrode. If all the assumptions of the Einthoven triangle hypothesis were correct, there would be no potential change at the central terminal. Because the assumptions are only approximately true, the potential changes at the central terminal are small, but not truly zero. No recording system can, strictly speaking, be 'unipolar' (since all voltage measurements reflect differences in potential) but the concept is a useful one because there is a very significant difference between those leads labelled 'unipolar' (aVR, aVL, aVF, and V_1–V_6) and those labelled 'bipolar' (I, II, III). The difference is that, in the unipolar leads, changes in potential at one connection (the central terminal) are very small so the voltage (potential difference) across the leads is almost entirely produced at the 'exploring' electrode, whereas in leads I, II and III the voltage changes observed are the result of significantly varying potentials at either or both connections.

Thus the right arm lead measures the potential difference (voltage) between the right arm (at the shoulder) and the central terminal. Such a recording lead is called 'VR', the 'V' standing for 'voltage' and the 'R' for 'right arm'. By convention the term 'VR' also stands for the voltage measured at such a lead, which is given by:

$$VR \quad = E_R - (E_R + E_L + E_F)/3 \qquad \text{Eq. 6}$$

$$= (3E_R - E_R + E_L + E_F)/3$$

Therefore:

$$VR \quad = (2ER + EL + EF)/3 \qquad \text{Eq. 7}$$

Similarly:

$$VL = E_L - (E_R + E_L + E_F)/3 \qquad \text{Eq. 8}$$

$$VF = E_F - (E_R + E_L + E_F)/3 \qquad \text{Eq. 9}$$

The precordial leads have 'exploring' electrodes situated close to the heart and use the Wilson central terminal as the 'indifferent' electrode. They are, therefore, also 'V' leads, hence their designation as 'V_1' – 'V_6'.

THE AUGMENTED LIMB LEADS

Later (1942), so called 'augmented' unipolar limb leads ('aVR', 'aVL' and 'aVF') were developed by Goldberger,[9] simply by omitting the relevant exploring limb connection from also being connected to the 'indifferent' lead. At first sight, this would appear to invalidate the concept of the central terminal; in fact, all it does is to increase the voltage of the recording by a factor of 50%. This is easily demonstrated. From Equation 6, if the right arm connection is now omitted from the indifferent lead, the resulting lead is referred to as 'aVR'. Again, by convention, the term 'aVR' also stands for the voltage measured at such a lead. Thus we obtain:

$$aVR = E_R - (E_L + E_F)/2 \qquad \text{Eq. 10}$$

$$= (2E_R - E_L - E_F)/2$$

Therefore:

$$aVR = 1/2 \, (2E_R - E_L - E_F) \qquad \text{Eq. 11}$$

From Equation 7, it follows that

$$VR = 1/3 \, (2E_R - E_L - E_F) \qquad \text{Eq. 12}$$

Comparing Equations 11 and 12, it is clear that aVR = 3/2 VR, aVL = 3/2 VL and aVF = 3/2 VF.

With modern operational amplifiers this augmentation is no longer necessary but it remains a conventional part of the ECG recording system.

INTER-RELATIONSHIP OF THE SIX LIMB LEADS

Thus there are six limb leads, three being bipolar (I, II and III) and three unipolar (aVR, aVL and aVF). The limb leads differ from the precordial leads in two important respects. First, the limb leads almost exclusively reflect voltage changes in the frontal plane of the body, whereas the precordial leads reflect changes in the horizontal plane. Second, the limb leads are remote from the heart. As a result of this latter feature, the limb leads reflect general, overall information relating to voltage changes (both depolarisation and repolarisation) rather than localised information of the type provided by the precordial leads (in which V_5 and V_6 preferentially reflect voltage changes associated with the left ventricle and V_1 and V_2 those associated with the right ventricle).

Furthermore, the limb leads are definitively inter-related so that, if any two are recorded simultaneously, the other four can be derived (in respect of the same time window). Thus, for example, if I and II have been recorded, aVR can be calculated.

From Equation 11:

$$aVR = 1/2 \, (2E_R - E_L - E_F)$$

$$= 1/2 \, (E_R - E_L) + 1/2 \, (E_R - E_F)$$

$$= 1/2 \, (-I) + 1/2 \, (-II)$$

$$= -1/2 \, (I + II)$$

In the same way, when any two limb leads are known, the other four can be calculated. This may sound unimportant to those seeking to interpret the ECG but it is, in fact, highly significant. Since all the information available from the limb leads can be obtained from any two of the leads it makes no sense, for example, to speak of 'T-wave inversion in lead I'. If the T-waves are abnormal in any limb lead, they are abnormal in all the limb leads (although simple pattern recognition procedures do not acknowledge this undeniable truth). Pattern recognition analyses will reveal most abnormalities and most of the time will also correctly identify normality (i.e. the absence of detectable abnormality), but pattern recognition techniques cannot be relied upon always to distinguish between normality and abnormality in respect of the frontal plane T waves. This approach will result in equivocation in borderline situations where the abnormality is just outside the limits of normal. It is, therefore, essential, in establishing the normality or otherwise of T-waves in the limb leads, to consider their overall relationship to the QRS complexes, for it is this relationship which determines whether the T-waves in the limb leads (collectively) are normal or not. Although, as indicated above, this relationship can be precisely defined from any two limb leads, the availability of six leads makes the process much simpler, as will be apparent from the technique (to be demonstrated) for determining the frontal plane axis of any electro-cardiographic deflection.

ORIENTATION OF THE LIMB LEADS IN THE FRONTAL PLANE

The orientation of the six limb leads in the frontal plane is shown in Figure 1. The arrangement of the leads as shown in Figure 1 follows the concepts of the Einthoven triangle hypothesis, but the leads can be adjusted to a more practical arrangement without any change in their orientation within the frontal plane, as shown in Figure 2.

CALCULATION OF THE ORIENTATION, IN THE FRONTAL PLANE, OF VECTORS REPRESENTING THE ECG DEFLECTIONS

From the arrangement of the limb leads as displayed Figure 2, one can produce the hexaxial reference system (Fig. 3) which permits description of the orientation of vectors within the frontal plane. The six primary radii formed by the six limb leads are produced through their joint centre giving rise to 12 diameters, which divide the frontal plane into 12 equal sectors of 30°. The orientation of lead I is arbitrarily assigned the value 0° and the remaining

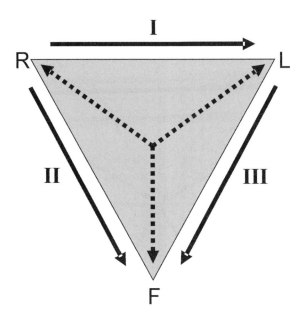

Fig. 1 Orientation, in the frontal plane, of the six limb leads.

positions are labelled (by convention) as shown. Using this template, the orientation within the frontal plane (the frontal plane axis) of any vector can be estimated to an accuracy of ±15°. Greater accuracy than this is not achievable (and should not be claimed) because the basic assumptions of the Einthoven triangle hypothesis are only approximately true. The frontal plane axis can be calculated in respect of any electrocardiographic deflections (QRS complex, T-wave, ST segment, P-wave, Ta-wave). It is most commonly used in relation to the QRS complexes and is most easily understood in this context, but knowledge of the relationship of the T-wave axis to the QRS axis is the key to the recognition of normal and of abnormal T-waves in the limb leads and

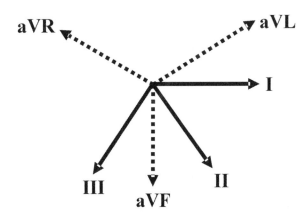

Fig. 2 A more practical way (than that used in Fig. 1) of displaying the orientation of the limb leads within the frontal plane.

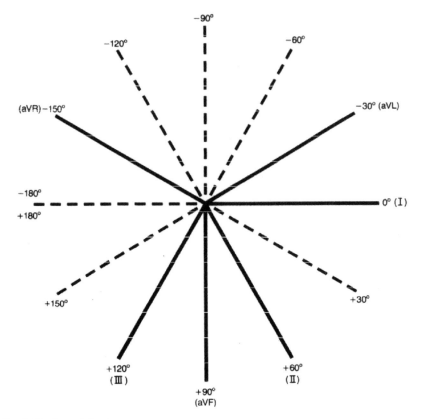

Fig. 3 The hexaxial reference system.

recent work has shown how important the frontal plane axis of the ST segment (vector orientation of the ST segment) is in relation to identifying: (i) the anatomical level of the block in cases of occlusion of the anterior descending branch of the left coronary artery; and (ii) the right coronary artery or the circumflex branch of the left as the site of block in acute inferior ST elevation infarction.

An example will help to clarify the use of the hexaxial reference system in measuring the frontal plane axis (*i.e.* the direction, as defined by the hexaxial reference system, of the mean vector) of any of the deflections on the ECG.

Consider the determination of the mean frontal plane QRS axis in the record shown in Figure 4, using the hexaxial reference system (Fig. 3). To determine the mean frontal plane QRS axis three items need to be addressed:

1. In which lead is the algebraic sum of QRS voltage deflections closest to zero? Clearly, the answer is lead I. It follows that the QRS axis is approximately at right angles to lead I and must therefore be +90° or −90° (approximately). [*It has been held that the area, rather than the voltage, of deflections should be measured. Such a process is, however, time consuming and, in general, the difference between the two approaches is small and not relevant bearing in mind that an accuracy exceeding ±15° cannot be claimed (by any technique). Furthermore, MacFarlane and Lawrie[2] found the area less reliable than the use of signed amplitudes (Chapter 13)*].

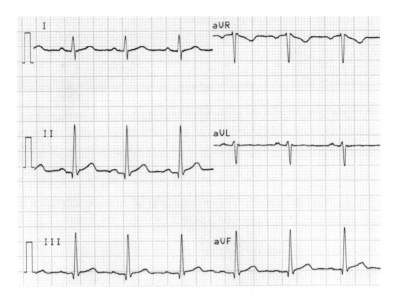

Fig. 4 To the nearest 30°, the mean frontal plane axis is +90°. To the nearest 15°, the axis is +75°.

2. Of these two possibilities, one (only) is aligned to another lead (in this case aVF). Inspection of the QRS in this lead shows it to be positive so, of the two options, the correct one must be +90° (approximately). This provides the axis to the nearest 30°.

3. Re-inspection of the lead with the algebraic sum of QRS voltage deflections closest to zero (lead I) shows the net QRS to be slightly positive (although close to zero). The estimate of the axis is, therefore, moved 15° towards lead I, and is thereby refined to +75°, to take account of the slight positivity in lead I. Had algebraic sum of QRS voltage deflections in lead I been slightly negative, the estimate of the axis would have been moved 15° away from lead I, and thereby refined to +105°, and had it been indistinguishable from zero the estimate of the axis would have remained at +90°. In each case, the updated estimate of the axis is correct to the nearest 15°. *(The 15° adjustment is in keeping with the scientific principle that the greatest accuracy one can claim in respect of any measurement is half the highest resolution of the measuring device. The 'measuring device' in this instance is the hexaxial reference system, the highest resolution of which is 30°).* The axis has, therefore, been calculated to the nearest 15°, which in any case is the greatest accuracy claimable in the light of the approximations involved in the assumptions of the Einthoven triangle hypothesis.

The technique described above in relation to determining the mean frontal plane QRS axis can be applied to any other part of the electrocardiographic waveform in which recognisable frontal plane deflections occur. In the normal, and in most abnormal, ECGs this applies to the P-waves, the QRS complexes and the T-waves. In cases where the ST segment is elevated or depressed, it also applies to the ST segments. It is only in respect of the QRS complexes, however, that one needs to determine the 'algebraic sum of deflections' since the P-waves, ST segments and T-waves have less complex shapes than the QRS complexes and in respect of these deflections, therefore, it is necessary in respect of item (1) above only to determine in which lead the smallest deflection is seen. The axis of the deflection is then known to be approximately (to the nearest 30°) at right angles to that lead. Following the principles in (2) and (3) above, the estimate of the axis can then be refined to an accuracy of ±15°.

When the axis of any deflection is known, the mean direction (positive or negative) of that deflection in all six limb leads is predictable. If the magnitude of a given deflection in one limb lead is known as well as the axis, both the direction and the magnitude of that deflection in all the limb leads is apparent.

PRACTICAL VALUE OF DETERMINING THE MEAN FRONTAL PLANE AXIS OF THE ELECTROCARDIOGRAPHIC DEFLECTIONS

MEAN FRONTAL PLANE QRS AXIS

The dominant direction of ventricular depolarisation in the frontal plane (mean frontal plane QRS axis) depends upon three separate items: (i) the physical position of the heart within the thorax; (ii) the properties and functioning of the intraventricular conduction tissue (predominantly the antero-superior and postero-inferior divisions of the left bundle branch system, but also the right bundle branch and the Purkinje network); and (iii) the electrical properties of the ventricular myocardium.

Normal range of frontal plane QRS axis

The mean frontal plane QRS axis, in the adult, lies within the range −30° to +90° (travelling clockwise with respect to the hexaxial reference system). Axes more negative than −30° indicate left axis deviation (LAD) and those more positive than 90° right axis deviation (RAD). When the axis is within the range −30° to +30° (travelling clockwise), the heart is said to be horizontal. When the axis is within the range +60° to +120° (travelling clockwise), the heart is said to be vertical. When the QRS complexes are approximately equiphasic in all six limb leads, the axis is indeterminate. This occurs when the vector loop (which is the locus of the instantaneous directions of ventricular depolarisation, within one QRS complex, in the given plane) is orientated approximately at right angles to the frontal plane. The finding of an indeterminate frontal plane QRS axis does not indicate abnormality.

RECOGNITION OF LEFT ANTERIOR FASCICULAR BLOCK (LEFT ANTERIOR HEMIBLOCK, LEFT SUPERIOR INTRAVENTRICULAR BLOCK)

The cardinal feature of left anterior fascicular block (LAFB) is an abnormal degree of left axis deviation. This means an axis more negative than −30° (which is the same thing as an axis of −45° or more negative', since the minimum axial resolution is 15°, so no points 'exist' between −30° and −45°). LAD alone is not sufficient for the diagnosis of LAFB since LAD can occur in extreme obesity, thoracic malformations, chronic lung disease and inferior infarction. The diagnosis of isolated LAFB requires, in addition to the demonstration of abnormal left axis deviation, the exclusion of: (i) the clinical

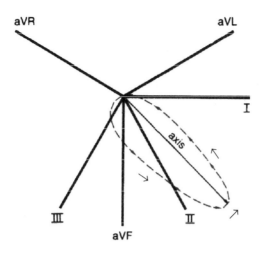

Fig. 5 The frontal plane vector loop with normal functioning of both divisions of the left bundle branch.

abnormalities listed above; and (ii) ECG evidence of inferior infarction; it also requires that the total QRS duration is not prolonged. It is commonly held that left ventricular hypertrophy (LVH) and left bundle branch block (LBBB) can give rise to left axis deviation. Whilst this is true, it is more accurate to say that these conditions may cause a left-ward shift of the existing axis by 15° or occasionally 30°. Thus LAD will result in these conditions only if the axis prior to the development of LVH or LBBB is −15° or more negative. In the case of LBBB, this truth is easily demonstrable when records are available prior to and following the development of the LBBB (Fig. 10).

When both the antero-superior (AS) and the postero-inferior (PI) divisions of the left bundle branch conduct normally, activation of the AS and PI parts of the left ventricular myocardium is near simultaneous. The resulting frontal plane vector loop is narrow and travels anticlockwise (Fig. 5). In the example shown in Figure 5 (and assuming normal conduction also in the right bundle branch), the QRS complexes would be narrow (≤ 0.10 s), there would be rs deflections in III, R in aVF, qR in II and in I, qr in aVL and QS in aVR.

When there is failure of conduction through the AS division of the left bundle, depolarisation of the posterior-inferior part of the left ventricle occurs normally but that of the antero-superior part is delayed and the vector loop travels counter-clockwise and appears as in Figure 6. In the example shown (and assuming normal conduction in the right bundle branch), the QRS duration would be within normal limits (≤ 0.10 s) although minimally longer than prior to the block, there would be rS deflections in III, aVF and II with qR deflections in I and aVL and an rS in aVR.

As can be seen from Figures 5 and 6, it is the *superior* rather than the *anterior* anatomical characteristic of the defect which produces the recognisable changes in the ECG. Current convention is to refer to the abnormality as 'left anterior fascicular block' or 'left anterior hemiblock', rather than the older, and clearly more appropriate, term 'left superior intraventricular block'.

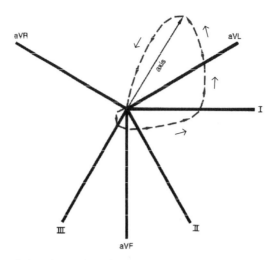

Fig. 6 The frontal plane vector loop in LAFB.

It is noteworthy that, in the absence of an anatomical abnormality, the commonest alternative cause of LAD is an established (Q-wave) inferior infarction, in which case the inferior wall is non-viable. There is, therefore, no deflection from the PI left ventricular myocardium and the frontal plane vector loop is directed superiorly. There is, therefore, LAD with q-waves in the inferior leads. The diagnosis of LAFB thus requires:[10] (i) QRS duration < 0.12 s (*i.e.* ≤ 0.10 s); (ii) LAD axis more negative than –30° (*i.e.* –45° or more negative); and (iii) rS in II, III, avF (*i.e.* no q-waves in these leads). An example is shown in Figure 7. The feature common to all cases of LAFB is abnormal left axis deviation.

RECOGNITION OF LEFT POSTERIOR FASCICULAR BLOCK (LEFT POSTERIOR HEMIBLOCK, LEFT INFERIOR INTRAVENTRICULAR BLOCK)

LPFB is much less common than LAFB because the posterior fascicle is thicker than the antero-superior fascicle and is less susceptible to fibrosis and ischaemia. The cardinal feature of left posterior fascicular block (LPFB) is an abnormal degree of right axis deviation.[10] This means an axis more positive than +90° (which is the same thing as 'an axis of +105° or more positive', since the minimum axial resolution is 15°, so no points 'exist' between +90° and +105°).

RAD alone is not sufficient for the diagnosis of LPFB since RAD can occur in right ventricular hypertrophy, chronic obstructive and acute pulmonary disease, emphysema, pulmonary embolism and extensive lateral infarction. The diagnosis of isolated LPFB therefore requires, in addition to the demonstration of abnormal right axis deviation, the exclusion of the clinical abnormalities listed above together with ECG evidence that the total QRS duration is not prolonged. It is commonly held that right bundle branch block (RBBB) can give rise to right axis deviation. Whilst this is true, it is more accurate to say that the development of RBBB may cause a right-ward shift of the existing axis by 15° or occasionally 30°. Thus, RAD will result only if the axis prior to the development of RBBB was +75° or more positive. This is easily

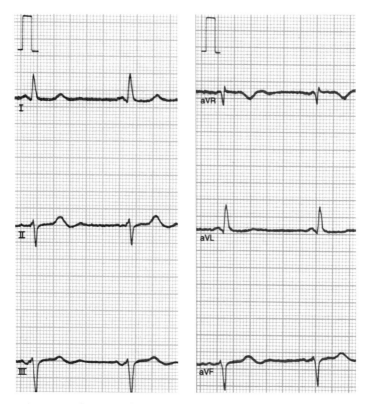

Fig. 7 Left anterior fascicular block. Only the limb leads are involved in the diagnosis. As expected from Figure 6, there are qR complexes in I and aVL and rS complexes in II, III and aVF.

demonstrable when records are available prior to and following the development of the RBBB (Fig. 10).

When there is failure of conduction through the PI division of the left bundle, depolarisation of the antero-superior part of the left ventricle occurs normally but that of the postero-inferior part is delayed and the vector loop travels clockwise and appears as in Figure 8. With the vector loop as shown in Figure 8 (and assuming normal conduction in the right bundle branch), the QRS duration would be within normal limits (≤ 0.10 s), there would be rS deflections in I and aVL with an Rs wave in II and qR patterns in aVF and III and a QR in aVR. This is, of course, not the only possible form of the frontal plane QRS loop in LPFB, so variations in the appearances in the individual limb leads will occur. **The feature common to all will be abnormal right axis deviation.**

An ECG showing LPFB is shown in Figure 9.

FRONTAL PLANE QRS AXIS IN BUNDLE BRANCH BLOCK, FASCICULAR BLOCK AND VENTRICULAR HYPERTROPHY

Right and left bundle branch block

It is widely held that the development of RBBB can give rise to RAD and that of LBBB to LAD. While these statements are true, they are potentially

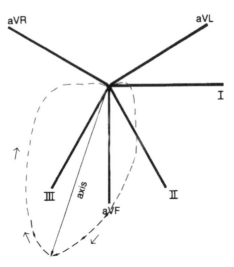

Fig. 8 The frontal plane vector loop in LPFB.

misleading for reasons already explained. For example, it is more accurate to state that the development of RBBB is sometimes associated with a shift of the axis to the right by 15° (and occasionally by 30°) and with the development of

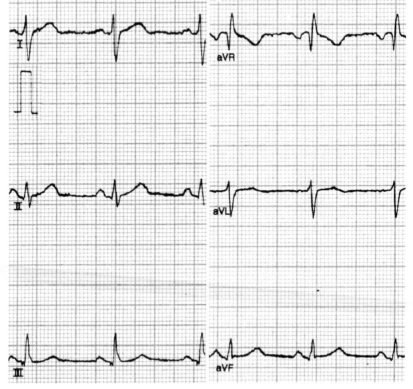

Fig. 9 Left posterior fascicular block. The diagnosis cannot be made on ECG criteria alone. Other causes of RAD must be excluded.

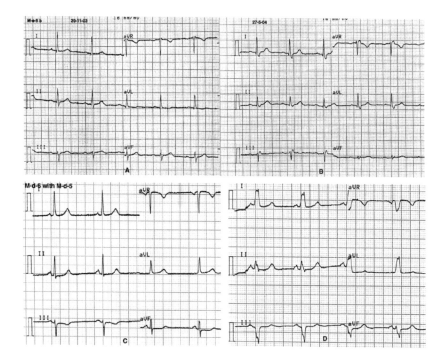

Fig. 10 Limb leads before and after the development of bundle branch block. (A) Before (axis 0°) and (B) after (axis 0°) the development of RBBB. (C) Before (axis 0°) and after (D) (axis –15°) development of LBBB. The P-waves and PR interval are identical in (A) and (B) and in (C) and (D), confirming that (A) and (B) are from the same subject as are (C) and (D).

LBBB the axis typically moves 15° (and occasionally 30°) to the left and that often there is no detectable axis change (Fig. 10). Thus, if the axis prior to the development of LBBB is in the region of –15° or –30°, a minor degree of left axis deviation may result (usually not more negative than –45°). Most often, however, the development of LBBB is not associated with the development of LAD, and, as indicated in the next section, the presence of an abnormal mean frontal plane QRS axis in association with bundle branch block is suggestive of additional intraventicular block.

Right bundle branch block plus fascicular block
RBBB plus LAH is indicated by the combination of RBBB with LAD (–45° or more negative).[11] An example is shown in Figure 11.

RBBB plus LPH is suggested by (there is also the requirement that other causes of RAD be excluded) the combination of RBBB with RAD (+90° or more positive). An example is shown in Figure 12.

Left bundle branch block plus right or left axis deviation
In the presence of LBBB, the finding of RAD (+105° or more positive; Fig. 12) or of LAD (–45° or more negative; Fig. 13) should lead to the suspicion a more diffuse intraventricular conduction abnormality than that indicated by LBBB alone (Fig. 13).[12]

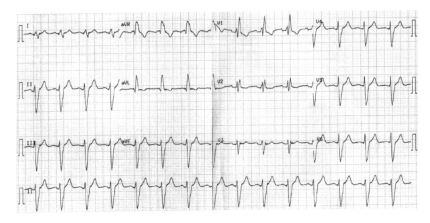

Fig. 11 RBBB plus LAH. The criteria for RBBB (total QRS duration ≥ 0.12 s plus rSR' in V_1) and for LAH (mean frontal plane QRS axis is more negative than −30° [in this case −90°] with initial r waves in II, III and aVF) are both fulfilled.

Right and left ventricular hypertrophy

As with LBBB, the frontal plane QRS axis moves slightly to the left in association with the development of left ventricular hypertrophy (LVH) but abnormal LAD only develops in such circumstances if the axis would have been towards the left side of the normal range in the absence of LVH. Since LVH most commonly occurs in older age groups within the population and since, in such groups, the heart is often horizontal, there clearly is an association between LVH and LAD. However, LAD is not amongst the Sokolow-Lyon[13] or the Cornell[14] criteria for LVH, although it is included in the Romhilt-Estes[15] scoring system.

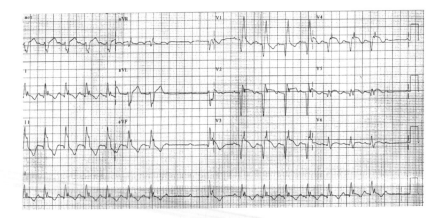

Fig. 12 RBBB plus RAD. The criteria for RBBB (total QRS duration ≥ 0.12 s plus rSr' in V_1) and for LPH (mean frontal plane QRS axis is more positive than −90° [in this case +120°]) are both fulfilled. The ECG cannot establish the diagnosis of LPH, it can only suggest the possibility, since there are numerous other causes of abnormal right axis deviation. In this case, the fact that there is occasional failure of atrioventricular conduction makes it virtually certain that there really is LPH as well as RBBB. This combination of blocks is highly likely to progress to complete block because the remaining fascicle is the least robust. In this case, there is also extensive anterior

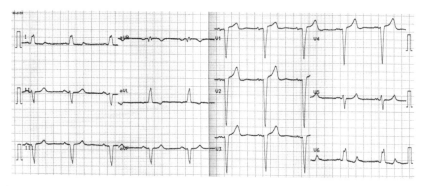

Fig. 13 LBBB with LAD. The frontal plane QRS axis is –60°. Abnormal LAD is not inevitable with LBBB (see Fig. 10C,D) The presence of a clearly abnormal frontal plane QRS axis indicates more diffuse intraventricular conduction than that indicated by LBBB alone.

The situation is different in respect of RVH. Abnormal RAD *is an essential* part of the diagnostic criteria for RVH.

In RBBB, LBBB and LVH, the frontal plane QRS axis determines the configuration of the QRS complexes in the limb leads (given their configuration in the precordial leads). Thus, when the heart is horizontal (axis –30° to +30°), appearances of the type seen in V_5 and V_6 will be reflected in I and aVL. When the heart is vertical (axis +60° to +120°), appearances of the type seen in V_5 and V_6 will be reflected in II, aVF and III.

SIGNIFICANCE OF Q-WAVES IN THE LIMB LEADS

An understanding of the frontal plane QRS axis is essential for distinguishing between normal and abnormal q-waves in aVL and III. Each of these leads can be a 'cavity lead', like aVR (which is orientated towards the cavities of the right and left ventricles). Cavity leads typically show dominantly negative QRS complexes and T-waves because the dominant direction of ventricular depolarisation is from endocardium to epicardium.

When the heart is vertical (axis +60° to +120°), aVL is a cavity lead and may have prominent q-waves or QS complexes, which, in this situation, cannot be considered to be abnormal.

When the heart is horizontal (axis –30° to +30°), III is a cavity lead and may have prominent q-waves or QS complexes, which, in this situation, cannot be considered to be abnormal.

FRONTAL PLANE T-WAVES

In the precordial leads, T-waves may reasonably be considered to be normal or to be abnormal in respect of any individual lead. This is because the precordial leads are close to the heart and the deflections from these leads are influenced more by subjacent parts of the myocardium than by more remote areas. Thus, in the adult ECG, it is acknowledged that the T-waves are usually upright in all the precordial leads, but that T-wave inversion in V_1 alone is not considered to be abnormal. T-wave inversion in V_2 in addition to V_1 can sometimes be normal but T-wave inversion in any other precordial lead is abnormal.

The same approach (*i.e.* declaring a T-wave to be normal or abnormal in respect of one particular lead) cannot be used in relation to the limb leads because these are remote from the heart. The T-waves in the limb leads reflect the direction of the vector of the later part of repolarisation in the frontal plane (*i.e.* the T-wave axis) just as the QRS complexes in the limb leads reflect the direction of depolarisation. If the T-waves are known in any two limb leads (or if the T-waves are known in any one lead and the T-wave axis is also known), the T-wave appearances in all the remaining limb leads can be predicted.

In normal circumstances, the direction of T-wave vector is the same as, or is close to, that of the QRS complex. Thus the net polarity of the T-waves in the frontal plane leads is generally the same as the net polarity of the preceding QRS complex in each lead; however, this generalisation does not permit of the clear delineation of normal from abnormal frontal plane T-waves in all situations. The most useful concept is that in the normal ECG the angle between the frontal plane T-waves and QRS complexes is less than 60° (*i.e.* ≤ 45°).[16] The frontal plane T-wave axis is calculated in the same way as for the QRS axis. When the frontal plane T wave axis is within the range ±45° with respect to the frontal plane QRS axis, the T-waves in the limb leads are within normal limits. When the angle between the two axes is 60° or more the T-waves in the limb leads are abnormal. This applies to all the limb leads since, as already explained, the limb leads are remote from the heart, and give an overall rather than a localised 'view' and the information content of all the limb leads given by any two leads.

ST SEGMENT IN ACUTE ST ELEVATION MYOCARDIAL INFARCTION

It is well recognised that, in acute ST elevation myocardial infarction (STEMI), elevation of the ST segments in the inferior leads (II, III and aVF) indicates inferior ischaemic damage and ST elevation in the precordial leads (V_1–V_6) indicates anterior ischaemic damage.[16a] An appreciation of the significance of the direction in the frontal plane of the dominant ST segment vector (*i.e.* the frontal plane ST axis) reveals considerably more, useful information. The direction of the ST vector is either: (i) (directly or almost directly) towards that lead with the greatest degree of ST elevation; or (ii) (directly or almost directly) away from the direction of that lead with the greatest degree of ST depression (and is, therefore, best assessed by using the lead with the greatest ST shift – up or down).

In the normal ECG, the ST segment is isoelectric in the frontal plane and no vector is detectable. With the development of ST shift (elevation or depression), a measurable frontal plane ST vector will be apparent and determination of the frontal plane ST segment axis provides useful information.

Recent studies have shown the importance of the frontal plane ST axis in predicting the site of occlusion in acute ST elevation myocardial infarction, not only in relation to inferior infarction but also in relation to anterior infarction.

Frontal plane ST segment vector in inferior infarction

In 1997, Herz *et al.*[17] demonstrated the significance of the finding of ST elevation more marked in lead III than in lead II, in inferior infarction when caused by occlusion of the right coronary artery (which accounts for 80% cases of inferior infarction). By contrast, they found that ST elevation more marked

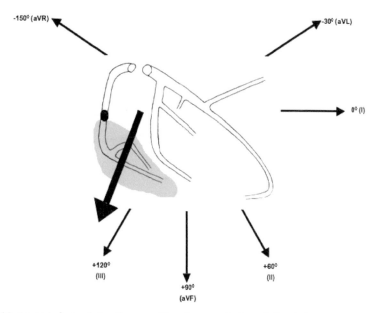

Fig. 14 Acute inferior infarction resulting from occlusion of the right coronary artery is associated with an ST segment vector close to +120°. This produces the greatest degree of ST elevation in III, with lesser ST elevation in aVF and less still in II. Leads I and aVL inevitably show ST depression. Lead aVR, being at right angles to the ST vector, shows little or no ST shift. Compare with Figure 15.

in lead II than in lead III was indicative of infarction caused by left circumflex artery occlusion. These findings were confirmed by Zimetbaum *et al.*[18] In a review article in 2003, Zimetbaum and Josephson,[19] in relation to the combination of (i) ST elevation in lead III exceeding that in lead II (which indicates an ST axis of +120°), and (ii) ST depression in I, aVL or both (inevitable when the ST axis is +120°), quoted a sensitivity of 90% and a specificity of 71% in the prediction of a right coronary occlusion. The positive and negative predictive values were, respectively, 94% and 70%. Inspection of Figure 14 shows why this distribution of ST segment change occurs. In inferior infarction resulting from right coronary occlusion, the ST segment vector is directed towards the damaged area, giving maximum ST elevation in lead III, with less ST elevation in aVF and II, and with ST depression in I, aVL. Figure 14 also shows that the greatest degree of ST depression will be in aVL, with a lesser amount in I. Even in the presence of dramatic ST depression in I and AVL, the ST segments in aVR will be close to isoelectric since this lead is virtually at right angles to the dominant direction of the ST vector. An example is shown in Figure 15.

Once it is recognised that the ST segment is close to zero in aVR and is greatest in III, it is clear that the ST vector is +120°. The appearances of the ST vector in the remaining four limb leads can be predicted from this information. Thus, an ST vector of +120° gives ST elevation in III and, inevitably, 'reciprocal' ST depression in aVL and I.

This again demonstrates the total inter-relationship between the six limb leads. If the ST segment measurement is known in any two limb leads, the

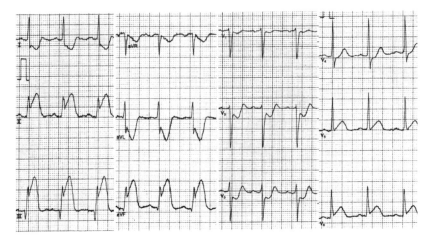

Fig. 15 Acute inferior infarction resulting from occlusion of the right coronary artery. ST elevation in III is greater than that in aVF which is greater than that in II, *i.e.* the frontal plane ST vector is directed at +120°. There is, therefore, very little ST shift in aVR but there is inevitably marked ('reciprocal') ST depression in I and aVL. Compare with Figure 14.

orientation of the ST segment vector (*i.e.* the ST segment axis) can be calculated; once this is known, the ST segment can be predicted in all the remaining limb leads. Furthermore, it is unnecessary to produce additional limb leads (such as '–aVR" at +30°, '–II' at –120°, '–aVF' at –90°, *etc.*) since these can all be predicted from (any two of) the conventional limb leads. (In the same way, although not strictly relevant here since this article relates exclusively to the [frontal plane] limb leads, Hurst[20] has pointed out that 'it is not necessary to record electrocardiograms from the right side of the chest searching for S-T segment elevation, because the deflections can be predicted from the standard 12-lead electrocardiogram').

By contrast, Figure 16 shows the direction of ST vector in relation to inferior infarction resulting from occlusion of the circumflex branch of the left coronary artery.

An example of a 12-lead ECG showing the results of occlusion of the circumflex branch of the left coronary artery is shown in Figure 17.

Since the ST segment in all the limb leads is completely defined once the vector is known, it is not necessary to specify the ST appearances in all the limb leads. Once the direction of the maximal ST vector in the frontal plane has been identified, the direction of the ST segment shift in all the other limb leads is totally predictable using the hexaxial reference system (as seen from Figs 14 and 16).

Frontal plane ST segment vector in anterior infarction
Perhaps surprisingly, in acute anterior STEMI, the limb leads give more information than the precordial leads concerning the site, within the anterior descending artery (LAD), of the acute coronary occlusion. In 1995, Tamura *et al.*[21] showed that ST segment depression of 1 mm or more in all of the inferior limb leads (II, III and aVF) – which implies an ST segment axis in the region of –90° – had a sensitivity of 77%, a specificity of 78%, a positive predictive value

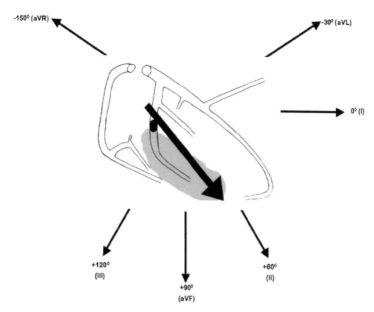

Fig. 16 Acute inferior infarction resulting from occlusion of the circumflex artery is associated with an ST segment vector close to +60°. This produces the greatest degree of ST elevation in II, with lesser ST elevation in aVF and in III. The ST segment in I will be slightly elevated, aVL will have an isoelectric ST segment and aVR will show ('reciprocal') ST depression. Compare with Figure 17.

of 73% and a negative predictive value of 77%, in relation to predicting the LAD occlusion to be proximal to the first septal perforating artery (S1) and the first diagonal artery (D1) in anterior infarction. In 1999, Engelen *et al.*[22] undertook a detailed study of 100 consecutive patients admitted to the

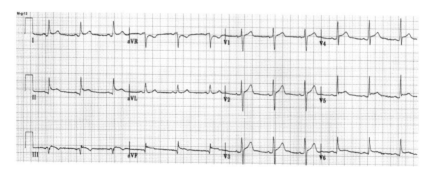

Fig. 17 Acute inferior infarction resulting from occlusion of the circumflex artery is associated with an ST segment vector close to +60°. The ST segment is isoelectric in aVL and must, therefore, be at right angles to that lead. This means the ST segment must be +60° or –120°. The ST segment is elevated in II, so the ST vector is +60°. One can predict from this that there will be ST elevation also in I, aVF and III, and that the ST elevation in aVF will be less than that in II. One can also predict that the degree of ST elevation in I will be similar to that in III (since both leads are at 60° to the ST vector) and that both will be less than that in II and aVF. One can also predict that the ST segment will be negative in aVR ('reciprocal' ST depression) and that it will be isoelectric in aVL, since this lead is at right angles to the ST segment vector. (In keeping with the occlusion in a dominant circumflex artery, there is also lateral involvement). Compare with Figure 16.

coronary care unit of the University Hospital, Maastricht with the diagnosis of acute anterior STEMI. They found that ST elevation in aVR had a specificity of 95% in indicating a block in the LAD proximal to S1. They stressed that the degree of ST elevation in aVR was small (usually < 1 mm) and that the sensitivity was low (43%) but also that, in the context of acute anterior STEMI, the finding of any ST elevation in aVR (which implies that the axis of the ST vector is more negative than –30°), is associated with LAD occlusion proximal to S1.

These descriptions are based on pattern recognition principles. It is, however, not necessary to specify the ST appearances in individual leads, once the ST segment axis has been determined, for this defines the ST appearances in all the limb leads. Figure 18 shows the direction of ST vector in relation to anterior STEMI resulting from occlusion of the LAD proximal to S1. Inspection of the direction of the ST segment vector in relation to the limb leads reveals the likely ST segment appearances in all the limb leads. Thus, with the ST vector as shown, there will be appreciable ST depression in II, aVF and III, isoelectric ST segments in I and some ST elevation in aVR and aVL.

A 12-lead ECG in a case of an LAD occlusion proximal to S1 is shown in Figure 19.

Yamaji et al.[23] further showed that, in cases of occlusion of the left main coronary artery, the findings were similar to those in LAD obstruction proximal to S1, but there was often a greater degree of ST elevation in aVR (0.16 ± 0.13 mV compared with 0.04 ± 0,10 mV) indicating a further negative shift of the axis of the ST vector (ST segment axis –105°).

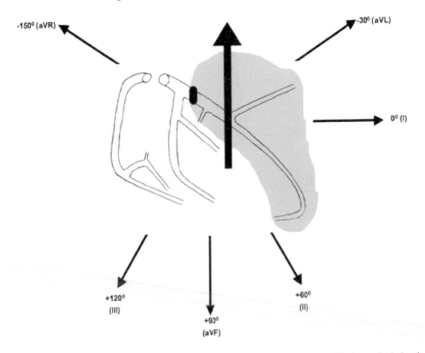

Fig. 18 Occlusion of the LAD proximal to S1. The dominant zone of ischaemia is in the anterobasal area of the left ventricle. This gives a superiorly orientated ST vector (arrow) with ST depression in III, aVF and II, and ST elevation (often quite minor but highly significant) in aVR and sometimes also in aVL. The ST segment is often isoelectric in lead I. Compare with Figure 19.

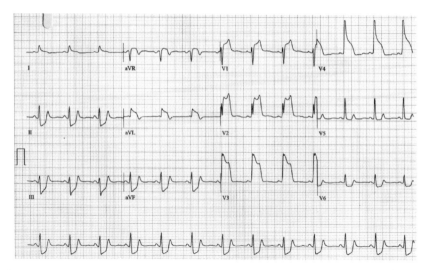

Fig. 19 Acute anterior STEMI due to occlusion of the LAD proximal to S1. The frontal plane ST segment vector is directed superiorly. There is, therefore, ST depression in II, III and aVF with an isoelectric ST in I. There is a minor degree of ST elevation in aVR (very highly significant since it indicates that the ST vector is more negative than –30°) and ST elevation in aVL. Compare with Figure 18.

When the LAD occlusion is distal to S1 and proximal to D1, there is no involvement of the most anterobasal part of the left ventricle and the ST segment vector is orientated upwards and to the left with an axis of about –30° (Fig. 20).

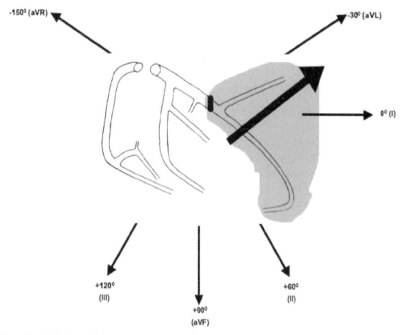

Fig. 20 Occlusion of the LAD distal to S1 and proximal to D1. The dominant zone of ischaemia is in the anterolateral area of the left ventricle. This gives an ST vector directed upwards and to the left (arrow) with ST elevation in aVL and I, ST depression in III, aVF, and isoelectric ST segments in II and aVR. Compare with Figure 21.

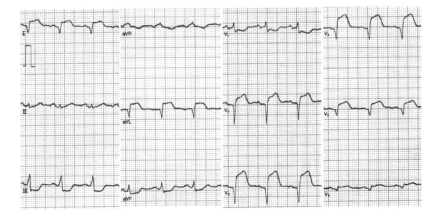

Fig. 21 Acute anterior STEMI due to occlusion of the LAD distal to S1 and proximal to D1. The ST segment vector is directed superiorly and to the left (–30°). There is, therefore, ST elevation in aVL and I, ST depression in III and aVF and minimal ST depression in aVR with an isoelectric ST in II. Compare with Figure 20.

An ECG showing the changes associated with occlusion at this site is shown in Figure 21.

When occlusion occurs distal to D1 the ST vector is directed more inferiorly than in Figure 20. It is then typically +60°, giving ST depression in aVR and isoelectric ST segments in aVL.

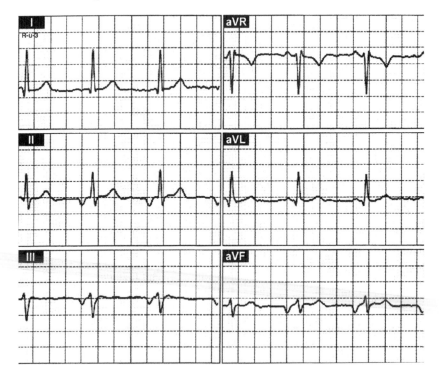

Fig. 22 The limb leads in a case of low atrial rhythm. The frontal plane P-wave vector is –90°.

When the rhythm is of sinus origin, the atrial depolarisation vector in the frontal plane is directed downwards and to the left. For that reason, the largest positive P-wave is most frequently to be found in lead II. The acceptable range for the P-wave axis in the presence of sinus rhythm is 0° to +90° (travelling clockwise).[24,25]

Figure 22 shows an example of an abnormal P-wave axis (−90°), clearly indicating that the origin of the rhythm is not the sino-atrial node. The rhythm is arising from an inferior location within the atria.

Key points for clinical practice

- The limb leads are definitively inter-related and the sum total of the information contained in all six leads is completely provided by any two of them. If any two are recorded simultaneously, the other four can be derived. In respect of each deflection (P, QRS, ST, T, Ta) if the axis of the deflection and the appearances in any one lead are known, the appearances of that deflection in all the limb leads is apparent.

- The limb leads provide overall, rather than localised, information about the heart; in the case of each electrocardiographic deflection, it is the direction of the vector of that deflection, within the frontal plane, which provides the diagnostic information.

- A simple technique, facilitated by the availability of all six limb leads, permits calculation of the mean frontal plane QRS axis to the nearest 15°. The mean frontal plane QRS axis, in the adult, lies within the range −30° to +90° (travelling clockwise). Precisely the same technique is used to determine the frontal plane axes of the T waves, P waves and (when there elevation or depression) of the ST segments.

- The cardinal feature of left anterior fascicular block (LAFB, LAH) is an abnormal degree of left axis deviation and that of left posterior fascicular block (LPFB, LPH) is an abnormal degree of right axis deviation.

- When the heart is horizontal (QRS axis −30° to +30°, travelling clockwise) lead III becomes a cavity lead and QS complexes are then acceptable. When the heart is vertical (QRS axis +60° to +120°, travelling clockwise) aVL becomes a cavity lead and QS complexes in this lead are then acceptable.

- RBBB does not consistently (or even frequently) give rise to RAD, nor do LVH or LBBB consistently (or even frequently) give rise to LAD. In each case, the axis moves 15° or occasionally 30° towards the respective side

- The mean frontal plane T-wave axis is normally within ±45° of the frontal plane QRS axis. When this angle is exceeded, the T-waves in (all) the frontal plane leads are abnormal.

(continued on next page)

Key points for clinical practice *(continued)*

- In sinus rhythm, the frontal plane P-wave axis lies within the range 0° to +90°. When the P-wave axis is outside this range, it is unlikely that the rhythm is of sinus origin.

- The normal ST segment is isoelectric and, therefore, subtends no significant angle on the frontal plane. When there is primary ST elevation, the direction of the ST vector indicates the major location of myocardial damage. Because of the inter-relationship of the six limb leads, those leads opposed to (*i.e.* at 180° to) the ones showing maximal ST elevation will inevitably show (reciprocal) ST depression.

- In acute inferior STEMI, an ST vector in the region of +120° (ST elevation most marked in III, less marked in aVF and less still in II) points to occlusion of the right coronary artery.

- In acute inferior STEMI, an ST vector in the region of +60° (ST elevation most marked in II, less marked in aVF and less still in III) points to occlusion of the circumflex coronary artery.

- In acute anterior STEMI, the direction of the frontal plane ST vector gives a better guide than the precordial leads to the location (within the anterior descending artery) of the coronary occlusion: (i) when the ST vector is directed at or close to –90° the occlusion is proximal to S1 and D1; (ii) when the ST vector –105° or more negative (which will usually imply ≥ 2 mm ST elevation in aVR) occlusion of the main stem is possible; (iii) when the ST vector is directed at or close to –30°, the occlusion is distal to S1 and proximal to D1; and (iv) when the ST vector is close to +60° the occlusion is distal to D1.

References

1. Kadish AH, Buxton AE, Kennedy HL *et al.* ACC/AHA clinical competence statement on electrocardiography and ambulatory electrocardiography: a report of the ACC/AHA/ACP-ASIM Task Force on Clinical Competence (ACC/AHA/ACP-ASIM Committee to Develop a Clinical Competence Statement on Electrocardiography and Ambulatory Electrocardiography) Endorsed by the International Society for Holter and Noninvasive Electrocardiology. *J Am Coll Cardiol* 2001; **38**: 2091–2100.
2. Macfarlane PW, Lawrie TDV. *Comprehensive Electrocardiology.* Oxford: Pergammon, 1989; Chapter 10.
3. Pipberger HV, Arzbaecher RC, Berson AS *et al.* Recommendations for standardisation of leads and of specifications for instruments in electrocardiography and vectorcardiography: report of the Committee on Electrocardiography. *Circulation* 1975; **52**: 11–31.
4. Hoff HE, Sekelj P. On the direction and manifest size of the variations of potential in the human heart and on the influence of the position of the heart on the form of the electrocardiogram. *Am Heart J* 1950; **40**: 163–211. (A translation from Einthoven W, Fahr GE, De Waart A. Über die Richtung und die manifeste Grosse der Potentialschwankungen im menschlichen Herzen und überden Einflus der Herzlage auf die Form des Elektrokardiogramms. *Pfluegers Arch* 1913; **150**: 275–315).
5. Burger HC, van Milaan JB. Heart-vector and leads Part I. *Br Heart J* 1946; **8**: 157–161.

6. Burger HC, van Milaan JB. Heart-vector and leads Part II. Geometrical representation. *Br Heart J* 1947; **9**: 154–160.
7. Burger HC, van Milaan JB. Heart-vector and leads Part III. *Br Heart J* 1948; **10**: 229–233.
8. Wilson FN, Johnston FD, MacLeod AG, Baker PS. Electrocardiograms that represent the potential variations of a single electrode. *Am Heart J* 1934; **9**: 447–458.
9. Goldberger E. A simple, indifferent electrocardiographic recording of zero potential and a technique of obtaining augmented, unipolar, extremity leads. *Am Heart J* 1942; **23**: 483–492.
10. Rowlands DJ. *Clinical Electrocardiography*. London: Gower Medical, 1991.
11. Willems JL, Demidena EO, Bernard R *et al*. World Health Organization/International Society and Federation of Cardiology Task Force. Criteria for intraventricular-conduction disturbances and pre-excitation. *J Am Coll Cardiol* 1985; **5**: 1261–1275.
12. Macfarlane PW, Lawrie TDV. *Comprehensive Electrocardiology*. Oxford: Pergammon, 1989; Chapter 14.
13. Sokolow M, Lyon TP. The ventricular complex in left ventricular hypertrophy as obtained by unipolar precordial and limb leads. *Am Heart J* 1949; **37**: 317–327.
14. Casale PN, Devereux RB, Alonso DR, Campo E, Kligfield P. Improved sex-specific criteria of left ventricular hypertrophy for clinical and computer interpretation of electrocardiograms: validation with autopsy findings. *Circulation* 1987; **3**: 565–572.
15. Romhilt DW, Estes Jr EH. A point-score system for the ECG diagnosis of left ventricular hypertrophy. *Am Heart J* 1968; **75**: 752–758.
16. Mirvis DM, Golberger AL. Electrocardiography. In: Zipes DP, LibbyP, Bonow RO, Braunwald E (eds) *Braunwald's Heart Disease*, 7th edn. Amsterdam: Elsevier Saunders, 2005; 117.
16a. Mirvis DM, Golberger AL. Electrocardiography. In: Zipes DP, Libby P, BonowRO, Braunwald E (eds) *Braunwald's Heart Disease*, 7th edn. Amsterdam: Elsevier Saunders, 2005; 134–136
17. Herz I, Assali AR, Adler Y, Solodky A, Sclarovsky S. New electrocardiographic criteria for predicting either the right or left circumflex artery as the culprit coronary artery in inferior wall acute myocardial infarction. *Am J Cardiol* 1997; **80**: 1343–1345.
18. Zimetbaum P, Krishnan S, Gold A, Carrozza II JP, Josephson M. Usefulness of ST-segment elevation in lead III exceeding that of lead II for identifying the location of the totally occluded artery in inferior wall myocardial infarction. *Am J Cardiol* 1998; **81**: 918–919.
19. Zimetbaum PJ Josephson ME. Use of the electrocardiogram in acute myocardial infarction. *N Engl J Med* 2003; **348**: 933–940.
20. Hurst JW. Letter to the Editor. *J Electrocardiography* 2007; **40**: 67.
21. Tamura A, Kataoka H, Mikuriya Y, Nasu M. Inferior ST segment depression as a useful marker for identifying proximal left anterior descending artery occlusion during acute anterior myocardial infarction. *Eur Heart J* 1995; **16**: 1795–1799.
22. Engelen DJ, Gorgels AP, Cheriex EC *et al*. Value of the electrocardiogram in localising the occlusion site in the left anterior descending coronary artery in acute myocardial infarction. *J Am Coll Cardiol* 1999; **34**: 389–395.
23. Yamaji H, Iwasaki K, Kusachi S *et al*. Prediction of acute left main coronary obstruction by 12-lead electrocardiography: ST elevation in aVR with less ST elevation in lead V_1. *J Am Coll Cardiol* 2001; **38**: 1348–1354.
24. Macfarlane PW, Lawrie TDV. *Comprehensive Electrocardiology*. Oxford: Pergammon, 1989; Chapter 22.
25. Spodick DH. Computer error and acceptable standards for electrocardiographic interpretation. *J Electrocardiol* 2006; **39**: 348–349.

Cara Hendry Farzin Fath-Ordoubadi

13

Percutaneous coronary intervention in acute coronary syndromes

The term 'acute coronary syndrome' encompasses a heterogeneous clinical spectrum, from the occurrence of escalating anginal chest pain at rest to acute ST elevation myocardial infarction. Unstable angina and non-ST elevation myocardial infarction account for in excess of 2.5 million hospital admissions world-wide each year, and present a significant burden in terms of morbidity and mortality.[1] Whilst recent years have witnessed a decline in the incidence of acute ST elevation myocardial infarction, the hospitalisation rate for chest pain and acute coronary syndrome has dramatically risen.[2] In this chapter, we discuss the non-ST elevation forms of acute coronary syndrome.

PATHOPHYSIOLOGY

The atheromatous plaque, once considered to be an inert structure, has been found over past years to be a metabolically active tissue which is subject to dynamic remodelling processes. The extracellular matrix is in a constant equilibrium of collagen synthesis and degradation. The regulation of matrix collagen turnover is provided by a variety of factors including matrix metalloproteinases and gelatinases. The collagen fibrils in the fibrous cap of the plaque provide mechanical strength; hence, the release of pro-inflammatory cytokines, which influence production of these factors, may cause the cap to weaken resulting in plaque instability. Denuded endothelium may also excite the thrombotic pathways.

The disruption of the unstable plaque results in a complex series of events. The highly thrombogenic, lipid-rich core contains tissue factor, which

Cara Hendry MB ChB MRCP
SpR in Cardiology, Manchester Heart Centre, Manchester Royal Infirmary, Manchester M13 9WL, UK

Farzin Fath-Ordoubadi BSc MB BCh MD FRCP
Consultant Cardiologist, Manchester Heart Centre, Manchester Royal Infirmary, Manchester M13 9WL, UK
E-mail: farzin.fath-ordoubadi@cmmc.nhs.uk

stimulates platelet activation and aggregation, and thrombus deposition on non-occlusive plaque. The clinical effects of this are dictated by the interaction of prothrombotic and fibrinolytic mechanisms at that time and result, ultimately, in the clinical event of the acute coronary syndrome. Partial or transient occlusion of the vessel lumen with thrombus results in acute coronary syndrome in the absence of ST elevation whilst complete occlusion results in acute ST elevation myocardial infarction.

CLINICAL FEATURES

Acute coronary syndromes are characterised clinically by the occurrence of prolonged (> 20 min) anginal chest pain, new onset of severe (Canadian Cardiovascular Society [CCS] class III) angina or recent deterioration in previously stable anginal symptoms to at least CCS III severity. It is almost impossible to differentiate clinically between the non-ST elevation and ST elevation forms of acute coronary syndrome.

DIAGNOSIS

Electrocardiography

Electrocardiography is an essential part of making the diagnosis of acute coronary syndrome and initiating appropriate treatment. It is mandatory to carry out electrocardiography as soon as possible after presentation with chest pain in order to identify those patients with ST segment elevation in whom prompt action may be required in the form of administration of thrombolytic therapy or primary angioplasty. Electrocardiography is not utilised solely for this purpose: electrocardiographic findings correlate strongly with the risk of subsequent myocardial infarction and death.[3-5] Additionally, ST segment depression on ECG at the time of presentation to hospital is associated with a 100% increase in the angiographic finding of either three vessel or left main stem disease than those without ST depression (45% versus 22%, respectively; $P < 0.001$).[6]

Detection of cardiac troponin

Recent changes to the guidelines for diagnosis of acute coronary syndrome and myocardial infarction issued jointly by the European Society of Cardiology and the American College of Cardiology emphasise the importance of the detection of cardiac troponins.[7] Troponin is located on the thin filament of the contractile apparatus of striated muscle and consists of three main subunits which are known as troponin T, C and I. Isoforms C and I are expressed exclusively on cardiac myocytes; therefore, their release into the circulation is specific for myocardial damage. The assays available for detection of these biomarkers vary markedly from one centre to another and this is reflected in the guidelines, with the diagnosis of myocardial damage being made as a troponin level which exceeds the 99th centile of levels in healthy subjects. Troponin release is first detected in the first 4–6 h after myocardial damage, and the level peaks between 14–18 h. The serum troponin may remain elevated for up to 14 days after the index episode. In clinical practice, troponin must be measured at least 12 h after the onset of the most recent episode of chest pain. The implementation of the new guidelines in accepting raised troponin as a central part in making the diagnosis of myocardial infarction may be, at least in part, responsible for the increase in incidence of non-ST elevation myocardial infarction; interestingly, data demonstrating its rise predate the release of the 2000 guidelines.[2]

Detection of cardiac troponin is a powerful indicator of prognosis in patients who present with chest pain.[8] The risk of death in patients diagnosed with non-ST segment elevation myocardial infarction at 30 days ranges from 3.6–26% based on a variety of clinical risk factors.[9,10] The risk of death exhibits a directly proportional, linear relationship with the troponin level.

Inflammatory biomarkers in acute coronary syndrome

Inflammation is central to the processes which underlie rupture of the atherosclerotic plaque. There has been much interest in the role of inflammation in determining prognosis in unstable coronary artery disease, and this has prompted investigation to identify novel biomarkers of cardiac risk.

The measurement at high-sensitivity of C-reactive protein in acute coronary syndrome in patients with myocardial damage has been found to impart an adverse prognosis.[11] This finding has driven further studies into measurement of cytokine levels, and other inflammatory markers. Recent trials have demonstrated that elevated levels of interleukin-6 and fibrinogen are clearly linked to long-term mortality.[11,12] Further investigation is required to evaluate fully the role of inflammation in coronary instability.

CLINICAL FEATURES ASSOCIATED WITH INCREASED RISK

The group of patients presenting with acute coronary syndromes is a heterogeneous population with a wide variation in risk of short- and long-term adverse events. In view of this, risk stratification is of key importance in tailoring patient management.

The major clinical trials in this patient group have utilised scoring systems to determine risk. The scores are based on similar well-known variables which have long been found to be associated with risk, but have a number of differences. Examples of these include the Thrombolysis In Myocardial Infarction (TIMI) scoring system which has been used in large-scale clinical trials to identify those patients at highest risk in both ST elevation and non-ST elevation forms of acute coronary syndrome. The TIMI risk scoring system correlates very closely with mortality at 30 days, with a more than 40-fold increase in mortality observed in comparing those with a score of 0 and those with a score > 8. The risk of mortality in those with a TIMI risk score of 0 was < 1%.[10,13] More recently, the PURSUIT and GRACE risk scores have also contributed to the understanding of which patients benefit most from revascularisation during the index admission.[14,15]

Key factors common to all algorithms used to predict risk are age, male sex, rest pain, presence of ST segment depression and elevated cardiac biomarkers. All are associated with a marked increase in the risk of subsequent morbidity and mortality (the last two listed being the most important adverse prognostic indicators).

Identification of those patients at the highest risk is essential in management of patients with chest pain. It is also of key importance to identify those patients with a good prognosis, in order to avoid exposing patients to the potential risks of unnecessary procedural complications. The lowest risk groups in the TIMI risk scoring system with negative troponin and normal electrocardiogram, with no other risk factors, had a risk of less than 1%.

TREATMENT OF ACUTE CORONARY SYNDROME

Treatment in all forms of acute coronary syndrome must be delivered as swiftly as possible in order for patients to derive maximum benefit. Additionally, all patients admitted with acute coronary syndrome should be treated with standard medical therapy, including aspirin, clopidogrel, β-blockade, low molecular weight heparin and aggressive lipid-lowering therapy (in the absence of contra-indications). In this chapter, we consider the terms angioplasty and percutaneous coronary intervention (PCI) interchangeably.

ANTIPLATELET AGENTS

Aspirin

The aggregation of platelets on the ruptured coronary plaque is central to the pathological process which underlies acute coronary syndrome. Aspirin acts by blocking the production of thromboxane A2, thus inhibiting platelet aggregation. Aspirin has been clearly established as beneficial in ST elevation myocardial infarction,[16,17] with vascular mortality reduction of 23% when given alone and 42% when combined with streptokinase. A substudy of the group noted above also showed a non-significant trend of 16% mortality reduction in patients given aspirin within 2 h of pain onset, compared with others receiving it within 5–12 h. Other forms of acute coronary syndrome also benefit from aspirin.[18,19]

The majority of physicians advocate an initial loading dose of 300–325 mg followed by maintenance dose of 75 mg daily. There does not appear to be any additional benefit in receiving a dose > 100 mg daily, despite this dose causing excess bleeding risk.[18] The first responder should initiate the loading dose of aspirin to maximise benefit.

Clopidogrel

Dual inhibition of platelet function is achieved using the thienopyridine clopidogrel in addition to aspirin. Clopidogrel causes irreversible blockade of the platelet P2Y12 receptor. In non-ST elevation acute coronary syndromes, addition of clopidogrel to aspirin has been demonstrated to reduce major adverse cardiovascular events, death, myocardial infarction and stroke, with a slight increase in the bleeding risk observed with all doses of aspirin.[20] Additionally, clopidogrel has recently been shown in cases of ST elevation myocardial infarction, when added to optimum reperfusion therapy including aspirin, to demonstrate a substantial additional mortality benefit after only 1 month of therapy.[21] The long-term effects of clopidogrel in ST elevation myocardial infarction have yet to be established. The recommended loading dose of clopidogrel is 300 mg, with a maintenance dose of 75 mg daily. Current recommendations for use in patients who have been treated with angioplasty are that clopidogrel should be continued for a minimum of 1 year post-procedure. Current research into clopidogrel is on-going, with trials assessing the roles of different dosing regimens and results in patients exhibiting resistance to its effects, and also into outcomes of patients receiving different loading doses in varying clinical situations.

Anticoagulation

Trials have demonstrated that, in combination with antiplatelet agents, the addition of anticoagulants is of clear benefit in the non-ST elevation acute coronary syndromes.[22] Initial investigations reviewed the role of unfractionated heparin, but subsequent trials have shown that weight-adjusted, low molecular weight heparin is superior to unfractionated heparin in reducing death, acute myocardial infarction and refractory anginal symptoms at both 30 days and 1 year[23,24] in this group of patients.

Thrombolytic therapy has also been studied in the non-ST elevation group, with disappointing results: there was no difference in death, myocardial infarction, or treatment failure with the use of tissue plasminogen activator (tPA). Fatal and non-fatal myocardial infarction occurred more frequently in the group treated with lytic therapy. There was also a trend to a higher number of intracranial haemorrhages in the lysis-treated group.[25]

Glycoprotein IIb/IIIa blockers

Activation of the platelet glycoprotein IIb/IIIa receptor is the final common pathway of the process leading to platelet aggregation and thrombus formation in acute coronary syndrome. The receptor binds fibrinogen and forms links between adjacent activated platelets, resulting in the formation and propagation of platelet thrombi. Potent inhibition of platelet action is, therefore, achieved by addition of platelet glycoprotein IIb/IIIa receptor antagonists to standard therapy as outlined above. Randomised, controlled trials in non-ST elevation acute coronary syndrome have studied the effects of a variety of these agents.[7,26–28] The entry criteria for the trials differ slightly but, overall, patients required the presence of ECG abnormality and/or positive cardiac biomarker. The drugs were commenced up to 12 h or 24 h after onset of pain and an intention to undertake early coronary angiography was not a prerequisite. A meta-analysis of these data involving 31,402 patients showed a significant benefit of antagonism of the glycoprotein receptor with a reduction in death or myocardial infarction at 30 days. Benefits were also maximal in the patient subgroups deemed to be at highest risk of complications. The bleeding risk was higher in the groups receiving glycoprotein IIb/IIIa blockers as would be expected (2.4 versus 1.4%; $P < 0.0001$) although the overall bleeding risk was low.[29]

The ACUITY trial recently published data on over 9000 patients with acute coronary syndrome, and assessed the importance of timing of initiation of glycoprotein IIb/IIIa blockers, and also compared the effects of bivalirudin plus glycoprotein IIb/IIa blockers with those obtained with standard heparin plus glycoprotein IIb/IIIa blocker. The trial demonstrated that the occurrence of ischaemia in the group who had glycoprotein receptor blockers deferred until time of angiography was not significantly increased; however, the rates of bleeding were significantly reduced. The combination of glycoprotein IIb/IIIa receptor blockers with bivalirudin carried a similar risk of ischaemia and bleeding to that of glycoprotein IIb/IIIa plus heparin, whilst that of bivalirudin alone compared to the heparin/glycoprotein IIb/IIIa antagonist carried a similar risk of ischaemia, and a significant reduction in the incidence of bleeding.[30]

In patients undergoing angioplasty in the setting of acute coronary syndrome, the prothrombotic pathways are also stimulated by mechanical disruption of the unstable plaque and the denuding of the endothelial surface of the coronary vasculature during PCI. The patients treated by angioplasty thereby derive additional early benefit by platelet receptor blockade, as seen in a number of trials.[26,31] The benefits are once again maximised in the highest risk patients undergoing PCI with elevated levels of troponin T or I, particularly in diabetics.[26,27] The large molecule glycoprotein IIb/IIIa inhibitor (abciximab) seems also to have added benefit in comparison to the other agents with smaller molecules.

Current recommendations for the use of glycoprotein IIb/IIIa antagonists suggest that all patients with non-ST elevation ACS (in the absence of contra-indication) undergoing percutaneous angioplasty should receive glycoprotein IIb/IIIa blockers, in addition to standard therapy as outlined above.[28]

THE ROLE OF PERCUTANEOUS CORONARY INTERVENTION

Overall, patients with a diagnosis of acute coronary syndrome or suspected non-ST elevation myocardial infarction carry a high risk of premature death, myocardial infarction and refractory ischaemia.[32,33] The most potent risk predictors are raised cardiac troponins and electrocardiographic abnormalities.

Percutaneous coronary intervention mechanically alters obstructing lesions within the coronary arteries, and improves coronary flow. This was, in early trials, achieved by use of balloon angioplasty; this practice has since been superseded by use of intracoronary stenting, which not only improves coronary flow but also maintains vessel integrity by means of scaffolding. Subsequent development of stents delivering drugs locally in the coronary arteries – drug eluting stents (DES) – has further reduced restenosis rates in target vessels.

Broadly speaking, the trials comparing invasive with conservative strategies in non-ST elevation acute coronary syndromes may be divided into two groups – those carried out before the advent of coronary artery stenting and glycoprotein IIb/IIIa therapy and those carried out after these treatments were established.

Initial trials pre-dating the use of stenting and blockade of the glycoprotein IIb/IIIa receptor underestimated the future value of interventional strategies. A summary of the trials is presented in Table 1.

The three landmark trials carried out prior to the above strategies were TIMI IIIb,[25] MATE[34] and VANQWISH.[35] Patients in all three studies were assigned to either early invasive or a conservative strategy. Common to all trials, including the later trials (with the exception of the later study ICTUS), was that the invasive strategy could include coronary artery bypass grafting where indicated, usually for left main stem or multivessel disease. Also

Table 1 Summary of randomised trials comparing invasive and conservative treatments

Trial (n)	Year	Patients	Entry criteria chest pain plus	Glycopro IIb/IIIa use (Inv/Cons)	Stent use (Inv/Cons)	Interv (Inv %)	Interv (Cons %)	CABG (Inv %)	CABG (Cons %)	Results (Inv vs Cons)	Favours Interv	Favours Cons
TIMI IIIb[25]	1995	1473	ECG changes or prior CAD	No	No	60	40	24	18	Death/MI/+ETT 18% vs 16% (P = NS)	+	+
MATE[34]	1998	201	History	No	No	58	37	16	8	Composite of recurrent ischaemia/death 13% vs 34% (P = 0.0002)	+	
VANQWISH[35]	1998	920	CKMB or CK+	No	No	44	33	23	21	Death/non-fatal MI 21 vs 6 pts (P = 0.007)	+	+
FRISC II[36]	1999	2457	ECG changes or trop/CKMB+	Yes	62/69%	78	37	35	19	Death/MI 19.9% vs 24.5% (P = 0.009) 5-year data	++	
TRUCS[39]	2000	148	History	96/95%	85/85%	77	38	25	8	Non-fatal MI/death 3.9 vs 12.5 (P = 0.053)	++	
TACTICS[38]	2001	2220	ECG abn/trop+/ prior CAD	94/59%	83/86%	61	37	20	13	Death/non-fatal MI/ rehospitalisation 16 vs 19.4% (P = 0.025)	++	
VINO[40]	2002	131	ECG abn AND trop/CKMB +	No	50/44%	73	39	35	30	Death/reinfarction 6.2 vs 22.3% (P < 0.001)	++	
RITA 3[41]	2002	1810	ECG abn/CAD on prev angios	25%*	88/90%	45	11	12	4	Death/non-fatal MI 16 vs 20% (P = 0.044), CV death/MI 12 vs 15% (P = 0.03)	++	
ICTUS[43]	2004	1200	Trop+ & either ECG abn/ETT+/ angios+	95/69%	Yes	79	53			Death/non-fatal MI/ rehospitalisation 22.7% vs 21.2% (P = 0.33)	+	+

*Denotes of all patients undergoing PCI.
Inv, invasive treatment; Cons, conservative treatment; Glycopro, glycoprotein; Interv, Intervention

common to many studies was the principle that elevation of cardiac biomarkers post-angioplasty was considered to meet the criteria for re-infarction. This accounts, at least in part, for the excess of cardiac events noted in some trials around the time of procedure. Conservative therapy patients were treated by optimal medical therapy, and symptom or functional test-driven coronary angiography and subsequent intervention by angioplasty or bypass as indicated by the findings at coronary angiography.

The first, large-scale, randomised study to evaluate this clinical dilemma was the TIMI IIIb study. The mean time to angiography in the invasive group was 1.5 days post randomisation, and in the conservative group 7.1 days. Those randomised to the invasive therapy had fewer re-hospitalisations within 6 weeks, and also received a lower number of anti-anginal medications per patient. The outcomes post-discharge were otherwise similar.[25] One could argue that routine early invasive strategy in this study did not demonstrate significant benefit in terms of mortality; however, in terms of quality of life, fewer medications and hospitalisations, and earlier return to work are important and have cost-saving benefits.

The results of VANQWISH show that the rate of death was higher within the first year for those patients undergoing the early invasive strategy. Closer analysis of the data, however, shows that there are a number of flaws of the trial. First, the trial selected relatively low-risk patients, only 34% of those screened were recruited for entry into the trial. The 9% of patients deemed to have the highest risk were actually managed invasively and were not randomised into the trial. Second, in the invasive arm, only 44% underwent a re-vascularisation procedure, compared to 33% in the conservative arm. Also, the increase in risk of death appears to be attributable to surgical intervention rather than percutaneous coronary intervention. Median time to angiography was 2 days and 14 days in the invasive and conservative groups, respectively.

The cross-over rates in all three early trials were high, and this has a strong confounding effect on the results.

The trials described subsequently were all carried out after usage of stents and glycoprotein IIb/IIIa receptor blocker therapy became widely available. In the FRISC II trial, approximately 60% of patients entering the study had a positive troponin result. The time scale of angioplasty in the invasive group was later than in previous trials, with 71% of patients having angiography within 10 days. At 1 year, there was a clear benefit seen in the invasive arm, with a reduction of the composite end-point of death or myocardial infarction.[36] The benefits of the invasive therapy were sustained at 5 years with a 4.6% absolute and 19% relative risk reduction in the composite end-point as noted above.[37]

The TACTICS TIMI 18 study involving 2220 patients further enhanced the understanding of this subject. Time to revascularisation in the invasive group, angioplasty or CABG, was 25 h and 89 h, respectively. The benefits were maximal in those patients with a positive troponin and benefits were borne out to 6 months. There was no clear benefit seen in those with a TIMI score of 0–1.[38]

RITA-3 in 2001 added further to the weight of evidence supporting an invasive strategy. The overlap of the treatments groups in RITA-3 was much less than that of earlier trials: only 11% of those assigned to conservative treatment underwent coronary angiography within the first 7 days. A clear benefit was seen in the invasive group in RITA-3 with a reduction in the combined primary end-point of death, non-fatal myocardial infarction or refractory angina at 1 year. Additional benefit was seen in terms of health-related quality-of-life assessments, and is largely attributable to a reduction in the number of anginal episodes and anti-anginal medications in the invasive group.[41] Long-term data from this study were released in 2005, and these clearly support the use of an early routine invasive strategy in patients with non-ST elevation acute coronary syndromes with a clear reduction in death and non-fatal myocardial infarction observed at mean of 5 years follow-up. The benefits, once again, were maximal in the high-risk patients – in the highest risk group, the interventional treatment was associated with a 56% reduction in the odds-of-death or myocardial infarction.[42]

The ICTUS study in 2005 recruited 1200 patients. The overall mortality in this trial was 2.5%, which is significantly lower than that of the other trials, and would suggest that the patients enrolled were low-risk patients and thus less likely to derive substantial benefit from angioplasty. Overall results of this trial did not show any clear difference in the outcomes between the two groups.[43] This is at odds with the previous trials of acute coronary syndromes.

More recently, the GUSTO IV ACS study, which had 7800 high-risk patients on the basis of troponin or ECG changes, and encouraged a conservative strategy, showed that the patients who had re-vascularisation had a clear mortality benefit, with a procedural risk of only 1.8%.[44] Meta-analysis involving the above studies confirms that PCI is the best treatment option, with a reduction in death/myocardial infarction from 14.4% to 12.2% with invasive therapy ($P = 0.001$).[45]

Registry data are also of use when assessing the utility of invasive strategies. There have been a number of publications in recent years which add considerably to our understanding of this subject. In many ways, the registry data reflect clinical practices more fully, and eliminates the issue of selection bias for entry into clinical trials. The GRACE registry, which contained almost 29,000 patients, demonstrated that not receiving in-hospital angioplasty in acute coronary syndrome was an independent predictor of mortality at 4 years.[46,47] Accordingly, the OASIS registry, which compared centres with varying proportions of in-patient angiography, assessed the effects of this on outcomes. Data on 4615 patients with acute coronary syndrome demonstrated that an improvement in the combined end-point of refractory angina, death, myocardial infarction and stroke was proportional to the utilisation of in-patient coronary angiography, 34.9% versus 46.8% (high rate versus low rate).[48]

A further proponent for early invasive therapy is the MITI registry, which contains long-term (mean, 3.2 years) follow-up data on 1635 patients with non-ST elevation ACS. These data demonstrate that patients from centres which undertake early angiography derive a significant mortality benefit,[49] implying that the early invasive strategy is beneficial.

An early invasive strategy is clearly the management of choice in acute coronary syndrome, and current recommendations by the joint committees of the American Heart Association/American College of Cardiology and the European Society of Cardiology reinforce this as noted below as a class Ia recommendation (Table 2).

Table 2 Recommendations of the joint committees of the American College of Cardiology/ American Heart Association and the European Society of Cardiology

---

ACC/AHA Guidelines

An early invasive strategy is recommended in patients with UA/NSTEMI and any of the following high-risk indicators

- Recurrent angina/ischaemia at rest or with low-level activities despite anti-ischaemic therapy
- Elevated troponin T or I
- New or presumed new ST segment depression at presentation
- Recurrent angina/ischaemia with CHF symptoms/S3 gallop, pulmonary oedema, worsening rales, or new or worsening mitral regurgitation
- High-risk findings on non-invasive stress testing
- Depressed LV systolic function (*e.g.* ejection fraction [EF] < 40% on non-invasive study)
- Haemodynamic instability or angina at rest accompanied by hypotension
- Sustained ventricular tachycardia
- PCI within 6 months
- Prior CABG

European Society of Cardiology Guidelines 2005

Characteristics of patients with NSTE ACS at high acute thrombotic risk for rapid progression to myocardial infarction or death who should undergo coronary angiography within 48 h

- Recurrent resting pain
- Dynamic ST segment changes: ST segment depression ≥ 0.1 mV or transient (< 30 min) ST elevation ≥ 0.1 mV
- Elevated troponin I, troponin T or CKMB level
- Haemodynamic instability during the observation period
- Major arrhythmias (ventricular tachycardia, ventricular fibrillation)
- Early post infarction unstable angina
- Diabetes mellitus

SUMMARY

The incidence of acute coronary syndromes without ST elevation is increasing in the UK. There are two main driving factors. First, the progressive improvement of diagnostic investigations, in particular biomarkers of myocardial necrosis (troponin I and T), has resulted in an increase in the diagnostic yield of individuals presenting to medical personnel with chest pain. Second, even allowing for this, the occurrence of non-ST elevation forms of ACS are increasing, whilst ST elevation infarction is falling, for undetermined reasons. Reasons for this include improved preventative therapy and increased survival of initial ST elevation myocardial infarction. Troponin release, indicating myocardial necrosis, is a marker of a high mortality and morbidity risk in this group.

The presence of electrocardiographic abnormality at time of presentation is a clear predictor of adverse outcome, and of multivessel or left main coronary artery disease. Conversely, the mortality risk in a patient with a normal electrocardiogram and a negative troponin test is less than 1%.

The advancement of adjunctive medical therapies has undoubtedly improved in recent years. More comprehensive platelet receptor blockade with the combination of aspirin and clopidogrel is a clearly beneficial in all forms of acute coronary syndrome.

Glycoprotein IIb/IIIa receptor antagonists have further reduced mortality in patients undergoing angioplasty in non-ST elevation acute coronary syndrome, and should be administered to all patients assigned to this therapy in the setting of acute coronary syndrome, as stated in current recommendations. The benefits are clear, and are greatest in high-risk patient groups such as diabetics.

Angioplasty techniques have also improved dramatically in recent years – stent technology has greatly reduced the need for target lesion revascularisation when compared to balloon angioplasty. Restenosis is the main limitation of angioplasty. The development of coronary stents eluting either paclitaxel or sirolimus (drug-eluting stents) in recent years has substantially reduced the need for repeat procedures compared with bare metal stents, and thus are rapidly superseding them in interventional cardiology with excellent results. There are two large trials investigating the use of drug-eluting stents in acute coronary syndrome – the TYPHOON study and the PASSION study. In TYPHOON, there was a non-significant trend in favour of the paclitaxel-eluting stent,[49] and similar finding for the sirolimus-eluting stent in PASSION.[50] Drug-eluting stents are, therefore, considered safe for use in acute coronary syndrome.

The clinical trials taking place after the introduction of these therapies for cardiological treatments have demonstrated very encouraging results, showing: (i) a reduced number of hospitalisations; (ii) fewer anti-anginal medications per patient with an early invasive strategy; and (iii) a reduction in end-points including death and myocardial infarction. These benefits exist beyond 1 year, and in some trials out to 5 years. These trials strongly support the use of angioplasty in non-ST elevation myocardial infarction. Registry data confirm these findings.

In summary, there is now an overwhelming body of evidence to support the use of in-patient angiography and early angioplasty in patients with moderate- and high-risk ACSs/NSTEMI (*i.e.* positive troponin or abnormal ECG or other indicator of high risk). This should be considered the treatment of choice in this group of patients.

Future developments may well include the adoption of bivalirudin as the thrombin inhibitor of choice in patients with acute coronary syndromes undergoing percutaneous coronary intervention, and there are further developments in drug delivery via drug-eluting stents, which remain to be assessed.

By far the most important challenge to clinicians will be in establishing dedicated angioplasty centres to optimise the delivery of angioplasty to the rising number of patients with this condition.

Key points for clinical practice

- An abnormal ECG is an independent predictor of risk of death and subsequent myocardial infarction in patients with non-ST elevation forms of acute coronary syndrome.

- A raised troponin level is associated with a poor prognosis.

- Risk stratification should be carried out in all patients with acute coronary syndromes to identify those at highest risk, who will benefit most from percutaneous intervention.

- Dual antiplatelet therapy with aspirin and clopidogrel should continue for at least 1 year after acute coronary syndrome and/or percutaneous coronary intervention.

- All patients with non-ST elevation acute coronary syndrome undergoing percutaneous coronary intervention should receive a glycoprotein IIb/IIIa receptor antagonist.

- In non-ST elevation acute coronary syndromes, an early invasive strategy is associated with better short-term and long-term results than conservative management.

References

1. Grech ED, Ramsdale DR. Acute coronary syndrome: unstable angina and non-ST segment elevation myocardial infarction. *BMJ* 2003; **326**: 1259–1261.
2. Murphy NF, MacIntyre K, Capewell S *et al*. Hospital discharge rates for suspected acute coronary syndromes between 1990 and 2000: population based analysis. *BMJ* 2004; **328**: 1413–1414.
3. Cannon CP, McCabe CH, Stone PH *et al*. The electrocardiogram predicts one-year outcome of patients with unstable angina and non-Q wave myocardial infarction: results of the TIMI III Registry ECG Ancillary Study. Thrombolysis in Myocardial Ischemia. *J Am Coll Cardiol* 1997; **30**: 133–140.
4. Savonitto S, Ardissino D, Granger CB et al. Prognostic value of the admission electrocardiogram in acute coronary syndromes. *JAMA* 1999; **281**: 707–713.
5. Mahadevan VS, Adgey AAJ. ST depression in ECG at entry indicates severe coronary lesions and large benefits of an early invasive treatment strategy in unstable coronary artery disease – the FRISC II ECG substudy. *Eur Heart J* 2002; **23**: 3–5.
6. Diderholm E, Andren B, Frostfeldt G *et al*. The prognostic and therapeutic implications of increased troponin T levels and ST depression in unstable coronary artery disease: The FRISC II invasive troponin T electrocardiogram substudy *Am Heart J* 2002; **143**: 760–767.
7. European Society of Cardiology/American College of Cardiology. Myocardial infarction redefined – A consensus document of The Joint European Society of Cardiology/American College of Cardiology Committee for the Redefinition of Myocardial Infarction. *Eur Heart J* 2000; **21**: 1502–1513.
8. Lindahl B, Venge P, Wallentin L. Relation between troponin T and the risk of subsequent cardiac events in unstable coronary artery disease. *Circulation* 1996; **93**: 1651–1657.
9. Cohen M, Stinnet SS, Weatherley BD *et al*. Predictors of recurrent ischemic events and death in unstable coronary artery disease after treatment with combination antithrombotic therapy. *Am Heart J* 2000; **139**: 962.
10. Wiviott SD, Morrow DA, Frederick PD, Anrman EM, Braunwald E. Application of the Thrombolysis In Myocardial Infarction Risk Index in non-ST-segment elevation

myocardial infarction: evaluation of patients in the National Registry of Myocardial Infarction. *J Am Coll Cardiol* 2006; **47**: 1553–1558.

11. Toss H, Lindahl B, Siegbahn A, Wallentin L for the FRISC Study Group. Prognostic influence of increased fibrinogen and C-reactive protein levels in unstable coronary artery disease. *Circulation* 1997; **96**: 4204–4210.

12. Lindmark E, Diderholm E, Wallentin L, Siegbahn A. Relationship between interleukin 6 and mortality in patients with unstable coronary artery disease: effects of an early invasive or noninvasive strategy.[see comment]. *JAMA* 2001; **286**: 2107–2113.

13. Morrow DA, Antman EWM, Charlesworth A *et al*. TIMI risk score for ST-elevation myocardial infarction: a convenient, bedside, clinical score for risk assessment at presentation: an Intravenous nPA for Treatment of Infarcting Myocardium Early II Trial Substudy. *Circulation* 2000; **102**: 2031–2037.

14. PURSUIT Investigators. Predictors of outcome in patients with acute coronary syndrome without persistent ST segment elevation. *Circulation* 2000; **101**: 2557–2567.

15. de Araujo Goncalves P, Ferreira J, Aguiar C, Seabra-Gomes R. TIMI, PURSUIT, and GRACE risk scores: sustained prognostic value and interaction with revascularization in NSTE-ACS. *Eur Heart J* 2005; **26**: 865–872.

16. Baigent C, Collins R, Appleby, Parish S, Sleight P, Peto R. ISIS-2: 10 year survival among patients with suspected acute myocardial infarction in randomised comparison of intravenous streptokinase, oral aspirin, both, or neither. BMJ 1998; **316**: 1337–1343.

17. ISIS-2 Collaborative Group. Randomised trial of intravenous streptokinase, oral aspirin or both or neither among 17,187 cases of suspected acute myocardial infarction. *Lancet* 1988; **ii**: 349–360.

18. Peters RJG, Mehta SR, Fox KAA *et al*. Effects of aspirin dose when used alone or in combination with clopidogrel in patients with acute coronary syndromes: observations from the Clopidogrel in Unstable angina to prevent Recurrent Events (CURE) Study. *Circulation* 2003; **108**: 1682–1687.

19. The RISC Group. Risk of myocardial infarction and death during treatment with low dose aspirin and intravenous heparin in men with unstable coronary artery disease. *Lancet* 1990; **336**: 827.

20. The CURE Trial Investigators. Effects of clopidogrel in addition to aspirin in patients with acute coronary syndromes without ST segment elevation. *N Engl J Med* 2001; **345**: 494–502.

21. COMMIT (ClOpidogrel and Metoprolol in Myocardial Infarction Trial) Collaboration. Addition of clopidogrel to aspirin in 45,852 patients with acute myocardial infarction: randomised placebo-controlled trial. *Lancet* 2005; **366**: 1607–1617.

22. Cohen M, Adams PC, Parry G *et al*. Combination antithrombotic therapy in unstable rest angina and non-Q-wave infarction in nonprior aspirin users. Primary end points analysis from the ATACS trial. Antithrombotic Therapy in Acute Coronary Syndromes Research Group. *Circulation* 1994; **89**: 81–88.

23. Cohen M, Demers C, Gurfinkel EP *et al*. A comparison of low-molecular-weight heparin with unfractionated heparin for unstable coronary artery disease. *N Engl J Med* 1997; **337**: 447–452.

24. Goodman SG, Cohen M, Bigonzi F *et al*. Randomized trial of low molecular weight heparin (enoxaparin) vs unfractionated heparin for unstable coronary artery disease. 1 year results of the ESSENCE study. *J Am Coll Cardiol* 2000; **36**: 693–698.

25. The TIMI III Investigators. Effects of tissue plasminogen activator and a comparison of early invasive and conservative strategies in unstable angina and non-Q-wave myocardial infarction. Results of the TIMI IIIB Trial. Thrombolysis in Myocardial Ischemia. *Circulation* 1994; **89**: 1545–1556.

26. PRISM-PLUS Study Investigators. The Platelet Receptor Inhibition in Ischemic Syndrome Management in Patients Limited by Unstable Signs and Symptoms Study. I. Inhibition of the platelet glycoprotein IIb/IIIa receptor with tirofiban in unstable angina and non-Q-wave myocardial infarction. *N Engl J Med* 1998; **338**: 1488–1497.

27. PURSUIT Trial Investigators. Inhibition of platelet glycoprotein IIb/IIIa with eptifibatide in patients with acute coronary syndromes. *N Engl J Med* 1998; **339**: 436–443.

28. Task Force of the ESC. Management of acute coronary syndromes in patients presenting without persistent ST segment elevation. *Eur Heart J* 2002; **23**: 1809–1840.

29. Boersma E, Harrington R, Moliterno D *et al*. Platelet glycoprotein IIb/IIIa inhibitors in acute coronary syndromes: a meta-analysis of all major randomised clinical trials. *Lancet* 2002; **359**: 189–198. Erratum appears in *Lancet* 2002; **359**: 2120.

30. Stone G. Bivalirudin for patients with acute coronary syndromes. *N Engl J Med* 2006; **355**: 2203–2216.

31. The EPIC Investigators. Use of a monoclonal antibody directed against the platelet glycoprotein IIb/IIIa receptor in high-risk coronary angioplasty. *N Engl J Med* 1994; **343**: 956–961.

32. Yusuf S, Pogue J, Hunt D *et al*. Variations between countries in invasive cardiac procedures and outcomes in patients with suspected unstable angina or myocardial infarction without initial ST elevation. *Lancet* 1998; **352**: 507–514.

33. Nicod P, Gilpin E, Dittrich H *et al*. Short- and long-term clinical outcome after Q wave and non-Q wave myocardial infarction in a large patient population. *Circulation* 1989; **79**: 528–536.

34. McCullough PA, O'Neill WW, Graham M *et al*. A prospective randomized trial of triage angiography in acute coronary syndromes ineligible for thrombolytic therapy. Results of the medicine versus angiography in thrombolytic exclusion (MATE) trial. *J Am Coll Cardiol* 1998; **32**: 596–605.

35. Boden WE, O'Rourke RA, Crawford MH *et al*. Outcomes in patients with acute non-Q-wave myocardial infarction randomly assigned to an invasive as compared with a conservative management strategy. *N Engl J Med* 1998; **338**: 1785–1792.

36. Wallentin L, Lagerqvist B, Husted S, Kontny F, Stahle E, Swahn E, for the FRISC II investigators. Outcome at 1 year after an invasive compared with a non-invasive strategy in unstable coronary-artery disease: the FRISC II invasive randomised trial. *Lancet* 2000; **356**: 9–16.

37. Bach RG, Lagerqvist B, Husted S *et al*. 5-year outcomes in the FRISC-II randomised trial of an invasive versus a non-invasive strategy in non-ST-elevation acute coronary syndrome: a follow-up study. *Lancet* 2006; **368**: 998–1004.

38. Cannon CP, Weintraub WS, Demopoulos LA, TACTICS-Thrombolysis in Myocardial Infarction 18 Investigators. Comparison of early invasive and conservative strategies in patients with unstable coronary syndromes treated with the glycoprotein IIb/IIIa inhibitor tirofiban [see comment]. *N Engl J Med* 2001; **344**: 1879–1887.

39. Michalis LK, Stroumbis CS, Pappas K *et al*. Treatment of refractory unstable angina in geographically isolated areas without cardiac surgery. Invasive versus conservative strategy (TRUCS study) [see comment]. *Eur Heart J* 2000; **21**: 1954–1959.

40. Spacek R, Widimsky P, Straka Z *et al*. Value of first day angiography/angioplasty in evolving Non-ST segment elevation myocardial infarction: an open multicenter randomized trial. The VINO Study [see comment]. *Eur Heart J* 2002; **23**: 230–238.

41. Fox KAA, Poole-Wilson P, Henderson RA *et al*. Interventional versus conservative treatment for patients with unstable angina or non-ST- elevation myocardial infarction: the British Heart Foundation RITA-3 randomised trial. *Lancet* 2002; **360**: 743–751.

42. Fox KAA, Poole-Wilson P, Henderson RA *et al*. 5-year outcome of an interventional strategy in non-ST-elevation acute coronary syndrome: the British Heart Foundation RITA 3 randomised trial. *Lancet* 2005; **366**: 914–920.

43. de Winter RJ, Windhausen F, Cornel JH *et al*. Early invasive versus selectively invasive management for acute coronary syndromes [see comment]. *N Engl J Med* 2005; **353**: 1095–1104.

44. Ottervanger JP, Armstrong P, Barnathan ES *et al*. Association of revascularisation with low mortality in non-ST elevation acute coronary syndrome, a report from GUSTO IV-ACS. *Eur Heart J* 2004; **25**: 1494–1501.

45. Mehta SR, Cannon CP, Fox KAA *et al*. Routine vs selective invasive strategies in patients with acute coronary syndromes. A collaborative meta-analysis of randomized trials. *JAMA* 2005; **293**: 2908–2917.

46. Van de Werf F, Gore JM, Avezum A *et al*. Access to catheterisation facilities in patients admitted with acute coronary syndrome: multinational registry study. *BMJ* 2005; **330**: 441.

47. Tang EWM, Wong C-KMD, Herbison PM. Global Registry of Acute Coronary Events (GRACE) hospital discharge risk score accurately predicts long-term mortality post acute coronary syndrome. *Am Heart J* 2007; **153**: 29–35.

48. Prabhakaran D, Yusuf S, Mehta S *et al*. Two-year outcomes in patients admitted with non-ST elevation acute coronary syndrome: results of the OASIS registry 1 and 2. *Indian Heart J* 2005; **57**: 217–225.
49. Scull GS, Martin JS, Weaver WD, Every NR, for the MITI Investigators. Early angiography versus conservative treatment in patients with non-ST elevation acute myocardial infarction. *J Am Coll Cardiol* 2000; **35**: 895–902.
50. Spaulding C, Henry P, Teiger E *et al*. Sirolimus eluting versus uncoated stents in acute myocardial infarction. *N Engl J Med* 2006; **355**: 1093–1104.
51. Laarman GJ, Suttorp MJ, Dirksen MT *et al*. Paclitaxel eluting stents versus uncoated stents in primary percutaneous coronary intervention. *N Engl J Med* 2006; **355**: 1105–1113.

J. Paul Miller

14

Are the benefits of statins confined to their lipid-lowering properties?

The term pleiotropic is used in genetics to describe genes that exert many phenotypic effects (πλειον, many; τροπη, turn or change). In recent years, it has also been widely used to describe effects of statin drugs which are not the result of reduction in low-density lipoprotein (LDL) concentration.[1–3]

Statins are inhibitors of the rate-limiting enzyme in cholesterol synthesis, β-hydroxy-β-methyl-glutaryl-coenzyme A reductase (HMG-CoA reductase). HMG-CoA reductase converts HMG-CoA to mevalonic acid, an early stage in the cholesterol synthetic pathway. As a result, HMG-CoA reductase inhibitors reduce the synthesis not only of cholesterol but also of the intermediates in the cholesterol synthetic pathway and its side branches.[4] Reductions in the many compounds involved have the potential for multiple metabolic (pleiotropic) effects, not directly mediated by reduction in LDL concentration. One might predict that, since these effects stem from the inhibition of a single rate-limiting enzyme, the effects of all statins would be qualitatively similar though there would be quantitative differences relating to the potency of the statin involved and the degree of enzyme inhibition. There is also the possibility of other biochemical effects of statins, not mediated by inhibition of HMG-CoA reductase, at sites yet to be elucidated, and which might vary qualitatively from one statin to another.

Postulated pleiotropic manifestations of statins at the cellular level include effects on endothelial function, inflammation, immunoregulation, plaque stability and thrombogenesis, though it is not always easy to dissect out to what extent these processes are independent of LDL reduction. It has also been suggested that statins might modify the course of a variety of diseases not generally thought to be disorders of cholesterol metabolism, including Alzheimer's disease, rheumatoid arthritis, sepsis and osteoporosis. It is

J. Paul Miller BM BCh MSc DPhil FRCP
Consultant Gastroenterologist, University Hospital of South Manchester NHS Foundation Trust, Wythenshawe Hospital, Manchester M23 9LT, UK
E-mail: jpmiller@btinternet.com

important to bear in mind the pitfalls of case-control data and the general superiority of the randomised controlled trial, a lesson exemplified by the apparent dramatic effects of oestrogen replacement in reducing coronary events in postmenopausal women[5] which was not in the end substantiated in randomised trials.[6]

Statins vary considerably in their water solubility with pravastatin and rosuvastatin being relatively hydrophilic whereas lovastatin, simvastatin, atorvastatin, and fluvastatin are lipophilic and should be able to enter peripheral cells more easily, theoretically leading to increased potential for pleiotropism and also for adverse effects. In clinical practice, this distinction between hydrophilic and lipophilic statins is not readily apparent.

Many pleiotropic effects of statins are thought to relate to reduction of metabolites in the cholesterol synthetic pathway downstream from HMG-CoA reductase particularly farnesyl-pyrophosphate and geranylgeranyl-pyrophosphate needed for the prenylation of proteins such as the Rho and Ras GTPases, important in

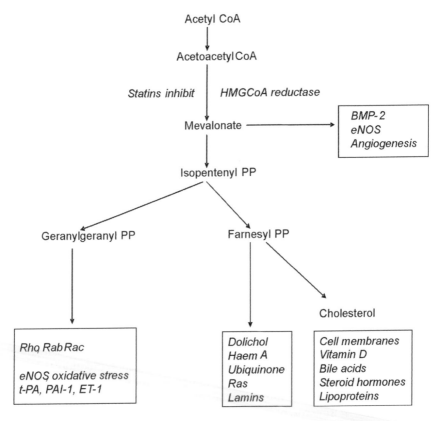

Fig. 1 Cholesterol synthetic pathway. Statins inhibit the rate-limiting enzyme HMG-CoA reductase. This also reduces the synthesis of several other downstream metabolites of mevalonic acid including farnesyl-pyrophosphate and geranylgeranyl-pyrophosphate which are important for the prenylation (lipid modification) of several proteins involved in intracellular signalling pathways. These have multiple actions including effects on leukocyte adhesion, fibrinolysis, apoptosis and cell division, and production of eNOS.
BMP-2, bone morphogenetic protein-2; eNOS, endothelial nitric oxide synthase; t-PA, tissue plasminogen activator; PAI-1, plasminogen activator inhibitor-1; ET-1, endothelin-1.

intracellular signalling (Fig. 1). *In vitro*, statins have been shown to suppress T-cell responses, reduce expression of class II histocompatability complexes and reduce chemokine synthesis in mononuclear cells. These effects are reversible by the addition of mevalonate to the medium and are, therefore, presumably the result of the down-regulation of HMG-CoA reductase.[3]

Independently of HMG-CoA reductase inhibition, some statins (simvastatin and lovastatin but not pravastain) have been shown to bind to, and modify the action of, lymphocyte function associated antigen-1 (LFA-1) with the potential to suppress the inflammatory process and lead to the development of orally-active compounds which may be valuable in the treatment of rheumatoid arthritis, psoriasis, transplant rejection and ischaemia-reperfusion injury.[7]

In many instances where an effect of a statin is reported but its mechanism is unclear, it is difficult to know whether or not it is a true pleiotropic effect. Much relevant work has been conducted in animals where it is easier to investigate these phenomena and their mechanisms, but the emphasis in this review is on studies in man.

STATIN END-POINT TRIALS

In a retrospective analysis of the West of Scotland Coronary Prevention Study (WOSCOPS), it appeared that treatment with pravastatin conferred benefit that could not be explained by reduction of LDL alone.[8] Risk of an event for patients in the placebo group was adequately explained by the Framingham risk equation whereas those on pravastatin fared better than predicted by the equation. Moreover, for a given in-trial LDL-cholesterol (LDL-C) concentration, those on pravastatin had fewer events than those on placebo. Intuitively, one would have predicted that the two groups would have done equally well or that those on the active drug might even have done less well if its full benefits took a significant time to become apparent. In another pravastatin trial, the benefits were also not clearly related to reduction in LDL-cholesterol.[9] In the Scandinavian Simvastatin Survival Study (4S), on the other hand, the benefits did appear to depend on the reduction in LDL-C.[10]

If there are benefits of pravastatin additional to those conferred by reduction in LDL-C, the question arises as to whether they are a class effect of statins or specific to this particular statin. Certainly, any additional benefit of pravastatin is not sufficient to outweigh, or even match, the impact of the greater reduction in LDL-C achieved with high-dose atorvastatin in terms of events[11] or coronary atheroma as judged by intravascular ultrasound (IVUS).[12]

Of major importance is the observation that in trials of cardiovascular end-points and cholesterol reduction, whether induced by statins or other means, there is a broadly linear relationship between reduction in events and reduction in LDL-C, consonant with the notion that the latter is of primary importance in determining the former. In the analysis of Robinson *et al.*,[13] trials of diet, bile acid sequestrating resins and partial ileal bypass seem to lie close to the same regression line as the statin trials suggesting that statins do not confer particular benefits beyond cholesterol reduction when it comes to preventing coronary events. The confidence limits for the point estimates in some of the individual trials are very wide especially for the non-statin trials where there is less reduction in LDL-C.

Liao and colleagues,[2,14] however, have pointed out that many of the statin trials lasted for about 5 years whereas benefits were slower to appear in the Lipid Research Clinics (LRC) trial of cholestyramine and in the Program on the Surgical Control of the Hyperlipidemias (POSCH) in which partial ileal bypass was used. These trials reported data after 7.4 years and 9.7 years, respectively. In Liao's analysis, if results are standardised at 4.5 years then for a given LDL-C reduction less benefit, in terms of reduction of non-fatal myocardial infarction or fatal coronary heart disease, is apparent in the non-statin trials. It is not immediately apparent why there is this difference in the conclusions of the analyses of Liao and of Robinson et al. which used 5-year data.[13] It is, however, an important difference when considering the underlying mechanisms for the clinical benefits of statins. The IMProved Reduction of Outcomes: Vytorin Efficacy International Trial (IMPROVE-IT, see <http://www.clinicaltrials.gov/ct/show/NCT00202878>) is comparing outcomes in patients with stabilised acute coronary syndromes randomised to simvastatin 40 mg daily with or without the addition of the cholesterol absorption inhibitor ezetimibe and may shed further light on the question of whether all the clinical benefits can be attributed to reduction in LDL-C.

ACUTE CORONARY SYNDROMES

The rapid separation of the Kaplan–Meier curves of event rates in some trials in patients with acute coronary syndromes (ACSs) compared to primary and secondary prevention trials using statins in stable patients[15] has been adduced as evidence of pleiotropism, and it may be. It needs to be remembered, however, that the nature of the patient population favours early detection of benefit with effective treatments because of the relatively high incidence of events in the short term in patients with ACSs, compared with secondary prevention studies in patients with stable disease.

In the recent PROVE IT-TIMI 22 trial (Pravastatin or Atorvastatin Evaluation and Infection Therapy – Thrombolysis in Myocardial Infarction 22), there is the suggestion that benefit was seen with atorvastatin 80 mg/day compared to pravastatin 40 mg/day within 30 days.[11] Although the difference between the event rates in the two groups was not significant at this stage, the point estimates suggested that the full benefit in relative risk was already apparent. The changes in LDL-C and CRP were also essentially complete by this time. The 30-day LDL-C concentration and CRP levels predicted event rates independently regardless of the drug with which they were achieved suggesting both LDL-dependent and independent effects. Patients on pravastatin and atorvastatin in PROVE-IT who achieved similar LDL-C and CRP levels had similar event rates.[16]

Not all studies of intensive statin treatment in ACSs show significant benefit. In the A to Z (Aggrastat to Zocor) trial,[17] early use of simvastatin did not yield a significant reduction in early cardiovascular events despite as great or greater initial reduction in LDL-C than in PROVE-IT[11] and MIRACL (Myocardial Ischemia Reduction with Aggressive Cholesterol Lowering)[18] relative to their respective comparator groups. Reduction in CRP, however, was only about half as great in A to Z as in PROVE-IT and MIRACL suggesting that in the short-term benefit may be more dependent on LDL-independent mechanisms.[19]

ENDOTHELIAL FUNCTION

It has been known for many years that children with familial hypercholesterolaemia and adults with coronary disease have impaired endothelial function[20] as judged by vasodilator responses to ischaemia or acetylcholine infusion. This is the result of impaired release of endothelium-derived relaxing factor (EDRF) subsequently identified as nitric oxide (NO). Exactly how important impaired endothelial dysfunction is in clinical vascular disease is not clear. Inappropriate vasospasm may play a part in acute coronary syndromes and NO also has effects on platelet aggregation and growth of vascular smooth muscle cells.[2,21]

Whether LDL reduction *per se* improves endothelial function is controversial. The observations that a single episode of LDL-apheresis improves vascular reactivity, both in the coronary[22] and forearm circulation,[23] suggests that it does. Combined treatment with diet and cholestyramine has also been reported to improve coronary endothelial function.[24] The situation is confused, however, as two recent studies failed to show an improvement of forearm blood flow in response to up to 3 months' treatment with ezetimibe despite improvements when LDL-C was reduced to a similar extent with statin treatment.[25,26] In one of these studies, statin treatment also led to an increase in the level of endothelium-bound superoxide dismutase activity and the number of functional endothelial progenitor cells whereas a similar reduction in LDL-C produced by ezetimibe did not.[26] In a further study, in patients with the metabolic syndrome, ezetimibe potentiated the effects of atorvastatin on forearm blood flow though the effect of ezetimibe monotherapy was not examined.[27] The latter authors concluded that there was unlikely to be a major effect of atorvastatin not mediated by cholesterol lowering because atorvastatin 10 mg/day combined with ezetimibe 10 mg/day had more pronounced effects on endothelium-dependent blood flow in response to acetylcholine infusion than atorvastatin 40 mg/day alone. This does not necessarily follow if most of any pleiotropic effect of atorvastatin on endothelial function is achieved with the 10-mg dose. Moreover, the ineffectiveness of ezetimibe monotherapy suggests that the statin effect is independent of reduction in LDL.

The effects of statins in improving endothelial function have been demonstrated many times. They have been shown to up-regulate endothelial nitric oxide synthase (eNOS) in *in vitro* systems[28] and the rapidity of the effect also suggests that it may be unrelated to LDL reduction. An endothelial-mediated vascular response is observed 1–3 days after the initiation of statin therapy before significant changes have occurred in circulating LDL-C. Even a single 40-mg dose of pravastatin is effective.[29,30] It is possible that these changes are mediated by reductions in other compounds derived from mevalonic acid such as the prenylated proteins derived from farnesyl- and geranylgeranyl-pyrophosphate,[3] though this would not explain the rapid improvement in endothelial function induced by LDL apheresis.[23] The mechanism for such a rapid action of pravastatin, which is hydrophilic and would not be expected to be taken up by peripheral cells in significant quantities,[31] is unclear.

INFLAMMATION

For many years, there has been a recognition that coronary events involve inflammatory and immunological processes[32] and not just lipid deposition leading to progressive atheromatous narrowing and occlusion of the artery. A variety of inflammatory cytokines and markers, including C-reactive protein (CRP), interleukin-6 (IL-6), serum amyloid A, P-selectin and adhesion molecules such as intercellular adhesion molecule-1 (ICAM-1) have been associated with increased cardiovascular risk. Although the degree of coronary narrowing may determine the development of stable angina, acute coronary syndromes including unstable angina and myocardial infarction are more dependent on the composition and the quality of the atheromatous plaque. Unstable plaques with a thin or weak connective tissue cap, which can be present in moderate or even in non-stenotic lesions (detectable by IVUS), are more likely to rupture, allowing blood into the vessel wall thus initiating the thrombotic process which leads to vascular occlusion. Plaque stability is a function of the relative proportions of macrophages and smooth muscle cells and their secretory products. The ability of statins to influence these processes by non-LDL dependent mechanisms is reviewed in detail by Schonbeck and Libby.[3]

In man, much interest over the last decade has been directed to the association of small changes in CRP (detectable only by a high sensitivity assay (hsCRP)), within what would clinically be regarded as the 'normal' range, and increased risk of CHD events[33] or adverse changes in vascular imaging. CRP is produced in the liver in response to IL-6 and other inflammatory cytokines. CRP may be more than just a marker of inflammation and may not be an innocent bystander in the genesis of atheromatous vascular disease.[34] It has been shown to activate complement, increase the levels of adhesion molecules, decrease expression of eNOS and induce plasminogen activator inhibitor.

A wide variety of drug treatments relevant to cardiovascular disease have been reported to influence CRP levels[35] including most classes of lipid-lowering agent. Statins, fibrates, ezetimibe, nicotinic acid and even bile acid-sequestrating agents, which are not systemically absorbed, have all been implicated in modifying CRP. Yet, in the case of statins, the reduction in CRP that is achieved is said to be little related to the reduction in LDL-C[36] and ezetimibe monotherapy seems to be without effect.

In the Reversal of Atherosclerosis with Aggressive Lipid Lowering (REVERSAL) trial,[37] progression of atherosclerosis judged by IVUS was significantly and independently related to both LDL-C and CRP. Patients who had better than average reductions in atherogenic lipoproteins (measured as LDL-C, non-HDL cholesterol and apolipoprotein B concentrations) as well as in CRP were least likely to show atheroma progression. Similarly, in the PROVE-IT trial,[16] least events were experienced by those patients who achieved the lowest LDL-C and CRP levels. Low levels of CRP conferred benefit independently of the concomitant concentration of LDL-C. In both studies, the correlation between CRP and LDL-C was weak confirming previous work which has suggested that LDL-C is not a major determinant of CRP.

Ezetimibe monotherapy has no significant effect on CRP; however, when added to simvastatin or atorvastatin across the dosage range, it produced an additional reduction in CRP.[38–40] Efrati et al.[41] also failed to see any reduction in CRP with ezetimibe alone and neither did the reduction they observed when ezetimibe was added to simvastatin reach statistical significance; however, numbers were small and this may represent type 2 error. Moreover, simvastatin decreased aortic stiffness determined by pulse-wave analysis whereas ezetimibe alone or when added to simvastatin had no effect.

Thus, although statin treatment reduces CRP, the mechanism for this does not appear to be closely dependent on the reduction in LDL or other atherogenic lipoproteins that is achieved. In addition, the clinical benefit that accrues from statin treatment relates both to the changes in atherogenic lipoproteins and in CRP (or a related variable) independently of each other.

Recent evidence has suggested that the relationship between CRP and vascular disease may be less strong and specific than had been previously thought.[42] The inflammatory effects seen in some in vitro work using human CRP have since been shown to be due to contaminants and not to CRP itself. The advent of specific CRP inhibitors should in due course enable more direct testing of any causal role.[43]

STROKE AND DEMENTIA

The strong epidemiological relationship between serum cholesterol and CHD events is not seen for stroke,[44] so it was not self-evident that statins would reduce the incidence of stroke. Thus the reduction in stroke seen in the statin trials[45] might, at first sight, be interpreted as a non-lipid effect. In the Multiple Risk Factor Intervention Trial (MRFIT), however, ischaemic stroke (which is much more common than haemorrhagic stroke) was positively correlated with serum cholesterol whereas low cholesterol levels, when associated with raised diastolic blood pressure, were found to be a risk factor for haemorrhagic stroke.[46] A recent, very large, Korean prospective cohort study confirms these observations and suggests that low cholesterol is only a risk factor for haemorrhagic stroke in heavy consumers of alcohol.[47]

Randomised clinical trials of statins have demonstrated a reduction in the incidence of first stroke and transient ischaemic episodes in trials of CHD prevention, which may be mediated, at least in part, by reductions in LDL.[13,45,48] The magnitude in the reduction of stroke incidence broadly parallels the reduction in LDL-C; however, the confidence intervals are wide for individual point estimates and it is not known whether lowering LDL by other methods would yield a similar or different relationship. Thus it remains unclear to what extent non-LDL mediated effects of statins might be involved.

There had been doubt about the ability of statin treatment to reduce the incidence of recurrent stroke but the recent publication of the SPARCL trial (Stroke Prevention by Aggressive Reduction in Cholesterol Levels)[49] showed a modest reduction in overall incidence of recurrent stroke with atorvastatin 80 mg/day at the cost of a small absolute increase in haemorrhagic stroke.

The data on statin use and stroke provide a basis for hoping that statins might also delay the development of dementia where this has a vascular basis. Although possession of the apolipoprotein-E4 polymorphism predisposes to the development of Alzheimer's disease,[50] the condition is not regarded primarily as a disorder of lipoprotein metabolism. Nevertheless, observational studies have suggested that statin use is associated with a lower prevalence of Alzheimer's disease. To date, a beneficial effect on cognitive decline has not been convincingly confirmed in prospective studies or randomised controlled trials[51,52] and it remains to be seen if any benefit will emerge with trials employing more detailed investigation of cognitive function.

SEPSIS

Sepsis has been defined as the systemic inflammatory response to the presence of infection. Among the putative pleiotropic actins of statins are anti-inflammatory, antioxidant and immunomodulatory effects which have been suggested as the basis of reported benefits for patients with rheumatoid arthritis and multiple sclerosis.[53,54] A recent large population-based cohort analysis from Canada[55] has suggested that hospital patients aged over 65 years with atherosclerosis on statins have a 19% lower incidence of sepsis. There should now be adequately powered controlled studies of statins both in the prevention and probably also the treatment of sepsis.

COLORECTAL CANCER

Statins have been shown to inhibit the growth of colon cancer cell lines *in vitro* and a recent case-control study from Israel showed a relative risk reduction of 47% for colon cancer.[56] A meta-analysis of more than 90,000 subjects in randomised controlled trials of statin use in the prevention of cardiovascular disease does not, however, show a reduction in gastrointestinal cancers overall;[57] neither is there a significant reduction in colorectal cancers (personal communication). A recent meta-analysis devoted to cancer risk suggests that statins are without effect.[58]

OSTEOPOROSIS

In 1999, Mundy *et al.*[59] showed that lovastatin and simvastatin had the ability to stimulate new bone formation in rodents and that this was associated with increased expression of the bone morphogenetic protein-2 (BMP-2) gene. It has subsequently been shown that pravastatin, perhaps because of its hydrophilicity, does not have the power to induce BMP-2 in osteoblasts.[60] The effects can be blocked by the addition of mevalonate and are, therefore, the result of HMG-CoA reductase inhibition. Several other sites of action for statins in bone metabolism have since been identified in animal and *in vitro* systems, reviewed in detail by Horiuchi and Maeda.[61]

Studies relating to bone turnover[61] and clinical fracture risk in humans, however, have to date yielded conflicting results. Some observational studies have shown a reduced incidence of bone fracture[62–64] in association with statin use whereas others have not.[65] Retrospective analyses of two of the cardiovascular end-point trials[66,67] have failed to show any effect on fracture incidence but these were probably not adequately powered for the purpose, given that the subjects were recruited to investigate cardiovascular benefits.

Moreover, in one of the trials, pravastatin was used and this seems to be less likely to have an effect on bone mineral metabolism based on *in vitro* work. The need for specific randomised controlled trials is clear.

CONCLUSIONS

There is no doubt that statin drugs exert multiple (pleiotropic) effects which are independent of reduction in LDL concentration but there is as yet no consensus as to the biological importance of these. Where pleiotropic effects are the result of inhibition of HMG-CoA reductase leading to reduction in metabolites downstream from mevalonic acid, they are likely to parallel the reduction in LDL concentration achieved and to differ quantitatively, but not qualitatively, between statins according to their potency. In this situation, LDL-C reduction can be both directly beneficial and a marker of potential indirect benefits from pleiotropic effects. There is, in addition, evidence of effects not mediated by suppression of HMG-CoA reductase activity and these effects may differ between statins but there is little evidence to date of their clinical importance. Suggestion of benefit in case-control studies in disorders not known to be related to abnormalities of cholesterol metabolism, such as osteoporosis, dementia and sepsis, should be regarded with some scepticism until confirmed in randomised trials.

A recent meta-analysis[13] suggests that clinical benefit in cholesterol-lowering trials relates principally to the reduction in LDL-C achieved and is independent of the means by which cholesterol is lowered. If this is correct, then there is little room for benefit mediated by pleiotropic effects of statins at least in primary prevention and in secondary prevention in patients with stable disease. Another analysis of the same data,[2,14] however, suggests that non-statin therapies are less effective, or at least are less rapidly effective, for a given cholesterol reduction; this distinction, if confirmed, may well be a manifestation of pleiotropism. The advent of ezetimibe, which like the statins predominantly lowers LDL-C but by a different mechanism, provides the opportunity to try to resolve this issue in clinical end-point trials.

For the moment, clinical judgements about risk should continue to be made on the basis of the traditional risk factors[68] with lipid treatment targets based on LDL or non-HDL cholesterol. It has been recommended by the American Heart Association and the US Centers for Disease Control[69] that hsCRP might be measured as an adjunct to risk estimation in primary prevention of CHD, but this has not been adopted in the UK. It currently seems premature, particularly when one considers that repeated measurements are necessary. Very small changes in hsCRP betoken substantial changes in risk and these small changes can be swamped by those which result from minor intercurrent inflammatory events.

The possibility of benefit from pleiotropic effects provides an additional reason to use statins as the first-line treatment whenever there is an indication to lower LDL-C, though the principal rationale for this is the enormous body of evidence showing reduction of cardiovascular events, and total mortality, in the context of both primary and secondary prevention of cardiovascular disease, whatever the mechanisms.

Key points for clinical practice

- Statins inhibit an early stage in cholesterol synthesis and, as a result, also reduce the synthesis of a large number of other active metabolites in the synthetic pathway leading to the potential for multiple metabolic effects not directly linked to reduction in low-density lipoprotein cholesterol (LDL-C). These are known as pleiotropic effects.

- The reduction in coronary events in long-term trials in stable patients is broadly linear, regardless of the means used to lower cholesterol, leading to the suggestion that benefit is mediated principally through the reduction in LDL-C and implying little scope for pleiotropism. This is controversial and an alternative analysis suggests that the benefits are seen sooner when statins are used to lower cholesterol.

- In shorter-term studies in acute coronary syndromes (ACSs), benefits are independently related to the reduction in both LDL-C and C-reactive protein (CRP). Patients with the lowest values of both these variables fare the best implying that anti-inflammatory effects of statins not directly resulting from reduction in LDL-C are important in this context.

- Because many, though not all, pleiotropic effects of statins are mediated through the inhibition of HMG-CoA reductase the reduction in LDL-C achieved is not only a measure of direct anti-atherogenic benefit, but also a marker for the likely magnitude of any pleiotropic advantage.

- Statins should usually be the first-line treatment when a decision is made to modify serum lipids, because of the vast body of clinical trial evidence showing reduction in coronary and cerebrovascular events and in total mortality. This will also ensure that any potential pleiotropic advantage, which may not be available from other classes of lipid-lowering drug, is obtained.

- Decisions about which patients should receive statin therapy should continue to be made according to existing guidelines based on global estimates of cardiovascular risk.

- For the present, targets for patients on statin treatment should continue to be based on lipid variables such as total cholesterol or preferably measures of atherogenic lipoproteins such as LDL-C or non-high density lipoprotein cholesterol.

ACKNOWLEDGEMENT

I am very grateful to Dr James K. Liao of the Brigham and Women's Hospital, Harvard Medical School for helpful discussion.

References

1. Almuti K, Rimawi R, Spevack D, Ostfeld RJ. Effects of statins beyond lipid lowering: potential for clinical benefits. *Int J Cardiol* 2006; **109**: 7–15.
2. Liao JK, Laufs U. Pleiotropic effects of statins. *Annu Rev Pharmacol Toxicol* 2005; **45**: 89–118.
3. Schonbeck U, Libby P. Inflammation, immunity, and HMG-CoA reductase inhibitors: statins as antiinflammatory agents? *Circulation* 2004; **109 (21 Suppl 1)**: II18–II26.
4. Goldstein JL, Brown MS. Regulation of the mevalonate pathway. *Nature* 1990; **343**: 425–430.
5. Stampfer MJ, Colditz GA, Willett WC et al. Postmenopausal estrogen therapy and cardiovascular disease. Ten-year follow-up from the nurses' health study. *N Engl J Med* 1991; **325**: 756–762.
6. Hulley S, Grady D, Bush T et al. Randomized trial of estrogen plus progestin for secondary prevention of coronary heart disease in postmenopausal women. Heart and Estrogen/progestin Replacement Study (HERS) Research Group. *JAMA* 1998; **280**: 605–613.
7. Weitz-Schmidt G, Welzenbach K, Brinkmann V et al. Statins selectively inhibit leukocyte function antigen-1 by binding to a novel regulatory integrin site. *Nat Med* 2001; **7**: 687–692.
8. Influence of pravastatin and plasma lipids on clinical events in the West of Scotland Coronary Prevention Study (WOSCOPS). *Circulation* 1998; **97**: 1440–1445.
9. Sacks FM, Moye LA, Davis BR et al. Relationship between plasma LDL concentrations during treatment with pravastatin and recurrent coronary events in the Cholesterol and Recurrent Events trial. *Circulation* 1998; **97**: 1446–1452.
10. Pedersen TR, Olsson AG, Faergeman O et al. Lipoprotein changes and reduction in the incidence of major coronary heart disease events in the Scandinavian Simvastatin Survival Study (4S). *Circulation* 1998; **97**: 1453–1460.
11. Cannon CP, Braunwald E, McCabe CH et al. Intensive versus moderate lipid lowering with statins after acute coronary syndromes. *N Engl J Med* 2004; **350**: 1495–1504.
12. Nissen SE, Tuzcu EM, Schoenhagen P et al. Effect of intensive compared with moderate lipid-lowering therapy on progression of coronary atherosclerosis: a randomized controlled trial. *JAMA* 2004; **291**: 1071–1080.
13. Robinson JG, Smith B, Maheshwari N, Schrott H. Pleiotropic effects of statins: benefit beyond cholesterol reduction? A meta-regression analysis. *J Am Coll Cardiol* 2005; **46**: 1855–1862.
14. Liao JK. Clinical implications for statin pleiotropy. *Curr Opin Lipidol* 2005; **16**: 624–629.
15. Ray KK, Cannon CP. Early time to benefit with intensive statin treatment: could it be the pleiotropic effects? *Am J Cardiol* 2005; **96**: 54F–60F.
16. Ridker PM, Cannon CP, Morrow D et al. C-reactive protein levels and outcomes after statin therapy. *N Engl J Med* 2005; **352**: 20–28.
17. de Lemos JA, Blazing MA, Wiviott SD et al. Early intensive vs a delayed conservative simvastatin strategy in patients with acute coronary syndromes: phase Z of the A to Z trial. *JAMA* 2004; **292**: 1307–1316.
18. Schwartz GG, Olsson AG, Ezekowitz MD et al. Effects of atorvastatin on early recurrent ischemic events in acute coronary syndromes: the MIRACL study: a randomized controlled trial. *JAMA* 2001; **285**: 1711–1718.
19. Nissen SE. High-dose statins in acute coronary syndromes: not just lipid levels. *JAMA* 2004; **292**: 1365–1367.
20. Celermajer DS, Sorensen KE, Gooch VM et al. Non-invasive detection of endothelial dysfunction in children and adults at risk of atherosclerosis. *Lancet* 1992; **340**: 1111–1115.
21. Meredith IT, Anderson TJ, Uehata A, Yeung AC, Selwyn AP, Ganz P. Role of endothelium in ischemic coronary syndromes. *Am J Cardiol* 1993; **72**: 27C–31C, discussion 31C–32C.
22. Igarashi K, Tsuji M, Nishimura M, Horimoto M. Improvement of endothelium-dependent coronary vasodilation after a single LDL apheresis in patients with hypercholesterolemia. *J Clin Apher* 2004; **19**: 11–16.
23. Tamai O, Matsuoka H, Itabe H, Wada Y, Kohno K, Imaizumi T. Single LDL apheresis improves endothelium-dependent vasodilatation in hypercholesterolemic humans. *Circulation* 1997; **95**: 76–82.

24. Leung WH, Lau CP, Wong CK. Beneficial effect of cholesterol-lowering therapy on coronary endothelium-dependent relaxation in hypercholesterolaemic patients. *Lancet* 1993; **341**: 1496–1500.

25. Fichtlscherer S, Schmidt-Lucke C, Bojunga S *et al*. Differential effects of short-term lipid lowering with ezetimibe and statins on endothelial function in patients with CAD: clinical evidence for 'pleiotropic' functions of statin therapy. *Eur Heart J* 2006; **27**: 1182–1190.

26. Landmesser U, Bahlmann F, Mueller M *et al*. Simvastatin versus ezetimibe: pleiotropic and lipid-lowering effects on endothelial function in humans. *Circulation* 2005; **111**: 2356–2363.

27. Bulut D, Hanefeld C, Bulut-Streich N, Graf C, Mugge A, Spiecker M. Endothelial function in the forearm circulation of patients with the metabolic syndrome – effect of different lipid-lowering regimens. *Cardiology* 2005; **104**: 176–180.

28. Laufs U, Fata VL, Liao JK. Inhibition of 3-hydroxy-3-methylglutaryl (HMG)-CoA reductase blocks hypoxia-mediated down-regulation of endothelial nitric oxide synthase. *J Biol Chem* 1997; **272**: 31725–31729.

29. Tsunekawa T, Hayashi T, Kano H *et al*. Cerivastatin, a hydroxymethylglutaryl coenzyme a reductase inhibitor, improves endothelial function in elderly diabetic patients within 3 days. *Circulation* 2001; **104**: 376–379.

30. Wassmann S, Faul A, Hennen B, Scheller B, Bohm M, Nickenig G. Rapid effect of 3-hydroxy-3-methylglutaryl coenzyme a reductase inhibition on coronary endothelial function. *Circ Res* 2003; **93**: e98–e103.

31. Hamelin BA, Turgeon J. Hydrophilicity/lipophilicity: relevance for the pharmacology and clinical effects of HMG-CoA reductase inhibitors. *Trends Pharmacol Sci* 1998; **19**: 26–37.

32. Libby P. Inflammation in atherosclerosis. *Nature* 2002; **420**: 868–874.

33. Ridker PM, Cushman M, Stampfer MJ, Tracy RP, Hennekens CH. Inflammation, aspirin, and the risk of cardiovascular disease in apparently healthy men. *N Engl J Med* 1997; **336**: 973–979.

34. Mazer SP, Rabbani LE. Evidence for C-reactive protein's role in (CRP) vascular disease: atherothrombosis, immuno-regulation and CRP. *J Thromb Thrombolysis* 2004; **17**: 95–105.

35. Prasad K. C-reactive protein (CRP)-lowering agents. *Cardiovasc Drug Rev* 2006; **24**: 33–50.

36. Albert MA, Danielson E, Rifai N, Ridker PM. Effect of statin therapy on C-reactive protein levels: the pravastatin inflammation/CRP evaluation (PRINCE): a randomized trial and cohort study. *JAMA* 2001; **286**: 64–70.

37. Nissen SE, Tuzcu EM, Schoenhagen P *et al*. Statin therapy, LDL cholesterol, C-reactive protein, and coronary artery disease. *N Engl J Med* 2005; **352**: 29–38.

38. Ballantyne CM, Houri J, Notarbartolo A *et al*. Effect of ezetimibe coadministered with atorvastatin in 628 patients with primary hypercholesterolemia: a prospective, randomized, double-blind trial. *Circulation* 2003; **107**: 2409–2415.

39. Sager PT, Capece R, Lipka L *et al*. Effects of ezetimibe coadministered with simvastatin on C-reactive protein in a large cohort of hypercholesterolemic patients. *Atherosclerosis* 2005; **179**: 361–367.

40. Sager PT, Melani L, Lipka L *et al*. Effect of coadministration of ezetimibe and simvastatin on high-sensitivity C-reactive protein. *Am J Cardiol* 2003; **92**: 1414–1418.

41. Efrati S, Averbukh M, Dishy V, Faygenzo M, Friedensohn L, Golik A. The effect of simvastatin, ezetimibe and their combination on the lipid profile, arterial stiffness and inflammatory markers. *Eur J Clin Pharmacol* 2007; **63**: 113–121.

42. Lowe GD, Pepys MB. C-reactive protein and cardiovascular disease: weighing the evidence. *Curr Atheroscler Report* 2006; **8**: 421–428.

43. Pepys MB, Hirschfield GM, Tennent GA *et al*. Targeting C-reactive protein for the treatment of cardiovascular disease. *Nature* 2006; **440**: 1217–1221.

44. Cholesterol, diastolic blood pressure, and stroke: 13,000 strokes in 450,000 people in 45 prospective cohorts. Prospective studies collaboration. *Lancet* 1995; **346**: 1647–1653.

45. Amarenco P, Labreuche J, Lavallee P, Touboul PJ. Statins in stroke prevention and carotid atherosclerosis: systematic review and up-to-date meta-analysis. *Stroke* 2004; **35**: 2902–2909.

46. Iso H, Jacobs Jr DR, Wentworth D, Neaton JD, Cohen JD. Serum cholesterol levels and six-year mortality from stroke in 350,977 men screened for the multiple risk factor

intervention trial. *N Engl J Med* 1989; **320**: 904–910.

47. Ebrahim S, Sung J, Song YM, Ferrer RL, Lawlor DA, Davey Smith G. Serum cholesterol, haemorrhagic stroke, ischaemic stroke, and myocardial infarction: Korean national health system prospective cohort study. *BMJ* 2006; **333**: 22.

48. Amarenco P. Effect of statins in stroke prevention. *Curr Opin Lipidol* 2005; **16**: 614–618.

49. Amarenco P, Bogousslavsky J, Callahan 3rd A *et al*. High-dose atorvastatin after stroke or transient ischemic attack. *N Engl J Med* 2006; **355**: 549–559.

50. Saunders AM. Apolipoprotein E and Alzheimer disease: an update on genetic and functional analyses. *J Neuropathol Exp Neurol* 2000; **59**: 751–758.

51. Miida T, Takahashi A, Ikeuchi T. Prevention of stroke and dementia by statin therapy: Experimental and clinical evidence of their pleiotropic effects. *Pharmacol Ther* 2007; **113**: 378–393.

52. Miida T, Takahashi A, Tanabe N, Ikeuchi T. Can statin therapy really reduce the risk of Alzheimer's disease and slow its progression? *Curr Opin Lipidol* 2005; **16**: 619–623.

53. McCarey DW, McInnes IB, Madhok R *et al*. Trial of Atorvastatin in Rheumatoid Arthritis (TARA): double-blind, randomised placebo-controlled trial. *Lancet* 2004; **363**: 2015–2021.

54. Vollmer T, Key L, Durkalski V *et al*. Oral simvastatin treatment in relapsing-remitting multiple sclerosis. *Lancet* 2004; **363**: 1607–1608.

55. Hackam DG, Mamdani M, Li P, Redelmeier DA. Statins and sepsis in patients with cardiovascular disease: a population-based cohort analysis. *Lancet* 2006; **367**: 413–418.

56. Poynter JN, Gruber SB, Higgins PD *et al*. Statins and the risk of colorectal cancer. *N Engl J Med* 2005; **352**: 2184–2192.

57. Baigent C, Keech A, Kearney PM *et al*. Efficacy and safety of cholesterol-lowering treatment: prospective meta-analysis of data from 90,056 participants in 14 randomised trials of statins. *Lancet* 2005; **366**: 1267–1278.

58. Dale KM, Coleman CI, Henyan NN, Kluger J, White CM. Statins and cancer risk: a meta-analysis. *JAMA* 2006; **295**: 74–80.

59. Mundy G, Garrett R, Harris S *et al*. Stimulation of bone formation *in vitro* and in rodents by statins. *Science* 1999; **286**: 1946–1949.

60. Sugiyama M, Kodama T, Konishi K, Abe K, Asami S, Oikawa S. Compactin and simvastatin, but not pravastatin, induce bone morphogenetic protein-2 in human osteosarcoma cells. *Biochem Biophys Res Commun* 2000; **271**: 688–692.

61. Horiuchi N, Maeda T. Statins and bone metabolism. *Oral Dis* 2006; **12**: 85–101.

62. Meier CR, Schlienger RG, Kraenzlin ME, Schlegel B, Jick H. HMG-CoA reductase inhibitors and the risk of fractures. *JAMA* 2000; **283**: 3205–3210.

63. Pasco JA, Kotowicz MA, Henry MJ, Sanders KM, Nicholson GC. Statin use, bone mineral density, and fracture risk: Geelong Osteoporosis Study. *Arch Intern Med* 2002; **162**: 537–540.

64. Wang PS, Solomon DH, Mogun H, Avorn J. HMG-CoA reductase inhibitors and the risk of hip fractures in elderly patients. *JAMA* 2000; **283**: 3211–3216.

65. van Staa TP, Wegman S, de Vries F, Leufkens B, Cooper C. Use of statins and risk of fractures. *JAMA* 2001; **285**: 1850–1855.

66. Pedersen TR, Kjekshus J. Statin drugs and the risk of fracture. 4S Study Group. *JAMA* 2000; **284**: 1921–1922.

67. Reid IR, Hague W, Emberson J *et al*. Effect of pravastatin on frequency of fracture in the LIPID study: secondary analysis of a randomised controlled trial. Long-term Intervention with Pravastatin in Ischaemic Disease. *Lancet* 2001; **357**: 509–512.

68. JBS 2: Joint British Societies' guidelines on prevention of cardiovascular disease in clinical practice. *Heart* 2005; **91 (Suppl 5)**: v1–v52.

69. Pearson TA, Mensah GA, Alexander RW *et al*. Markers of inflammation and cardiovascular disease: application to clinical and public health practice: a statement for healthcare professionals from the Centers for Disease Control and Prevention and the American Heart Association. *Circulation* 2003; **107**: 499–511.

J. Andreas Hoschtitzky Daniel J.M. Keenan

15

Mitral valve repair

Mitral valve repair has become the established primary treatment for mitral regurgitation from degenerative disease around the world. The shift from replacing the mitral valve to repairing it, and doing this earlier in the course of the disease, has taken place over the past 30 years. This development has paralleled the improvement in outcomes for cardiac surgery, whereby most established surgical units in the Western world now achieve mortality figures for most procedures between 0.5–10% depending on age, co-morbidities and complexity of the operation.[1]

AETIOLOGY AND PATHOLOGICAL FINDINGS

Mitral regurgitation is caused by a multitude of abnormalities. The clinically prevailing causes are degenerative mitral valve disease, rheumatic disease, ischaemic heart disease, infective endocarditis, congenital abnormalities and rare causes like trauma. In the Western world, degenerative disease forms the dominant aetiology, whereas in poorer healthcare economies, rheumatic disease still prevails as the most important cause of mitral regurgitation.

DEGENERATIVE MITRAL VALVE DISEASE

This consists of a group of conditions with confusing and overlapping terminology including myxomatous degeneration, fibro-elastic deficiency, mitral

J. Andreas Hoschtitzky MSc MRCS(Ed)
SpR in Cardiothoracic Surgery, Manchester Heart Centre, Manchester Royal Infirmary, Oxford Road, Manchester M13 9WL, UK

Daniel J.M. Keenan BSc MB BCh FRCS (for correspondence)
Consultant Cardiothoracic Surgeon, Manchester Heart Centre, Manchester Royal Infirmary, Oxford Road, Manchester M13 9WL, UK
E-mail: daniel.keenan@cmmc.nhs.uk

valve prolapse (MVP), Barlow's disease, floppy leaflets, billowing leaflets, and leaflet prolapse. Connective tissue disorders like Marfan's syndrome show similarities.

Myxomatous degeneration

This is a heterogeneous group of conditions. The histological features consist of focal disruption of the fibrous layer of the valve associated with loss of collagen, accompanied by thickening of the spongiform layer by proteoglycan deposition, weakening the leaflet. The leaflets and endocardium of the left ventricle develop fibrous thickening subsequently, the posterior annulus along the base of the leaflet tends to calcify and there is a tendency to chordal thickening and fusion occasionally, but mostly the chordae will lengthen and or rupture with time.

Mitral valve prolapse

Either or both of the leaflets may be enlarged, and the enlarged leaflet(s) prolapse(s) into the atrium during ventricular systole. The pathological features include: posterior annular dilation, poor coaptation of thickened leaflet tissue, and interchordal ballooning of predominantly the posterior mitral valve leaflet, with or without elongated, thinned, or ruptured cords. In young patients, it appears to be associated with a competent and minimally distorted valve and is more prevalent in women, whereas in older patients it is associated with severe mitral regurgitation in a deformed valve, and occurs more often in men. Only a small proportion of young people with MVP will, as they grow older, develop severely distorted mitral valves with gross regurgitation.

Fibro-elastic deficiency and Barlow's disease

These two conditions are at two ends of a spectrum of this degenerative process. Fibro-elastic deficiency occurs in older patients and is characterised by an area of degenerative disease coupled with others with thin leaflets. Barlow's disease, on the other hand, is seen in younger patients (less than 60 years old) and is characterised by marked billowing, mainly of the anterior leaflets, and a substantial amount of excess tissue. The normal reference points used for repair of the valve are lost and this produces a challenging condition for repair. It has histological similarities to Marfan's syndrome and fibro-elastic deficiency. The leaflets are fragile and the stress on them appears to lead to redundancy and stretching. Most patients lie in the middle of this spectrum.

Connective tissue disorder

Marfan's syndrome and Ehlers–Danlos syndrome have valvar abnormalities similar to myxomatous degeneration, suggesting an analogous connective tissue problem.

INFECTIVE ENDOCARDITIS

This is characterised by colonisation with or without destruction of the heart valves, endocardium, and major vessels, resulting in vegetations laden with micro-organisms (most frequently bacteria, but also viruses or fungi), fibrin and inflammatory cells. It can be divided into acute and subacute forms.

Staphylococcus aureus is the leading cause of acute endocarditis (including for intravenous drug users) and produces a very destructive valvar infection often in previously normal heart valves, with mortality up to 50%. The subacute form is more indolent in nature, can take weeks to months before diagnosis and is usually caused by α-haemolytic Streptococci and other less virulent micro-organisms. These valves are often already abnormal to start with, secondary to previous rheumatic fever, myxomatous degeneration or congenital abnormalities of either the septum or the mitral valve. There is also a group called culture-negative endocarditis (5–10% of cases), who often already will have had previous antibiotic treatment, where no organism can be isolated from the blood.

The Duke criteria provide a standardised assessment of patients with suspected infective endocarditis, describe blood-culture evidence of infection, echocardiographic findings, predisposing factors, and clinical and laboratory information.[2] The previously important clinical findings of immunological and microvascular embolic sequelae are now uncommon, as earlier antibiotic therapy has shortened the clinical course significantly. With guided antibiotic therapy, vegetations often sterilise and organise with fibrosis. Complications include congestive heart failure, mitral regurgitation (rarely stenosis), fistulation, annular abscess formation, suppurative pericarditis, heart block and embolisation. Regurgitation occurs either because of leaflet perforation, chordal rupture, or fistulation from annular abscesses. Annular abscesses are often due to virulent organisms, and are surgically challenging to deal with.

ISCHAEMIC MITRAL REGURGITATION

The primary underlying pathology here is the abnormal ventricle. Due to ischaemic heart disease and either previous infarction or stunning, the left ventricular cavity dilates and splays the papillary muscles open. This results in malcoaptation of the leaflets secondary to leaflet tethering (typically the posterior leaflet), volume overload to the ventricle, loss of systolic annular contraction and annular dilatation, and mitral regurgitation. Acute myocardial infarction can also cause papillary muscle rupture with gross regurgitation. This is a life-threatening emergency.

RHEUMATIC MITRAL VALVE DISEASE

Rheumatic valve disease accounts for the majority of mitral valve disease; however, in the West, it now accounts for many less cases of mitral valve surgery than previously. The inflammatory process is a progressive one affecting all components of the mitral valve and is, therefore, much less amenable to conservative techniques than with degenerative disease. Repair in the setting of rheumatic valve disease produces disappointing results with a high rate of re-operation. Accordingly, we do not advocate mitral valve repair procedures in this setting.

ANATOMY

When considering mitral valve pathology, one has to evaluate all components of the mitral valve. These include the leaflets, annulus, chordae tendineae, papillary muscles, and the left ventricle (Fig. 1).

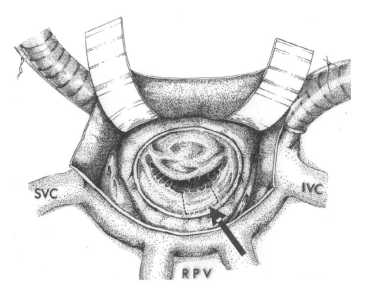

Fig. 1 Surgeon's view of the mitral valve following opening of the left atrium through the inter-atrial groove, with retraction of the right atrium away from the surgeon. The prolapsing segment (P2) is indicated (arrow). SVC (superior vena cava), IVC (inferior vena cava), RPV (right pulmonary veins).

The mitral valve has two leaflets, anterior and posterior, attached to the annulus, papillary muscles and left ventricle by means of primary, secondary and tertiary chordae tendineae. Each leaflet receives chordae tendineae from both the antero-lateral (A-L) and postero-medial (P-M) papillary muscles. The anterior mitral valve leaflet (AMVL) is in fibrous continuity with the aortic valve and attaches to one-third of the annular circumference and hinges between the two fibrous trigones. This part of the annulus does not contract. The posterior portion of the annulus is muscular and contracts during systole to reduce asymmetrically the area of the orifice. This causes the valvar orifice to go from elliptical during ventricular systole to circular during late diastole, increasing leaflet coaptation during systole and maximising orifice area during diastole. This explains why dilation of the annulus occurs posteriorly with mitral regurgitation. The A-L papillary muscle has a dual blood supply from the left anterior descending coronary artery and either a diagonal branch or an obtuse marginal branch of the left circumflex artery. The P-M papillary muscle is fed by a single vessel, either the left circumflex artery or the right coronary artery and is, therefore, much more susceptible to infarction. The circumflex coronary artery runs laterally and the coronary sinus medially around the mitral annulus through the atrio-ventricular groove. The bundle of His is located near the postero-medial trigone.

The valvar orifice is D-shaped, and its annulus saddle-shaped in a horizontal plane. The posterior mitral valve leaflet (PMVL) is rectangular and its free margin divided into three scallops, the largest being the middle one. They are named P1, P2 and P3. Analogous to this, the reciprocal parts of the AMVL are also divided into three scallops – A1, A2, and A3. The leaflets meet in or below the plane of the orifice during systole with apposition to about 50% of the depth of the posterior leaflet and 30% that of the anterior leaflet.

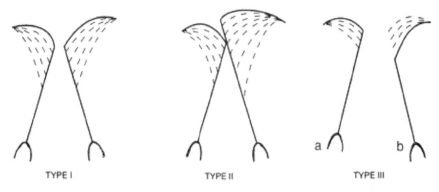

TYPE I   TYPE II   TYPE III

Fig. 2 Mechanism of mitral regurgitation according to Carpentier.[3] [Reprinted from *Journal of Thoracic and Cardiovascular Surgery*, vol. **86**, Carpentier A. Cardiac valve surgery: the 'French correction', pp. 323–337. Copyright © 1983 Elsevier with permission]

CLASSIFICATION OF MECHANISM

A better way to describe regurgitation than that by means of its aetiology is by using the standardised description of the mechanism of regurgitation as proposed by (see Fig. 2).[3] This consists of:

Type I   Annular dilatation or leaflet perforation, but normal leaflet motion.

Type II   Excessive leaflet motion or prolapse.

Type III   Restrictive leaflet motion, which is subdivided in type a (mainly during diastole), and type b (during systole).

NATURAL HISTORY

DEGENERATIVE MITRAL REGURGITATION

Isolated, mild-to-moderate mitral regurgitation tends to be tolerated for a long time without becoming symptomatic. However, if the mitral regurgitation is due to structural valve abnormalities, it tends to progress with time as the effective orifice area increases. The left ventricle (LV) and left atrium (LA) start to increase in size once severe mitral regurgitation occurs. The mitral regurgitation remains compensated for a variable amount of time, but it is usually a few years before the chronic volume-overload takes it toll on the LV and dysfunction of the LV occurs. The LV ejection fraction (EF) decreases somewhat, but manages to remain compensated for some time still despite the severe structural abnormalities of both mitral valve and LV. Symptoms of LV dysfunction tend to develop once severe mitral regurgitation occurs over the course of 6–10 years. Numerous studies indicate that patients with chronic severe mitral regurgitation have a high likelihood of developing ventricular dysfunction.[4,5]

Severe mitral regurgitation due to a flail posterior leaflet has a malignant course with a mortality rate of 7% per year; at 10 years' follow-up, 90% of patients are dead or have had mitral valve surgery. This is mainly influenced by symptoms and LV function (Fig. 3).

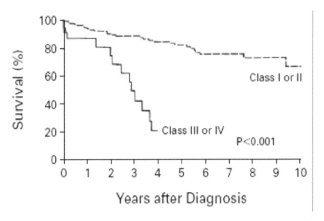

Fig. 3 Kaplan–Meier survival curves for patients with flail mitral leaflet treated medically: impact of symptomatology. (Reproduced from Ling, Enriquez-Sarano, Seward *et al*[4] with permission – copyright © 1996 Massachusetts Medical Society)

ISCHAEMIC MITRAL REGURGITATION

Patients with ischaemic mitral regurgitation have a substantially bleaker outlook than patients with regurgitation from other causes,[6–8] with 5-year survival figures of 50%. This is because the underlying mechanism of mitral regurgitation is usually caused by LV dysfunction resulting from myocardial infarction, with often a relatively normal mitral valve, and mitral regurgitation is secondary to papillary muscle displacement and tethering of the mitral leaflet(s) or annular dilatation.

CLINICAL MANAGEMENT

Patients may be asymptomatic, breathless or have symptoms relating to congestive heart failure. They may also present with palpitations due to new onset atrial fibrillation (AF), which may be associated with emboli. There may be symptoms of angina. Patients with endocarditis may or may not have additional signs such as hepatosplenomegaly, splinter haemorrhages and other signs of infection and embolisation. Findings during examination may reveal atrial fibrillation in some patients, signs of congestive heart failure, and cardiomegaly. Auscultation will reveal murmurs typical of mitral regurgitation and/or mitral stenosis and, in patients who develop secondary tricuspid regurgitation, an additional murmur associated with this.

Chest X-ray findings may include cardiomegaly and pulmonary vascular plethora, whereas on the electrocardiogram (ECG) a multitude of abnormalities can sometimes be found including AF, ventricular hypertrophy, axis deviation, p-wave abnormalities, intraventricular conduction delay, heart block, and ischaemic changes.

ECHOCARDIOGRAPHY

Transthoracic echocardiography (TTE) will provide the physician with a definitive diagnosis of mitral regurgitation. This test will not only evaluate the severity of mitral regurgitation, but sometimes also lends itself to establishing a mechanism. Furthermore, LA size and thrombus, LV function, tricuspid valve

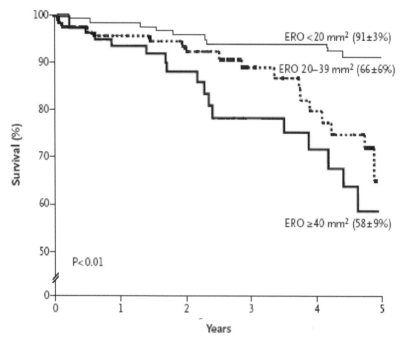

Fig. 4 Kaplan–Meier survival curve for patients with asymptomatic mitral regurgitation who were medically managed, according to effective regurgitant orifice (ERO) values measured by echocardiography, demonstrating that regurgitant orifice areas are strongly correlated to survival. Values are described as mean ± SE. (Reproduced from Enriquez-Sarano *et al*[11] with permission – copyright © 2005 Massachusetts Medical Society)

function and pulmonary artery (PA) pressure can be assessed. However, to establish repairability of the mitral valve, a transoesophageal echocardiogram (TOE) is necessary.[9] This will establish the morphology of the mitral valve and, using colour Doppler, the severity of the regurgitation. Experienced sonographers will also assess the width of the vena contracta[10] and obtain quantitative values (*e.g.* regurgitant volume, regurgitant fraction and regurgitant orifice area). Colour-flow estimation of mitral regurgitation may poorly estimate the degree of mitral regurgitation though; therefore, the proximal isovelocity surface area (PISA) method is most commonly used today for quantification.

In order to assess the mechanism of mitral regurgitation by TOE, the regurgitant jet direction is commonly used. In degenerative disease, the direction of the jet is usually opposite to the leaflet that prolapses in about 80% of patients, *i.e.* PMVL prolapse causes an anteriorly directed jet, and AMVL prolapse a posteriorly directed jet. In bi-leaflet prolapse, there may be two or more jets within the atrium or a broad, central jet. In ischaemic/functional mitral regurgitation restricted leaflet motion or annular dilatation occur, causing a central jet. In endocarditis with leaflet perforation and in regurgitation at the level of the commissures, an eccentric jet can occur.

The current American Heart Association guidelines[10] state that severe mitral regurgitation (3–4+) is defined as:

1. **Qualitatively** – the vena contracta width has to be greater than 0.7 cm with a large central mitral regurgitation jet (area greater than 40% of the

LA area) or with a wall-impinging jet of any size, swirling in the LA, and the Doppler vena contracta width is ≥ 0.70 cm.

2. **Quantitatively** – the regurgitant volume has to be ≥ 60 ml/beat, the regurgitant fraction ≥ 50%, and the regurgitant orifice area ≥ 0.4 cm^2 (see Fig. 4).

INTRA-OPERATIVE TRANSOESOPHAGEAL ECHOCARDIOGRAM

Once a decision to operate has been made, the TOE is used again by the anaesthetist during the operation (Fig. 5) to confirm the pathology, and the mechanism, but also to assess the atrial septum for shunting which would need correction, and estimate the risk of systolic anterior motion (SAM) caused by the coaptation plane being too close to the outflow tract of the left ventricle. This risk is low, if the distance between the crest of the septum and the coaptation point is greater than 2.5 cm on a mid-oesophageal view in long-axis, but increased if the distance is shorter. This may influence the type of repair the surgeon performs.

The necessity for concomitant tricuspid valve repair is also assessed according to its annular dimensions and regurgitation. After the repair has been performed, the quality of the repair is intricately tested and assessed by various manoeuvres, including volume loading and increasing the afterload if necessary. Anything more than mild mitral regurgitation would not be accepted and re-repaired or, if the repair was too difficult, the valve replaced sparing the posterior leaflet to preserve ventricular function. Regional wall motion abnormalities are also assessed alongside of any residual air bubbles in the heart. In the future, 3-D echocardiography may become established as the preferred method to quantify regurgitation and assess anatomy even more accurately.

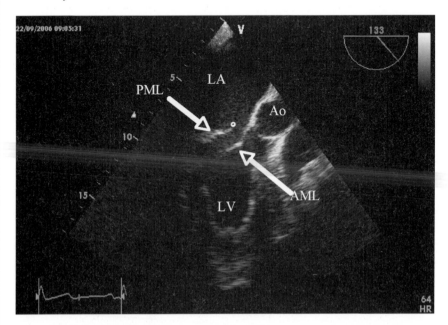

Fig. 5 TOE image demonstrating prolapse of the posterior leaflet. AML anterior mitral leaflet, PML posterior mitral leaflet, Ao ascending aorta, LV left ventricle, LA left atrium.

CARDIAC CATHETERISATION

Pre-operative coronary angiography is recommended in all patients over 40 years of age and any patient with a history or clinical presentation suggesting the presence of coronary artery disease. While left ventriculography may demonstrate mitral regurgitation, much more information is gleaned from echocardiography. Mitral annular calcification visible on fluoroscopy indicates that mitral valve surgery will be complex. Furthermore, right- and left-sided chamber pressures can be measured.

CARDIAC MAGNETIC RESONANCE

This is currently not the standard method of functional and anatomical assessment, but may have a more important role in the future in assessing regurgitant volume, concomitant coronary artery disease and other myocardial or valvular problems.

MITRAL VALVE REPAIR

INDICATIONS

An updated, joint, consensus statement on the management of valvular heart disease by the American Heart Association and American College of Cardiology, was published in 2006.[10] Table 1 summarises those situations indicating surgery in degenerative mitral regurgitation.

The major change with these guidelines is the recommendation that asymptomatic patients with chronic severe mitral regurgitation and good LV function should be offered surgery. This reflects the growing ability of surgeons,

Table 1 Situations indicating surgery in degenerative mitral regurgitation

Class I – Indication
- Symptomatic acute severe mitral regurgitation
- Symptomatic severe chronic mitral regurgitation and moderate-to-good LV (EF > 30% or end-systolic dimension > 55 mm)
- Asymptomatic chronic severe mitral regurgitation with mild-to-moderate LV dysfunction (EF 30–60% or end-systolic dimension > 40 mm)
- Mitral valve repair rather than replacement is the operation of choice, and patients should be referred to surgical centres with expertise in this

Class II – Indication
- Asymptomatic chronic severe mitral regurgitation with preserved LV function where the likelihood of repair is > 90%
- Asymptomatic chronic severe mitral regurgitation with preserved LV function, with new onset AF or systolic PA pressures > 50 mmHg (rest) or > 60 mmHg (exercise)
- Symptomatic class III–IV chronic severe mitral regurgitation, poor LV function (EF < 30% or end-systolic dimension > 55 mm) where it is a primary valvar problem and mitral valve repair is likely or if the mitral regurgitation is due to severe LV dysfunction despite optimal therapy for heart failure (including cardiac resynchronisation therapy).

Table 2 Impact of CABG alone on moderate ischaemic regurgitation. Postoperative TTE was performed within 6 weeks of surgery.[6]

Mitral regurgitation severity	Pre-operative (n = 136)	Intra-operative TEE (n = 38)	Post operative TTE (n = 68)	Patients with both intra- and postoperative TEE (n = 18)
0+	0	29	4	6
1+	0	8	4	6
2+	0	53	51	56
3+	100	11	37	33
4+	0	0	3	0
Mean[a]	3.0 ± 0.0	1.4 ± 1.0^{b}	2.3 ± 0.8^{b}	2.2 ± 0.8^{b}

[a]Mean mitral regurgitation grade ± SD
[b]$P < 0.001$ versus pre-operative value.

in most situations, to repair effectively rather than to replace the valve, and at low mortality and morbidity. This requires networks of cardiologists, surgeons and anaesthetists working closely together so that patients and their echocardiograms can be discussed and optimum timing for surgery agreed. It will also foster an environment where the next generation of these professionals can be trained.

If the primary pathology is ischaemic mitral regurgitation, the indications are different. If acute rupture of the papillary muscle is the cause of the mitral regurgitation, surgery on an emergency basis is indicated with either valve repair or replacement.[12] If papillary muscle dysfunction is the primary mechanism, surgery is considered if haemodynamic stabilisation with an intra-aortic balloon pump and aggressive medical therapy does not improve the clinical condition. Valve surgery in the acute setting is usually in addition to revascularisation.

The indication for mitral valve surgery in the patient who undergoes coronary artery bypass grafting (CABG) with mild-to-moderate mitral regurgitation is still controversial. Mitral regurgitation is an independent negative prognostic indicator in this group. Some data suggest benefit of mitral valve repair in such patients. CABG alone may improve LV function and reduce ischaemic mitral regurgitation in selected patients,[13–15] although often it may be insufficient and significant residual mitral regurgitation is left (Table 2). These patients may benefit from concomitant mitral valve repair with an annuloplasty ring at the time of the CABG.[8,14,16] The benefits of performing mitral valve surgery in this patient group have not yet unequivocally been established though we would advocate liberal use of repair techniques in such patients who suffer from breathlessness.

In those with endocarditis, patients should undergo repair, if possible, for cardiac complications, heart failure and persistent infections.[10]

TECHNIQUES OF MITRAL VALVE REPAIR

The predominant technique followed by a majority of surgeons around the world follows the principles of repair developed by . These have clear, long-

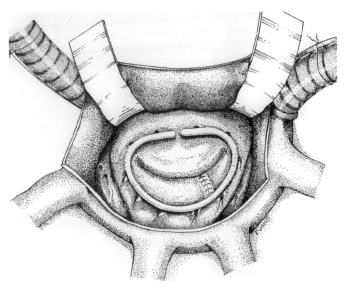

Fig. 6 Appearance of the mitral valve following excision of P2 and implantation of an annuloplasty ring.

term, established and reproducible results. Operative techniques will systematically address the various components of the mitral valve apparatus after intricate assessment by the surgeon of the mechanism of mitral regurgitation. These may include leaflet procedures *e.g.* quadrangular resection of P2 with or without a sliding annuloplasty, triangular resection of A2, partial leaflet transfers, leaflet plication, and leaflet patching or reconstruction with xenograft or autograft material if destroyed by infection, and commisurotomy. If chordal rupture or elongation is part of the pathology, chordal shortening or transposition of chordae or artificial chordae may be used to bring the leaflets back into the correct coaptation plane. Annular procedures may include annular plication and sliding annuloplasty. All repairs should be completed by using an annuloplasty ring though to prevent future dilatation and to support the repair for longevity.[17] This will simultaneously address the often-dilated mitral valve annulus. The alternative technique used by some surgeons is called the edge-to-edge repair or Alfieri-suture. This has been associated with variable results in the ischaemic group of patients,[18,19] but has not produced as consistently good results as the -style repairs overall.

As far as annuloplasty rings are concerned, there is a multitude to choose from including rigid and flexible rings, complete and incomplete rings, and special rings for ischaemic pathology. None have shown superiority to others in specific pathologies; therefore, the choice of rings is mostly due to a surgeon's preference.

The majority of the reconstructive work on the mitral valve consists of dealing with posterior leaflet pathology and the commonest procedure for P2 prolapse (commonest pathology) is quadrangular resection of P2 (see Fig. 6). This consists of resection of the middle scallop of the posterior leaflet, repair of the remaining posterior leaflet, with or without sliding annuloplasty, and an annuloplasty ring. The sliding annuloplasty and resection of posterior leaflet tissue decreases the height of the posterior leaflet and ensures a decreased risk of SAM induced by the repair, as the annuloplasty transfers the plane of coaptation closer to the left ventricular outflow tract (LVOT).

If the coaptation plane is further than 2.5 cm from the LVOT then P2 can be preserved and instead artificial chordae used to increase the depth of coaptation, which increases success and durability of the repair. These are sutured to the head of the closest papillary muscle and sutured as replacement primary chordae to the edge of the leaflets after judging their required length.

With the advent of less invasive approaches to surgery, various techniques have evolved and are slowly being established in some centres.[20,21] These include endoscopic mitral valve repair through the video-assisted thoracoscopic route, robotic repairs, mini-thoracotomy, mini-sternotomy or partial sternotomies. All of these techniques employ cardiopulmonary bypass, some of it through the femoral route. These methods have not all been uniformly adopted, but are slowly gaining more acceptance and popularity. They are not applicable when simultaneous CABG is required.

RESULTS OF MITRAL VALVE REPAIR

Mitral valve repair has demonstrated various advantages over replacement, including improved long-term survival, better preservation of left ventricular function, and greater freedom from endocarditis, thrombo-embolism, and anticoagulant-related haemorrhage.[22–26]

Operative mortality for most degenerative mitral repairs is around 1%, increasing with different aetiologies and depressed ventricular function, to 4–5%. Long-term results have been studied in depth and have demonstrated excellent durability of repairs beyond 20 years using the techniques for non-rheumatic pathology. Long-term survival in patients undergoing repair being similar to that of the general population (Fig. 7).[22] Elderly patients undergoing mitral repairs have more pre-operative risk factors, and have a higher operative risk than younger patients. However, restoration of life expectancy after surgery is independent of age. Therefore, elderly patients with mitral regurgitation should be carefully considered for surgery before heart failure develops.[27]

Edge-to-edge repair

Results of this technique have been reported for a multitude of mitral pathologies, with a low risk of creating mitral stenosis. In ischaemic mitral regurgitation, however, a significant number of patients undergoing repair with this technique progress to severe mitral regurgitation after surgery.[28] Furthermore, an annuloplasty ring appears mandatory, in view of otherwise suboptimal results, particularly in the presence of annular calcification, and if done as a rescue procedure.[29] As far as leaflet pathology is concerned, it appears that some groups are able to obtain similar long-term results in the setting of anterior leaflet prolapse as when posterior leaflet prolapse appears to be the main culprit.[30] Patients with end-stage dilated cardiomyopathy can undergo repair with this technique with low hospital mortality and important

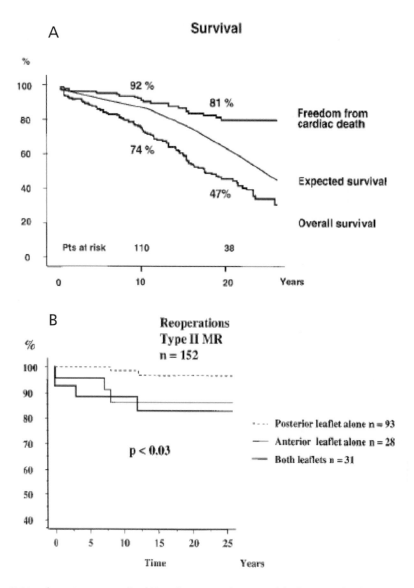

Fig. 7 Very long-term mortality (A) and re-operation rates (B) after mitral valve repair for mainly type II (increased leaflet mobility) mitral regurgitation. This demonstrates a near-normal restored life-expectancy in these patients.[22]

symptomatic improvement.[19] It also eliminates SAM if at risk of this, but does not appear to be a good technique for the prevention of long-term recurrent mitral regurgitation if performed for residual mitral regurgitation after complex mitral repair.[18]

Chordal repair techniques
Use of artificial chordae, rather than leaflet resection has been associated with excellent short-term results in myxomatous degeneration, although long-term results are unclear.[31,32]

Leaflet type

Repair durability appears to be best for posterior leaflet prolapse where part of the posterior leaflet was resected and an annuloplasty with a ring was performed. Some groups have reported that chordal shortening procedures, annuloplasty alone, and leaflet resections without annuloplasty jeopardise late results, but this appears dependent on experience and learning.[17,26,32]

FAILURE OF THE MITRAL REPAIR

Recurrent, severe mitral regurgitation after previous repair of the mitral valve can be treated with a repeat mitral repair in selected cases with low operative mortality and durable results in the medium term.[33]

ANTICOAGULATION

Patients who undergo mitral valve repairs all need anticoagulation with warfarin or synthrome for at least 3 months. Depending on risk factors for thrombo-emboli (*e.g.* AF), anticoagulation ought not to continue beyond 3 months. Aspirin should be prescribed if anticoagulation ceases.

CONCOMITANT CARDIAC PROCEDURES

AORTIC VALVE REPLACEMENT

In double-valve pathology, one has to determine which valve is worse and treat according to that lesion. In aortic regurgitation, both lesions will produce LV dilatation; if aortic stenosis predominates, there will generally be modest systemic systolic hypertension and a mild increase in LV wall thickness. In severe aortic valve disease and severe mitral regurgitation with symptoms, LV dysfunction or pulmonary hypertension aortic valve replacement with mitral repair should be planned. If the mitral regurgitation is less severe, this may improve after isolated aortic valve replacement, particularly if the mitral valve is structurally normal. TOE and exploration of the mitral valve may be helpful in the decision-making. If a patient is undergoing mitral surgery for severe mitral regurgitation but has concomitant moderate aortic stenosis, assessment may be difficult due to reduced cardiac output through the valve. Mean valve gradients of greater than 30 mmHg are then used as an indication for a double-valve procedure. When the gradient is less, examination of the valve and TTE are helpful in decision-making. Either way, if a double-valve procedure is performed, the mitral valve should be repaired.

TRICUSPID VALVE REPAIR

Surgery on the tricuspid valve for TR is regularly performed at the time of mitral valve surgery. TR associated with dilatation of the tricuspid annulus should be repaired, because tricuspid dilatation is an on-going process that may progress to severe TR if left untreated. Patients with severe TR of any cause have a poor long-term outcome because of RV dysfunction and/or systemic venous congestion. The AHA/ACC guidelines suggest that repair is beneficial for severe TR in patients with mitral valve disease requiring mitral valve surgery (Class I recommendation), and also for less than severe TR in patients undergoing mitral valve surgery when there is pulmonary hypertension or tricuspid annular dilatation (Class IIb recommendation).[10]

ATRIAL FIBRILLATION ABLATION

Performing concomitant Cox-Maze III procedures or pulmonary vein isolation with alternative energy sources cures atrial fibrillation in 80–100% of patients and, therefore, may prevent future thrombo-embolic events by restoring normal sinus rhythm. Of patients presenting for mitral valve surgery, 30–50% have atrial fibrillation. In such patients, an important goal of the procedure is ablation of AF in addition to mitral valve repair. When AF has been present for less than 1 year, mitral valve repair alone is likely to cure the AF. In contrast, when AF has been present for more than 1 year, 80% of patients will remain in AF. Therefore, surgical ablation of atrial fibrillation is indicated in patients having mitral valve surgery who have a history of more than 1 year of paroxysmal, persistent, or permanent atrial fibrillation. An important part of this adjuvant procedure is excision of the left atrial appendage with the associated reduction in the risk of thrombo-embolism.

LEFT VENTRICLE REMODELLING

There is a greater understanding nowadays regarding the dynamic relationship between the ventricular septum, ventricular cavities, mitral valve and coronary arteries. This has generated much interest in the investigation of patients with substantial heart failure. Various techniques have evolved over the past 10 years that complement mitral repair techniques in selected patients. These techniques include the left ventricular endoaneurysmorraphy or surgical ventricular restoration for patients with a substantial ventricular aneurysm, and cardiac resynchronisation therapy for those with prolonged QRS duration, substantially reduced EF and symptoms of heart failure. Apical restriction devices, such as the Acorn device, which try to alter the stresses in the ventricular myocardium and change its shape are also currently under investigation.[34] The incremental value of the individual subprocedures when combined is subject to further investigation.

NON-SURGICAL TECHNIQUES

Nothing stands still in cardiological and surgical practice. Two percutaneous valve repair procedures for mitral regurgitation have been proposed. Both use some of the principles learned at surgery. The first simulates the Alfieri edge-to-edge repair with clips and the second an annuloplasty by placing ring devices in the coronary sinus.[35] The first technique has been tested and shown to work in a small selected group; it continues to be evaluated. For the second, human experience is still awaited. This might be limited by the lack of a complete coronary sinus in a significant minority of patients. It remains to be seen if the results from this limited application of the surgical principles will suffice to reverse symptoms and/or prevent deterioration in LV function consequent on mitral regurgitation, and not be associated with a significant complication rate.

Key points for clinical practice

- Severe mitral valve regurgitation is associated with a significantly reduced life expectancy.

- The predominant reason for severe mitral regurgitation in the Western world is degenerative mitral valve disease.

- All patients with a pan-systolic murmur, irrespective of symptomatology, should undergo an echocardiogram; if that indicates mitral regurgitation, they need periodic evaluation by a cardiologist.

- Symptomatic patients, patients with ventricular dysfunction, pulmonary hypertension or recent onset of atrial fibrillation should be referred for mitral surgery.

- Selected patients with asymptomatic severe mitral regurgitation should be referred for mitral surgery, providing the likelihood of the valve being repaired is > 90% in expert centres.

- Mitral valve repair is preferable to replacement; therefore, patients should be referred to centres with a demonstrated expertise in mitral repair.

- Mitral valve repair is associated with low operative mortality, and excellent durability of the repair long-term.

- Mitral valve repairs should be supported by an annuloplasty ring.

References

1. Keogh B, Kinsman R. *The Society of Cardiothoracic Surgeons of Great Britain and Ireland. Fifth National Adult Cardiac Surgical Database Report 2003: Improving outcomes for patients.* Henley-on-Thames; Dendrite Clinical Systems, 2003.
2. Durack DT, Lukes AS, Bright DK. New criteria for diagnosis of infective endocarditis: utilization of specific echocardiographic findings. Duke Endocarditis Service. *Am J Med* 1994; **96**: 200–209.
3. Carpentier A. Cardiac valve surgery: the 'French correction'. *J Thorac Cardiovasc Surg* 1983; **86**: 323–337.
4. Ling LH, Enriquez-Sarano M, Seward JB *et al.* Clinical outcome of mitral regurgitation due to flail leaflet. *N Engl J Med* 1996; **335**: 1417–1412.
5. Rosen SE, Borer JS, Hochreiter C *et al.* Natural history of the asymptomatic/minimally symptomatic patient with severe mitral regurgitation secondary to mitral valve prolapse and normal right and left ventricular performance. *Am J Cardiol* 1994; **74**: 374–380.
6. Aklog L, Filsoufi F, Flores KQ *et al.* Does coronary artery bypass grafting alone correct moderate ischemic mitral regurgitation? *Circulation* 2001; **104 (Suppl I)**: I-68–I-75.
7. Connolly MW, Gelbfish JS, Jacobowitz IJ *et al.* Surgical results for mitral regurgitation from coronary artery disease. *J Thorac Cardiovasc Surg* 1986; **91**: 379–388.
8. Akins CW, Hilgenberg AD, Buckley MJ *et al.* Mitral valve reconstruction versus replacement for degenerative or ischemic mitral regurgitation. *Ann Thorac Surg* 1994; **58**: 668–675.
9. Enriquez-Sarano M, Freeman WK, Tribouilloy CM *et al.* Functional anatomy of mitral

regurgitation: accuracy and outcome implications of transesophageal echocardiography. *J Am Coll Cardiol* 1999; **34**:1129–1136.

10. Bonow RO, Carabello BA, Chatterjee K *et al.* ACC/AHA 2006 practice guidelines for the management of patients with valvular heart disease: executive summary. A Report of the American College of Cardiology/American Heart Association Task Force on Practice Guidelines (Writing Committee to Revise the 1998 Guidelines for the Management of Patients With Valvular Heart Disease) developed in collaboration with the Society of Cardiovascular Anesthesiologists endorsed by the Society for Cardiovascular Angiography and Interventions and the Society of Thoracic Surgeons. *J Am Coll Cardiol* 2006; **48**: 598–675.

11. Enriquez-Sarano M, Avierinos J-F, Messika-Zeitoun D *et al.* Quantitative determinants of the outcome of asymptomatic mitral regurgitation. *N Engl J Med* 2005; **352**: 875–883.

12. Tavakoli R, Weber A, Vogt P *et al.* Surgical management of acute mitral valve regurgitation due to post-infarction papillary muscle rupture. *J Heart Valve Dis* 2002; **11**: 20–25.

13. Lam BK, Gillinov AM, Blackstone EH *et al.* Importance of moderate ischemic mitral regurgitation. *Ann Thorac Surg* 2005; **79**: 462–470.

14. Schroder JN, Williams ML, Hata JA *et al.* Impact of mitral valve regurgitation evaluated by intraoperative transesophageal echocardiography on long-term outcomes after coronary artery bypass grafting. *Circulation* 2005; **112**: I293–I298.

15. Duarte IG, Shen Y, MacDonald MJ, Jones EL, Craver JM, Guyton RA. Treatment of moderate mitral regurgitation and coronary disease by coronary bypass alone: late results. *Ann Thorac Surg* 1999; **68**: 426–430.

16. Grossi EA, Goldberg JD, LaPietra A *et al.* Ischemic mitral valve reconstruction and replacement: comparison of long-term survival and complications. *J Thorac Cardiovasc Surg* 2001; **122**: 1107–1124.

17. Gillinov AM, Cosgrove DM, Blackstone EH *et al.* Durability of mitral valve repair for degenerative disease. *J Thorac Cardiovasc Surg* 1998; **116**: 734–743.

18. Brinster DR. Midterm results of the edge-to-edge technique for complex mitral valve repair. *Ann Thorac Surg* 2006; **81**: 1612–1617.

19. De Bonis M. Mitral valve repair for functional mitral regurgitation in end-stage dilated cardiomyopathy: role of the 'edge-to-edge' technique. *Circulation* 2005; **112 (9 Suppl)**: I402–I408.

20. Felger JE, Chitwood WR, Nifong LW, Holbert D. Evolution of mitral valve surgery: toward a totally endoscopic approach. *Ann Thorac Surg* 2001; **72**: 1203–1209.

21. Vanerman H, Wellens F, DeGeest R *et al.* Video-assisted port-access mitral valve surgery from debut to routine surgery. Will trocar-port-access cardiac surgery ultimately lead to robotic cardiac surgery? *Semin Thorac Cardiovasc Surg* 1999; **3**: 223–234.

22. Braunberger E, Deloche A, Berrebi A *et al.* Very long-term results (more than 20 years) of valve repair with Carpentier's techniques in non-rheumatic mitral valve insufficiency. *Circulation* 2001; **104 (Suppl I)**: I8–I11.

23. Mohty D, Orszulak TA, Schaff HV *et al.* Very long-term survival and durability of mitral valve repair for mitral valve prolapse. *Circulation* 2001; **104 (Suppl I)**: I1–I7.

24. Enriquez-Sarano M, Schaff HV, Orszulak TA *et al.* Valve repair improves the outcome of surgery for mitral regurgitation: a multivariate analysis. *Circulation* 1995; **91**: 1022–1028.

25. Lee EM, Shapiro LM, Wells FC. Superiority of mitral valve repair in surgery for degenerative mitral regurgitation. *Eur Heart J* 1997; **18**: 655–663.

26. Suri RM. Survival advantage and improved durability of mitral repair for leaflet prolapse subsets in the current era. *Ann Thorac Surg* 2006; **82**: 819–826.

27. Detaint D, Sundt TM, Nkomo VT *et al.* Surgical correction of mitral regurgitation in the elderly: outcomes and recent improvements. *Circulation* 2006; **114**: 265–272.

28. Bhudia SK, McCarthy PM, Smedira NG *et al.* Edge-to-edge (Alfieri) mitral repair: results in diverse clinical settings. *Ann Thorac Surg* 2004; **77**: 1598–1606.

29. Maisano F, Caldarola A, Blasio A *et al.* Midterm results of edge-to-edge mitral valve repair without annuloplasty. *J Thorac Cardiovasc Surg* 2003; **126**:1987–1997.

30. De Bonis M, Lorusso R, Lapenna E *et al.* Similar long-term results of mitral valve repair for anterior compared with posterior leaflet prolapse. *J Thorac Cardiovasc Surg* 2006; **131**: 364–370.

31. Nigro JJ, Schwartz DS, Bart RD *et al*. Neochordal repair of the posterior mitral leaflet. *J Thorac Cardiovasc Surg* 2004; **127**: 440–447.

32. Lim E, Ali ZA, Barlow CW *et al*. Determinants and assessment of regurgitation after mitral valve repair. *J Thorac Cardiovasc Surg* 2002; **124**: 911–917.

33. Cerfolio RJ, Orzulak TA, Pluth JR, Harmsen WS, Schaff HV. Reoperation after valve repair for mitral regurgitation: early and intermediate results. *J Thorac Cardiovasc Surg* 1996; **111**: 1177–1183, discussion 1183–1184.

34. Grossi EA, Crooke GA. Mitral valve surgery in heart failure: insights from the Acorn clinical trial. *J Thorac Cardiovasc Surg* 2006; **132**: 455–456.

35. Alfieri O, Maisano F, Colombo A. Percutaneous mitral valve repair procedures. *Eur J Cardiothorac Surg* 2004; **26**: S36–S38.

Index

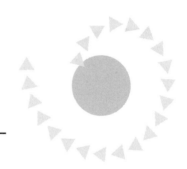